Design, Development, and Optimization of Bio-Mechatronic Engineering Products

Kaushik Kumar
Birla Institute of Technology, India

J. Paulo Davim
University of Aveiro, Portugal

A volume in the Advances in Mechatronics and Mechanical Engineering (AMME) Book Series

IGI Global
DISSEMINATOR OF KNOWLEDGE

Published in the United States of America by
IGI Global
Engineering Science Reference (an imprint of IGI Global)
701 E. Chocolate Avenue
Hershey PA, USA 17033
Tel: 717-533-8845
Fax: 717-533-8661
E-mail: cust@igi-global.com
Web site: http://www.igi-global.com

Library of Congress Cataloging-in-Publication Data

Names: Kumar, K. (Kaushik), 1968- editor. | Davim, J. Paulo, editor.
Title: Design, development, and optimization of bio-mechatronic engineering products / Kaushik Kumar and J. Paulo Davim, editors.
Description: Hershey, PA : Engineering Science Reference, [2019] | Includes bibliographical references.
Identifiers: LCCN 2018052155| ISBN 9781522582359 (hardcover) | ISBN 9781522582366 (ebook)
Subjects: LCSH: Prosthesis. | Orthopedic apparatus.
Classification: LCC RD130 .D47 2019 | DDC 617.9--dc23 LC record available at https://lccn.loc.gov/2018052155

This book is published in the IGI Global book series Advances in Mechatronics and Mechanical Engineering (AMME) (ISSN: 2328-8205; eISSN: 2328-823X)

British Cataloguing in Publication Data
A Cataloguing in Publication record for this book is available from the British Library.

All work contributed to this book is new, previously-unpublished material.
The views expressed in this book are those of the authors, but not necessarily of the publisher.

For electronic access to this publication, please contact: eresources@igi-global.com.

Advances in Mechatronics and Mechanical Engineering (AMME) Book Series

ISSN:2328-8205
EISSN:2328-823X

Editor-in-Chief: J. Paulo Davim, University of Aveiro, Portugal

MISSION

With its aid in the creation of smartphones, cars, medical imaging devices, and manufacturing tools, the mechatronics engineering field is in high demand. Mechatronics aims to combine the principles of mechanical, computer, and electrical engineering together to bridge the gap of communication between the different disciplines.

The **Advances in Mechatronics and Mechanical Engineering (AMME) Book Series** provides innovative research and practical developments in the field of mechatronics and mechanical engineering. This series covers a wide variety of application areas in electrical engineering, mechanical engineering, computer and software engineering; essential for academics, practitioners, researchers, and industry leaders.

COVERAGE

- Micro and nanomechanics
- Nanomaterials and nanomanufacturing
- Computational Mechanics
- Biologically Inspired Robotics
- Vibration and acoustics
- Bioengineering Materials
- Control Methodologies
- Autonomous Systems
- Control Systems Modelling and Analysis
- Tribology and surface engineering

IGI Global is currently accepting manuscripts for publication within this series. To submit a proposal for a volume in this series, please contact our Acquisition Editors at Acquisitions@igi-global.com or visit: http://www.igi-global.com/publish/.

The Advances in Mechatronics and Mechanical Engineering (AMME) Book Series (ISSN 2328-8205) is published by IGI Global, 701 E. Chocolate Avenue, Hershey, PA 17033-1240, USA, www.igi-global.com. This series is composed of titles available for purchase individually; each title is edited to be contextually exclusive from any other title within the series. For pricing and ordering information please visit http://www.igi-global.com/book-series/advances-mechatronics-mechanical-engineering/73808. Postmaster: Send all address changes to above address.

Titles in this Series

For a list of additional titles in this series, please visit:
https://www.igi-global.com/book-series/advances-mechatronics-mechanical-engineering/73808

Handbook of Research on Green Engineering Techniques for Modern Manufacturing
M. Uthayakumar (Kalasalingam University, India) S. Aravind Raj (Vellore Institute of Technology, India) Tae Jo Ko (Yeungnam University, South Korea) S. Thirumalai Kumaran (Kalasalingam University, India) and J. Paulo Davim (University of Aveiro, Potugal)
Engineering Science Reference • ©2019 • 403pp • H/C (ISBN: 9781522554455) • US $275.00

Non-Conventional Machining in Modern Manufacturing Systems
Kaushik Kumar (Birla Institute of Technology, India) Nisha Kumari (Birla Institute of Technology, India) and J. Paulo Davim (University of Aveiro, Potugal)
Engineering Science Reference • ©2019 • 303pp • H/C (ISBN: 9781522561613) • US $215.00

Advanced Fuzzy Logic Approaches in Engineering Science
Mangey Ram (Graphic Era University (Deemed), India)
Engineering Science Reference • ©2019 • 488pp • H/C (ISBN: 9781522557098) • US $245.00

Recent Advancements in Airborne Radar Signal Processing Emerging Research...
Amir Almslmany (Independent Researcher, Egypt)
Engineering Science Reference • ©2018 • 190pp • H/C (ISBN: 9781522554363) • US $145.00

Stochastic Methods for Estimation and Problem Solving in Engineering
Seifedine Kadry (Beirut Arab University, Lebanon)
Engineering Science Reference • ©2018 • 275pp • H/C (ISBN: 9781522550457) • US $205.00

Design and Optimization of Mechanical Engineering Products
K. Kumar (Birla Institute of Technology, India) and J. Paulo Davim (University of Aveiro, Portugal)
Engineering Science Reference • ©2018 • 347pp • H/C (ISBN: 9781522534013) • US $235.00

For an entire list of titles in this series, please visit:
https://www.igi-global.com/book-series/advances-mechatronics-mechanical-engineering/73808

IGI Global
DISSEMINATOR OF KNOWLEDGE

701 East Chocolate Avenue, Hershey, PA 17033, USA
Tel: 717-533-8845 x100 • Fax: 717-533-8661
E-Mail: cust@igi-global.com • www.igi-global.com

Table of Contents

Section 2
Scaffolds and Tissue Engineering

Section 3
Prosthesis: Design, Machining, and Optimization

Detailed Table of Contents

created a new site in advanced tissue engineering and scaffolds manufacturing area. Another important thing is that, with the use of CAD file software, any complex design can be prepared (i.e., this technology does not have any limited sites). But here it is very much essential to study and analyze machine printability characteristics, cross-linking time and biocompatibility of printing objects as well as bio-ink. However, mechanical properties like shear thinning, mechanical elasticity are also required. In this chapter, different types of scaffold-preparing methods and the bio-printing process are discussed, which are used in scaffold and tissue engineering.

Section 3
Prosthesis: Design, Machining, and Optimization

Nature has, over a large span of geological time, engineered near perfect solutions to most problems humans face today. Motion of the limbs is one such area, and the cutting edge in the development of effective prostheses is biomimetics. Limb prostheses have been used by mankind for the better part of known history, and most of the technology currently available in prosthetics is not exclusively new. However, modern prosthetics either are uncomfortable—and the lack of flexion affects the gait of the patient—or too expensive for a large segment of the populace. This chapter seeks to study the mimicry of physiological systems through the design for an ankle prosthesis that includes a passive damper and mimics the shape and behavior of the natural ankle joint.

Electrochemical micromachining is an advanced technology of recent trends of machining of hard and electrically conductive materials in micrometer and sub-micrometer scale. This manufacturing technique finds application in many technologically demanding industries: locomotive, biomedical, electronics, etc.

machining. These parameters can be achieved by proper modeling and simulation. In this chapter, a model for flow analysis of electrolytes in inter-electrode gaps is designed to obtain optimal process parameters for machining. The geometric model used in this simulation consists of cylindrical workpiece, an inlet allowing the flow of sodium nitrate solution as electrolyte to the machining zone, and a cylindrical tool with a flat end. Electrolytic flow simulation is incorporated using computational fluid dynamics by ANSYS–CFX 15.0 for finding pressure variation, streamline velocity pattern, turbulent energy, and temperature contour in IEG. According to the CFD analysis, the passivation effect, stagnation effect, pressure, and temperature zone are studied.

Preface

The editors are pleased to present the book *Design, Development, and Optimization of Bio-Mechatronic Engineering Products* under the book series book series *Advances in Bioinformatics and Biomedical Engineering (ABBE)*. Book title was chosen as it converge upcoming technologies in biomedical engineering for the next decade. In present time of interdisciplinary research environment, "Biomechanics" is the key word for all major disciplines and many scholars are working in these areas. This book provides an insight for all researchers, academicians, post graduate or senior undergraduate students working in the area.

Utilising the principles and theories of mechanical engineering to biological systems is a multi disciplinary area known as Biomechanical engineering. It is a bioengineering subdiscipline, which stems from the scientific discipline of biomechanics. Biomechanics, specifically, is the study of biological systems such as the human body, combined with the study of mechanics, or mechanical applications. Using the skills learned from biology, engineering and physics for research and development of components for health care, such as organs that have been made from artificial materials, or new advances with prosthetic limbs. The creation of biomaterial, which is an artificial material that can be integrated into living tissue or can live in sync with biological material, is one of the biggest advances in medicine to this day. Those in this field might also hold the job of not only installing, but also adjusting, maintain, repairing, and providing technical help for all the biomaterial. Biomechanical Engineering is involved with creating and producing a variety of products in everyday use, from environmentally safe plastics to various foods, fabrics and medicines. A combination of engineering and biology, it's a fast-growing field with many new and exciting opportunities in genetic engineering and biotechnology. Students who love science, are good with design and appreciate tough analytical challenges are ideally suited to Biomechanical Engineering.

Preface

With advances in science and technology, the efforts to replicate natures work have been bolstered over the years. There are numerous techniques and technologies available today. Mechanical engineering with the aid of electronics contributes towards advancement of bio-mechatronics products like pacemakers, artificial kidney replacement, artificial hearts, and even new joints or limbs and also new advancement for hospital monitoring systems, to better and more accurately monitor human health. The replacement of ailing organs and lost limbs is now a reality. Bio-Mechatronic Engineering Products generally comes under three categories:

Prosthesis (plural: prostheses; from Ancient Greek prosthesis, "addition, application, attachment") is an artificial device that replaces a missing body part, which may be lost through trauma, disease, or congenital conditions.

Orthosis (plural: orthoses; Greek: Ορθός, translit. ortho, lit 'to straighten, to align') is "an externally applied device used to modify the structural and functional characteristics of the neuromuscular and skeletal system"

Replacement is a surgical procedure in which the affected body part is replaced by an implant i.e. dental implant, heart valve etc. Replacement surgery can be performed as a total replacement or a hemi (half) replacement.

Bio-Mechatronic Engineering Products are today playing an important and ever more effective role in improving the quality of life of people who otherwise would not have been able to lead a normal, healthy life. The words prosthetics', 'orthosis' etc. bring to the mind visualizations of plastic legs and arms without any form of articulation. Some even think of the wooden stump which would be used by seafarers as prosthetic legs and the hooks used in place of lost arms. While the history of Bio-Mechatronic Engineering Products does include these, today they could not be further from these popular images. This is a growing field, with new developments and advances being made almost every day. Advances in the fields of medicine and engineering have today given the world a new breed of Bio-Mechatronic Engineering Products which not just look and feel like the physiological part but also resemble them strongly in function.

The chapters in the book have been provided by Researchers and Academicians working in the field and have gained considerable success in the field.

The chapters in the book have been categorized in four sections, namely, Section 1: Review of the State of the Art; Section 2: Scaffold and Tissue Engineering; Section 3: Prosthesis: Design, Machining, and Optimization; and Section 4: Orthotics.

Section 1 contains Chapter 1 to Chapter 3, whereas Section 2 has Chapter 4, Section 3 consists of Chapter 5 to Chapter 8, and Section 4 with Chapters 9 and 10.

Section 1 of the book starts with Chapter 1 which provides a systematic survey of realm of biomechanics with the eyes of a mechanical engineer. A survey may help a beginner to have a general look on the broader aspects of the sub-domains of biomechanics. The chapter overviews the realm of biomechanics and provide an introduction to various areas with mention to researches carried out from a mechanical engineer's perspective. Prominent areas like biomechanics of human motion; bone and joint biomechanics; biomechanics of spine; biomechanics of head, shoulder and muscles; biomechanical analysis of heart and lungs; biomechanical analysis of arteries and veins and MEMS in biomechanics are explored. As the field is a subject in itself so the chapter focuses primarily on few prominent researches made in the last two decades in various domains.

In Chapter 2, a review of development of prosthetics and orthotics of lower body has been summarized. The history of these items is exhaustive yet very colourful. In this chapter, history and development of prosthetics and orthotics of the lower body has been elaborated for better understanding of the current state of the art in the fields. Due to enormous vast field, a historical perspective is provided followed by enumeration of the types of devices and techniques available without going into the form and function of individual products.

Chapter 3, the last chapter of the section, discusses about bioresorbable composites and Implants. The domain of medical sciences is flooded with different biomaterials in the form of ceramics, metal alloys, composites, glasses, and polymers etc. which have gained wide range acceptance. Bio-implants from such biomaterials have been constructed and used widely for different clinical applications. With the continual progress, biomaterials that may be resorbed inside the body have been developed. These have done away with the major challenge of removal of an implant after it has served its intended function. Important factors that are taken into consideration in design and development of implants from such biomaterials are mechanical properties, degradation rate, surface modification, rate of corrosion, biocompatibility and non-toxicity. Given the importance of such materials in clinical applications, the present chapter presents an overview of the bioresorable composites and their implants. The related properties and the functions served have been outlined briefly. Further, the challenges associated and the remedies to overcome them have also been delineated.

Section 2 is dedicated to Scaffolds and Tissue Engineering Applications and contains a single chapter: Chapter 4. The chapter discusses a revolutionary manufacturing process namely 3D bio-printing which is currently being used in medical fields specially in preparing of bone scaffolds and tissue engineering area. With the help of new biocompatible material like polymers, bio-gels, ceramics, this technology have created a new site in advanced tissue engineering and scaffolds manufacturing area. Moreover the beauty of the system is that, with the use of CAD file software, any design can be prepared irrespective of its complexity. The chapter not only discusses the novel technique but also describes and analyses machine's printability characteristic, cross-linking time and biocompatibility of printing objects as well as bio-ink. In this chapter, different types of scaffold preparing methods, bio-printing process are discussed which are used in scaffold and tissue engineering area.

From here the book starts with Section 3 which groups the Prosthesis part.

The first chapter of the section, Chapter 5, illustrates the design of a prosthetic ankle complex. Nature has, over a large span of geological time, engineered near perfect solutions to most problems humans face today. Motion of the limbs is one such area and the cutting edge in the development of effective prostheses is biomimetics. Limb prostheses have been used by mankind for the better part of known history and most of the technology currently available in prosthetics is not exclusively new. However, modern prosthetics either are uncomfortable and the lack of flexion affects the gait of the patient or too expensive for a large segment of the populace. This chapter seeks to study the mimicry of physiological systems through the design for an ankle prosthesis which includes a passive damper and mimics the shape and behaviour of the natural ankle joint.

The real challenge after the design is manufacturing of a prosthetic component. In Chapter 6 a non-traditional machining technique electrochemical micromachining (ECMM) has been introduced to create a proper component which can be used clinically. This chapter aims at developing an optimized model for flow analysis of electrolyte in inter-electrode gap to obtain optimal process parameter for machining. Experimentation has been done to associate the findings of optimized output in ECMM such as material removal rate (MRR), overcut and depth. Influence of voltage, feed rate, concentration, pulse on/pulse off ratio and inter-electrode gap (IEG) was investigated and finally optimized using response surface method. The outcome was validated using ANOVA.

On producing a component for prosthetic application, it is required to ascertain excellent surface finish which is usually in microns. The most sophisticated instrument for identification and measurement for the same is Atomic Force Microscope. But acquisition of experimental data from atomic force microscopy (AFM) sometimes has artefacts that distort the information contained in the image. Such artefacts can be very delirious especially for sensitive applications such as in biomedical and microelectronics. Chapter 7 deals with correction of artefacts and optimization of Atomic Force Microscopy imaging. In order to elaborate the subject a case of thin aluminium films has been considered. The chapter illustrates the correction of the artefacts resulting from tapping mode imaging. It also shows the application of Taguchi optimization technique for reducing artefacts during AFM imaging. Using AFM images of Al films Fourier filtering is illustrated as a useful technique for the correction. Taguchi optimization was employed to determine the optimal scan rate, scan size, integral and proportional gains in minimizing the size and number of artefacts at the imaging stage. The correction technique was shown to improve the morphological information of the AFM images while the Taguchi method was effective for determining the best imaging conditions for AFM analysis.

The next chapter and last chapter of the section, Chapter 8, elaborates another hindrance in the biomechanical product development, the induced stress. During production, machining etc. generally stresses are induced which requires to be minimised for effective service and life span. In this chapter, the induced stress concentrations are minimised via the optimisation of tab design configurations. Stress concentration obtained via finite element analysis were used to develop a full factorial design for statistical analysis and compared with a Taguchi, Taguchi- multi response and Taguchi-genetic algorithm optimisations. The chapter concludes that in order to minimise the stress concentrations, low values of tab stiffness, thickness and taper angle were required while the adhesive thickness was increased. The conclusion was supported with neumerical data.

From here the book starts with Section 4 which groups the Orthosis part.

The section starts with Chapter 9 which reviews the processing and characterization of materials for Orthotic Devices. The recent utilization of fibre reinforced composites as bio-material in fabrication of orthoses have accelerated the research in finding the most favourable and compatible combinations of bio-polymeric composites. The strength, flexibility, biological compatibility, wear strength, durability and fatigue strength can be easily altered considering different combinations of polymers and their reinforced structures. The major drawback presently faced by researchers is the degree of mimicking the behavioural and functional aspects of body muscles and bones, by the synthetic polymeric composites more appropriately. In this chapter, a thorough review of the presently used various types of polymeric composites employed as materials for orthotic implants, their properties, and their applications based on their availability for common people (cheap cost), availability for wide variety of specialized functions and for the best quality and compatibility factor. The common orthotic products mainly used on patients to support their weak joint or limb and their most favourable material properties or material of choice was discussed in details. A few characteristic determination tests for polyethylene composites performed for material properties like ultimate tensile strength, elastic modulus, thermal degradation properties, bending strength and surface resistance are taken into consideration to validate the usability of polyethylene composites and their improvement trend in modification of the combination of fibres and matrix.

Chapters 10, the last chapter of the section and the book, discusses the application of electrochemical micromachining for machining in micro level devices required for orthotic products which are usually made of harden materials. In present chapter a model for flow analysis of electrolyte in inter electrode gap is designed to obtain optimal process parameter for machining. The geometric model used in this simulation consists of cylindrical workpiece, an inlet allowing the flow of sodium nitrate solution as electrolyte to the machining zone and a cylindrical tool with flat end. Electrolytic flow simulation is incorporated using computational fluid dynamics by ANSYS–CFX for finding pressure variation, streamline velocity pattern, turbulent energy, and temperature contour in inter electrode gap (IEG).

First and foremost, the editors would like to thank God. In the process of putting this book together it was realized how true this gift of writing is for anyone. You have given the power to believe in passion, hard work and pursue dreams. This could never have been done without the faith in You, the Almighty. The Editors would also like to thank all the Chapter Contributors, the Reviewers, the Editorial Advisory Board Members, Book Development Editor and the team of Publisher IGI Global for their availability for work on this editorial project.

Kaushik Kumar
Birla Institute of Technology, India

J. Paulo Davim
University of Aveiro, Portugal

Section 1

Review of the State of the Art

Chapter 1
A Systematic Survey of the Realm of Biomechanics:
A Mechanical Engineer's Perspective

Deepak Mahapatra
National Institute of Technology Raipur, India

Shubhankar Bhowmick
https://orcid.org/0000-0001-9799-8724
National Institute of Technology Raipur, India

Shubhashis Sanyal
National Institute of Technology Raipur, India

ABSTRACT

The area of biomechanics is challenging and broad as it involves multidisciplinary concepts of engineering together with functional knowledge of biosciences. The area is rapidly evolving and new additions to it are being made daily. A survey that may help a beginner to have a general look on the broader aspects of the sub-domains of biomechanics is not available. The chapter aims to overview the realm of biomechanics and provide an introduction to various areas with mention to researches carried out. A broad survey of various areas of biomechanics from a mechanical engineer's perspective is reported in this chapter. Prominent areas like biomechanics of human motion; bone and joint biomechanics; biomechanics of spine; biomechanics of head, shoulder, and muscles; biomechanical analysis of heart and lungs; biomechanical analysis of arteries and veins; and MEMS in biomechanics are explored. Though it is difficult to include all the developments relevant to the above areas, the authors have focused primarily on a few prominent studies made in the last two decades in various domains.

DOI: 10.4018/978-1-5225-8235-9.ch001

INTRODUCTION

Biomechanics involves the study of living organisms and processes relevant to human body with an engineer's perspective. This means the physical, anatomical and other functional characteristics of human body are studied under the umbrella of engineering concepts, for example-the concepts of engineering mechanics in the study of motion of human beings (especially for athletes), flow properties of blood using fluid dynamics and many more. Statics, dynamics, kinematics and kinetics of biological systems are used to study their response to mechanical forces. The studies relevant to biological systems has been an area of interest for researchers since medieval era but it has gained considerable attention in 20th century, and the specialist area of bio-medical engineering has evolved. Till the last decade of 20th century the studies of biomechanics were mainly focused on researches of simulations of cardiac, respiratory and/or skeletal systems as a whole; but with the rapid advancement in computational capabilities, the modeling of basic biological entities like tissues, cells etc. is possible in today's era; thus accuracy of prediction related to functioning of biological systems has improved considerably. The need for development of devices that work on micro- or nano- levels and compatible to biological processes is more pertinent.

The area of biomechanics is very challenging and broad as it involves multidisciplinary concepts of engineering sciences together with functional knowledge of biosciences, to provide necessary solutions. The non-linearity associated with biological systems make the problems too complex, further adding to the difficulties. In spite of the tremendous challenges, there is rapid advancement in the field of biomechanics research as a result of which a number of reports/ findings on the biomechanical processes are published as journal papers and textbooks of repute. Due to the large volume of literature relevant to various areas of biomechanics, it is very difficult to include or summarize all the developments, the present report highlights some of the prominent researches made in the last two decades. The contents are arranged such that the study is classified into seven sections; each section focuses primarily on a particular system- biomechanics of i) human motion, ii) bone, joint and muscle, iii) spine, iv) head, neck and shoulder, v) heart and lungs, vi) arteries and veins, vii) MEMS in biomechanics. As such the following report will greatly help a beginner to – a) know the basic terminologies associated, b) relate the biological processes with engineering concepts and c) the latest findings in the area.

SURVEY

Biomechanics of Human Motion

Kinesiology (Kinetics + Physiology) is an area under biomechanics specific to human movement. It is the study of human movement with a closer and finer view. Thorough knowledge of human anatomy is a prerequisite as it provides essential labels for musculoskeletal structure and joint motion relevant to human motion. Before proceeding to the survey part it is customary to have an overview of the nomenclature/ notations used to describe human movement. Figure 1 and 2 give a sufficient exposure of the notations generally used. A number of books (Hall, 2011; Kundson, 2007; Tozeren, 2000; Nigg et al, 1999; Peterson et al, 2008; Andris, 2004) can be referred for an in depth study. In (Manal et al, 2004) authors have categorized study of human movement according to their application in five groups viz. motion control (as in a humanoid robot), pathological treatment (design improvements in prosthetic and orthopedic devices), sports/athlete improvisation, ergonomics, and computer animation/simulation. Researchers are working widely in each of these specific areas.

Biomechanics of Bone, Joint and Muscle

Bones

Bones are the structural members of our skeleton i.e. a range of sizes of bones attached to each other in a constructive way so as to give the body shape as it is; thereby providing a shield for the soft tissues and organs. From an engineer's point of view the structure of bones that give them strength is of considerable importance; and the way bones are connected at joints to give a constrained motion using the muscle forces is also significant. Bone's strength is owing to its composition and specialized structure that provides it with naturally tailored properties. It can sustain huge loads considering its aspect ratio maintaining its flexibility and strength in tension. Minerals contribute to a bone's hardness and compressive strength, and collagen provides its flexibility and tensile strength. A frontal view of human skeleton showing all major bones with respective name and classification of each is presented in Figure 3 adapted from. Figure 4 represents a schematic representation of longest bone of human body-femur; the nomenclature of bone and its

Figure 1. Representation of a person through reference section planes- a) The sagittal plane divides the front view into left and right half, b) The frontal plane divides the top view into anterior(towards chest) and posterior(towards back) portions, c) The transverse (horizontal) plane divides the front view into two parts- superior(top) and inferior(bottom)
(OpenStax College, n.d.)

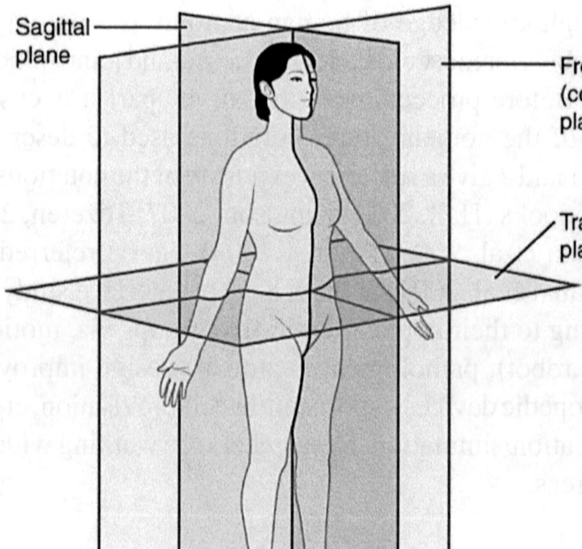

constituents may be studied through this figure. Figure 5a and 5b represents the strength of the bone; its comparison with other engineering materials and its strength at different locations. A number of research publications on mechanical properties and testing of bones is available in literature. An introduction to bone material composition and properties can be referred in (Peterson et al, 2008).

In order to predict the behavior of bones under different loading conditions (existing in different bones according to their function and those can be of very high order), the mechanical properties like elasticity, strength, rigidity/ flexibility, time dependency of strength i.e. visco-elasticity, plasticity, fracture, fatigue strength, creep strength etc. must be precisely known a priori. Reilly and Cleveland have exhaustively reviewed the publications to explore mechanical properties of bones. In (Jones et al, 2003) authors discuss about the technical requirements, precision, calibration and reproducibility of loading systems for mechanical testing of trabecular bone. An excellent review on fracture mechanisms in bones especially of children is illustrated in. Authors (Pierce et al, 2004). have compiled the fracture patterns according to various types of loading so as to assist the physician to better assess the causes of the injury and medication thereafter.

As the cost of experimentation is very high both on the part of equipment specifications or collection of specimen for test, computational testing using Finite Element Analysis (FEA) is highly appreciated. Accurate virtual bone or bone implant can be generated using images obtained from Computed Tomography (CT) or Magnetic Resonance Imaging (MRI) technique to provide patient specific data which can be processed and analyzed. A large number of publications on FE analysis of bones and implants are available. The authors (Raji et al, 2011) have studied the finite element analysis of thigh bone called femur (Figure 4, which is the largest bone of human body) using the geometry imported from CT scan data and analysis in ANSYS. Another long bone below femurcalled tibia (Refer Figure 3) supports the entire load of human body and is subjected excessive compressive stress. In many accidental cases it is seen that this bone gets fractured. To only remedial action that can be performed is to join the fractured parts by an external supporting plate which is screwed within. The modeling and analysis of such plates and screws so as to tailor the exact specification required for patient specific need, will be of considerable use. A similar work in which an FEA model of tibial screw has been established by experimental verification by Sheng-Muo et al (2004).

Joints

Joints are largely responsible for directional capabilities of human body. Each bone of body performs its specific function by the directed muscle forces. In this regard the motion of the bones has to be constrained in a systematic way that is controlled by the joint function. Hence the flexibility of joints to perform a specified function thereby maintaining its stability is largely required. The different joints of human body and their analogues used in engineering analysis are presented in Figure 6. It can be clearly assessed that the principles of joints used in mechanism synthesis and analysis can be applied to biomechanics as well. Moreover these principles can be used

Figure 2. A-f terminologies used to describing rotations at various joints (OpenStax College, n.d.)

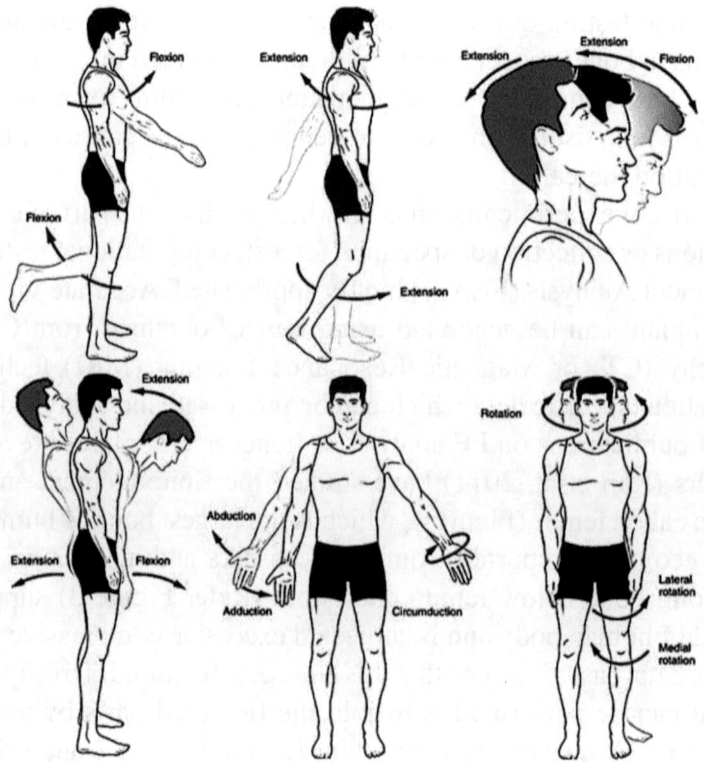

in the synthesis of prosthetic implants in case of any abnormality in joint functioning.

Thus if the joint functioning and its mobile characteristics are neatly characterized then it will greatly suffice not only the diagnosis and surgery but also aid in synthesis of customized prosthetic devices needed for patient specific need. In (Peterson et al, 2008) authors have presented a detailed analysis of motion characteristics of joints of human body. Joint lubrication is a separate area of research and bio-tribology concepts may be required/ applied for successful joint prosthetics. Arthroplasty or prosthetic implant is common for remedy of joint abnormalities. The motion characteristics of joints in part and body as whole can be accessed through the biomechanical gait analysis. In this method the human motion is minutely observed using cameras and analyzed by computers using a 3D trajectory. Different mechanical techniques for implants to cure arthritis are dealt in (Giuse et al, 2011; Lester, 2009).

Figure 3. Frontal and rear view of the human skeleton
(OpenStax College, n.d.)

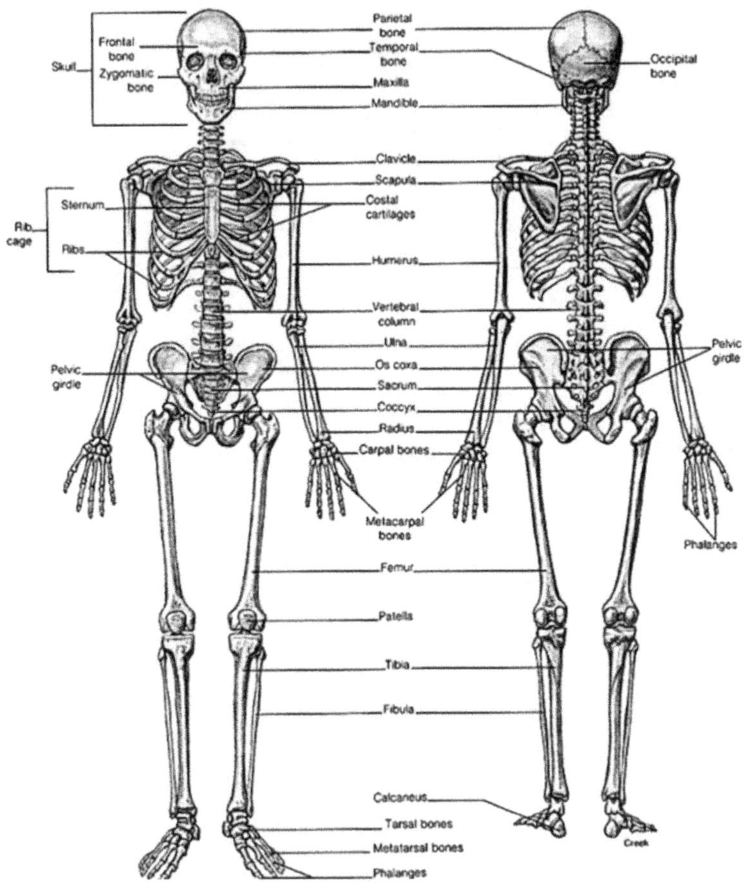

Muscle

Determination of muscle forces has been a big challenge for researchers since long time. Muscles are activated by neural commands and quantifying them is quite complex. Instead if muscle forces are determined, neural commands may be obtained from it. Figure 7 represents the progressie organization of a muscle fiber- the hierarchy follows like actin/myosin –sacomeres-myofibrils-myofibrils-muscle fibre-fascicles. It is clearly observed that the behaviour of muscle fibre is the agglomerated efforts of its constituents (actin/myosin). There are quite a number of reports that model the muscle behaviour, out of which the most preferred model is that of viscoelastic behaviour similar

Figure 4. Diagram of a long bone (femur) shown in longitudinal view (OpenStax College, n.d.)

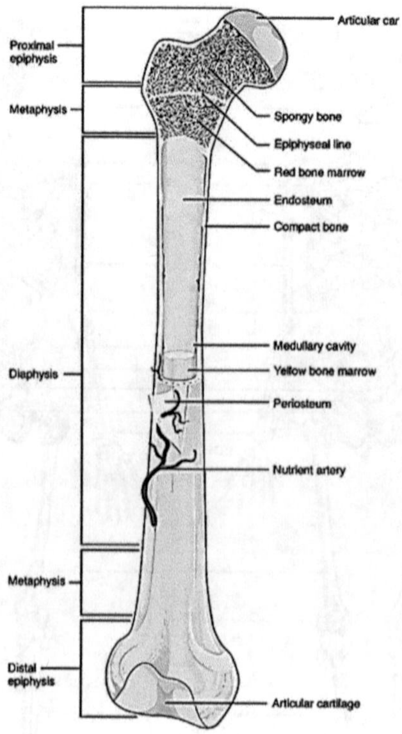

to a standard linear solid. A summary of study of Muscle Force-length and Muscle Force-Velocity relations are reported in (Peterson et al, 2008; Reilly et al, 1974). Need for computational models have compelled a number of researches in this area. A review of the latest works on relationships between muscle force, its length, velocity and their activation is reported in (Ahmet et al, 2007). An excellent review on computational modelling of ligaments and tendon is reported in. Both the structure and function of ligaments have been covered in (Weiss et al, 201 with main focus on their constitutivemodelling.

Biomechanics of Spine

Spine or backbone (in laymen terms) or vertaebra is an assembly of significant segments resulting in a complex maneuver of bones, muscle and fibers intervoven to give its functional characteristics. It can move in all the three planes and it connects the upper and lower part of the body. Moreover

Figure 5. a) Stress–strain curves for cortical bone tested in tension in four different orientations; b) Stress–strain curves for bone and other materials in tension

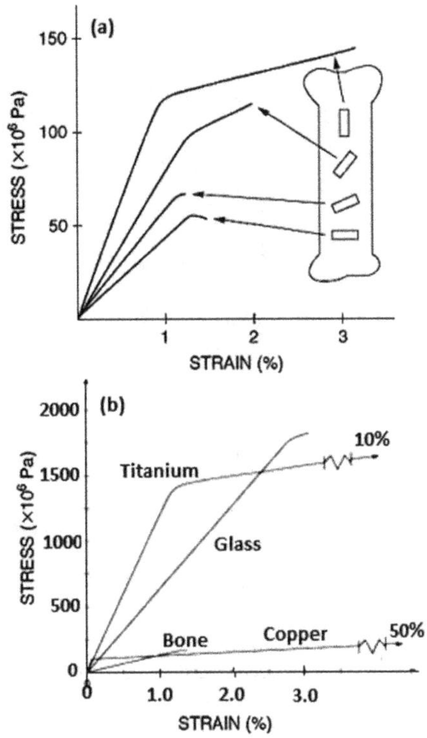

it contains and hence protects the delicate spinal cord therby helping in smooth functioning of nervous system. Due to its significance, even a small malfunctioning of any of its components results in fatal injuries needing costly medications. This makes spine to be one of the most challenging areas under biomechanical research. In Figure 8 the classification of spine is diagramatically represented as five distinct parts, with each part sustaing a specific function. Cervical is closest to head while coccygeal is closest to feet. Cervical spine consists of seven neck bones, thoracic contains twelve bones of chest/ribs, lumbar consists of five bones of lower back, sacral is single bone made from five fused sacral segments attached to pelvis and finally coccyx (whose extension become tail in animals). It has been observed through clinical studies that the lumbar part of spine is the most succeptible to injury (back pain and slip disc are common ailments related to it). Hence the exact modeling and analysis of spine components may provide considerable support to the clinicians.

Figure 6. Synovial (Freely movable) joints of human body and their analogues in mechanics
(OpenStax College, n.d.)

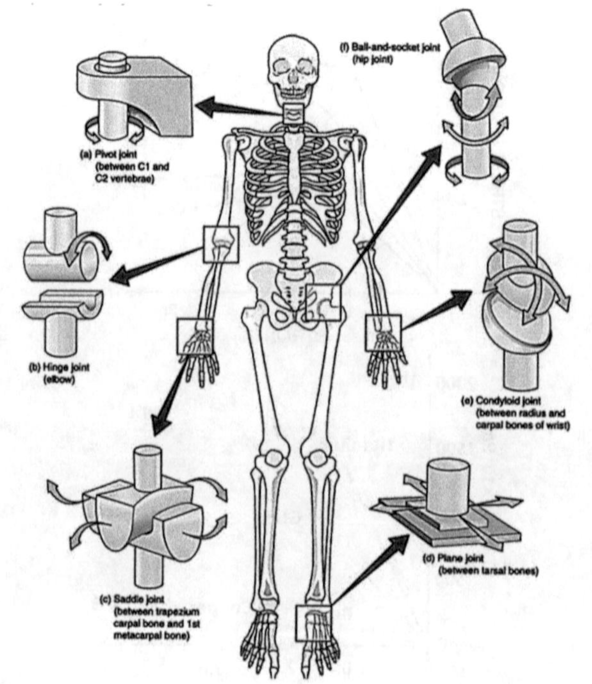

Researchers have focused on formulating techniques to model the mechanical behavior of spine since long time. Mechanism of injury and body's response to it if modeled correctly will help patients and doctors for appropriate recovery. A detailed survey of cervical spine mathematical modeling is reported in reference (huelke et al, 1986) along with experimental validations. Excellent review of lumbar spine is reported in references (Behrsin et al, 1988) A survey of applied numerical techniques and their experimental validation of biomechanics of the lumbar part of spine to improve efficiency of traction is reported in (Fonet, 2006). Another review is presented in (Thomas et al, 204) that take into account the effect of degeneration of disc and joints of spine on its load-bearing and kinematic behavior.

From the above it is clear that the modeling and analysis and their validation can prove to be quite effective for medical treatments. Many researches on computational study of the understanding of the mechanical behavior of a spine segments has been reported. Numerous models of spine and vertebrae have been developed and are in use in research today to investigate almost every

Figure 7. a) Macro-Skeletal muscle organized progressively from myofibrils-muscle fibre-fascicles ;b)Micro-Skeletal muscle organized progressively from actin/myosin –sacomeres-myofibrils
(OpenStax College, n.d.)

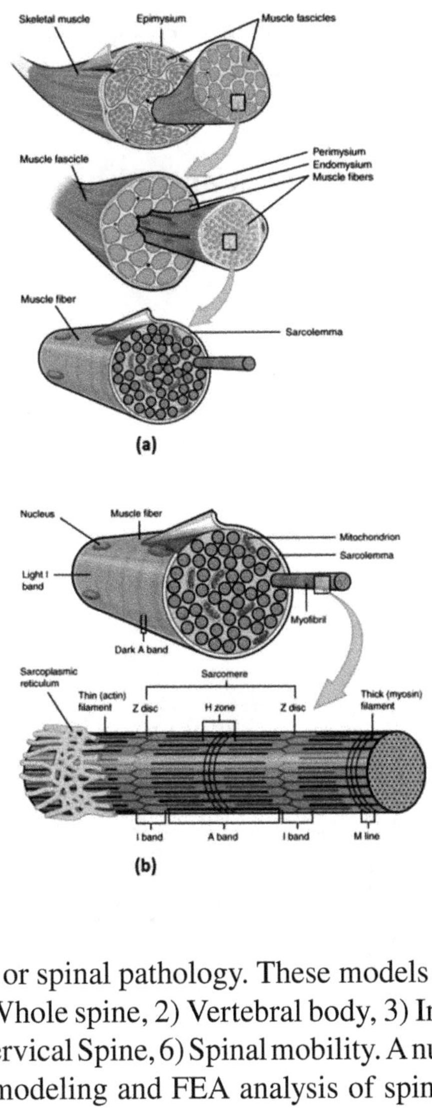

physical movement or spinal pathology. These models can be characterized into six groups- 1) Whole spine, 2) Vertebral body, 3) Inter-vertebral disc, 4) Lumbar Spine, 5) Cervical Spine, 6) Spinal mobility. A number of publications are devoted to the modeling and FEA analysis of spine parts and implants (Jang et al, 2010; Kuo, Coombs et al, 2012) . An extensive discussion on various types of loading on spinal constituents is reported in (Hall, 2011).

To alleviate the lower back pain researchers are constantly in search of new synthetic materials that are effective for nucleus replacement and compatible to spine topology. Testing of various materials (titanium base alloys Ti6Al4V, super alloys of Ti-Ni) for their adaptability and suitability is relevant in this sense. Hydrogel nucleus implants made up of Polyvinyl alcohol (PVA) or Polyvinyl pyrollidone (PVP) were prepared of different sizes and shapes and tested in human lumbar inter-vertebral discs (IVDs) (Joshi et al, 2005; Joshi et al, 2006) FEA simulations can again be an effective tool in testing the biomechanical compatibility. In (Vena et al, 2005) a computational study of L4-L5 lumbar spine both for a healthy and implanted spine (using U shaped super-alloy) has been investigated.

Biomechanics of Head, Neck and Shoulder

Head and Neck

Three types of injuries of head/neck viz. diffuse injury, focal injury or injury resulting from relative motion between brain and skull may lead to traumatic injuries and must be accounted (Peterson et al, 2008). Knowledge on the

Figure 8. Two views (lateral and posterior) of human spine
(OpenStax College, n.d.)

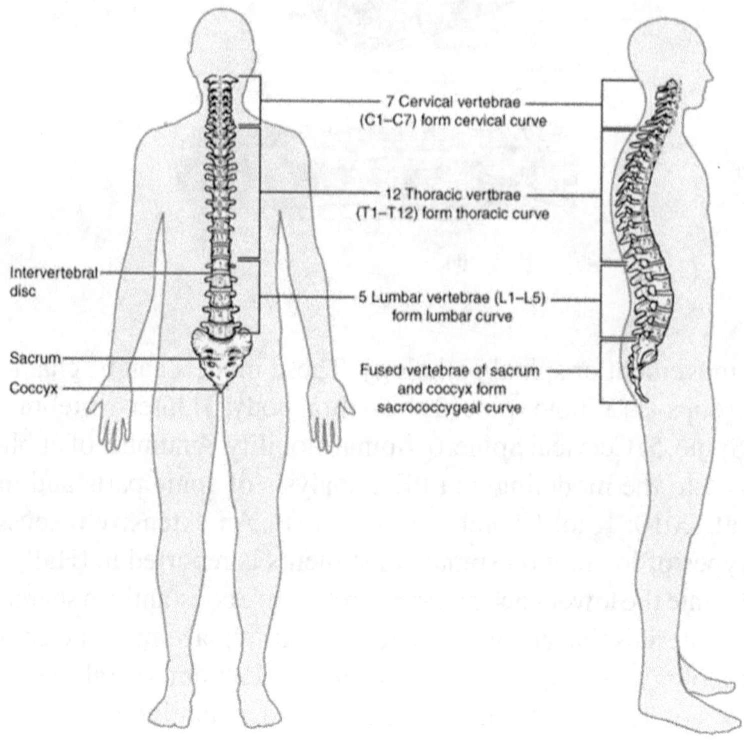

mechanisms by which an impact load results in injury is still incomplete and exhaustive research on modeling and analysis of brain injuries is in progress. A separate research area called 'Brain Injury Biomechanics' has been initiated to track such developments. A detailed review on Traumatic brain injuries (TBI) from biomechanical point of view is reported in (Namjoshi et al, 2013). In (El Sayed et al, 2008) authors have utilized a constitutive model for soft tissue to calculate the mechanical damage due to TBI in terms of volumetric and shear loss. Finite element modeling and analysis is again a wide area of application and research under this umbrella. Wide range of publications on both modeling of human head and analysis is available. A review of the various literatures can be referred in (Samaka et al, 2013). FEA simulations for effect of impact i.e. contact forces and coup pressure on head in (Horgan et al, 2003; Kleiven et al, 2002) while in (Pinnoji et al, 2007) a comparison of helmeted and non-helmeted head for impact is investigated

Shoulder

Another significant functional part of this category which is an assembly of five articulated joints(Hall, 2011) as shown in Figure 9 is Shoulder. Each of the joint of shoulder assembly maneuvers a specific function owing to its typical orientation. The upper shoulder joint is called glenohumeral joint, which helps in 3D rotation of hands as it is a ball-and-socket joint. The sternoclavicular (SC) joint is a modified ball and socket, that permits the free motion of the frontal and transverse plane accompanied by rotation of saggital plane(Figure 9).

The shoulder being a complex assembly of joints is subjected to injuries of different kinds, the most injuries are seen in athletes of various sports. The dislocation of glenohumeral joint is the most common type of injury (Hall, 2011). Another common injury called rotator cuff impingement syndrome or subacromial impingement syndrome, or shoulder impingement syndrome among workers or athletes who engage in overhead works like painting, lifting, swimming, tennis, etc., such that result in narrowing of the space between acromion and rotator cuff due to which they rub against each other resulting in pain and irritation. If not taken care of this may result in disability of the shoulder. A detailed review on anatomical and biomechanical mechanisms of this syndrome is published in (Michner et al, 2003).

Biomechanical Analysis of Heart and Lungs

Cardiovascular (Heart) diseases are the major cause of death in almost all parts of the world. As such it is one of the major challenges for a bio-mechanist to open new paradigms for preventing/ curing such diseases. Biomechanical analysis of heart is very challenging due to its immense complexities. Hence it is one of the most crucial areas under biomechanical research. The cardiac system consists of heart, arteries and veins. In this subsection our focus will primarily be on heart in general and its valves in particular. (Arteries and veins will be dealt in next subsection). Figure 10 shows the nomenclature of heart and its constituents, while Fig-11a represents the sectioned view of the heart to explore its inner anatomy.The anatomy of heart comprises of four chambers, two on each side, and there are two pumps located in such a way that they sync each other perfectly and with the body. The circulation of blod through the heart is carried in two steps- one is systemic and other is pulmonary. The left chambers of heart participate in systemic while the right work during pulmonary. The flow of blood through the heart is regulated by four valves as shown in Figure 11b. The functioning of the heart is astonishing display of flexibility with strength jointly carried by all the four valves. The mitral and tricuspic valves in the upper chambers let the blood flow into the ventricles while the pulmonary and aortic valve release blood out of ventricle. The mitral valve is having two leaves while the others have three. The valves must operate in such a way that the opening/ closing operation must not interrupt in the blood flow and even the slightest of resistance may cause fatal heart malfunctioning. It can be observed that the leaves of the valves can be modeled as cantilever plates/ beams subjected to fluid interaction and would be a FSI problem. The development of effective and accurate numerical simulation can be great help to medical community (Peterson et al, 2008). A review that covers various computational models is reported in (Weinberg et al, 2010). Fluid structure Interaction between heart valves and blood has been a topic of interest to many researchers and a number of publications can be found in recent literature (Wuarteroni et al, 2002; Voose et al, 2003; Loon et al, 2004; Torii et al, 2004; Loon et al, 2005; Loon et al, 2006; Santos, 2007; Nobili et al, 2008; Griffith et al, 2009). References (Port, 2008; Sitijen et al, 2004) are dedicated to mitral valve analysis while (Hart et al, 1998; Hart, 2002; Astorino et al, 2008) are devoted to aorta valve.

Figure 9. A) Various articulations of shoulder joint (OpenStax College, n.d.) b) Different views of clavicle (collar bone) (OpenStax College, n.d.)

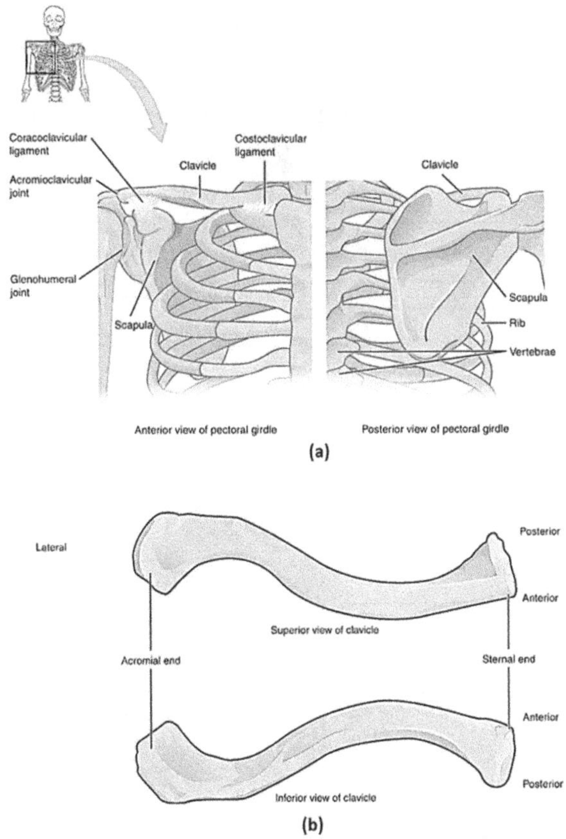

Continuing with the modeling techniques, literature on interaction between cardiac system and the respiratory system has also been established. In (Lee et al, 2011) authors have developed a non-linear dynamic models simulation and analysis of heart-lung interactions. The relevance of fluid structure interaction (FSI) in modeling the lung dynamics has inspired new research in recent times. In (Malve et al, 2011) FSI techniques are applied to simulate and analyze the behavior of human trachea before and after implantation thereby suggesting the possibilities of improvement.

A number of publications on stent artery interaction and thereby modelling of healthy, diseased and stented arteries are published. In (Gasse, 2007) authors have analyzed mechanically the damage in arteries due to plaque and intervention due to stent and this analysis can be used for an optimum

Figure 10. Heart anatomy
(OpenStax College, n.d.)

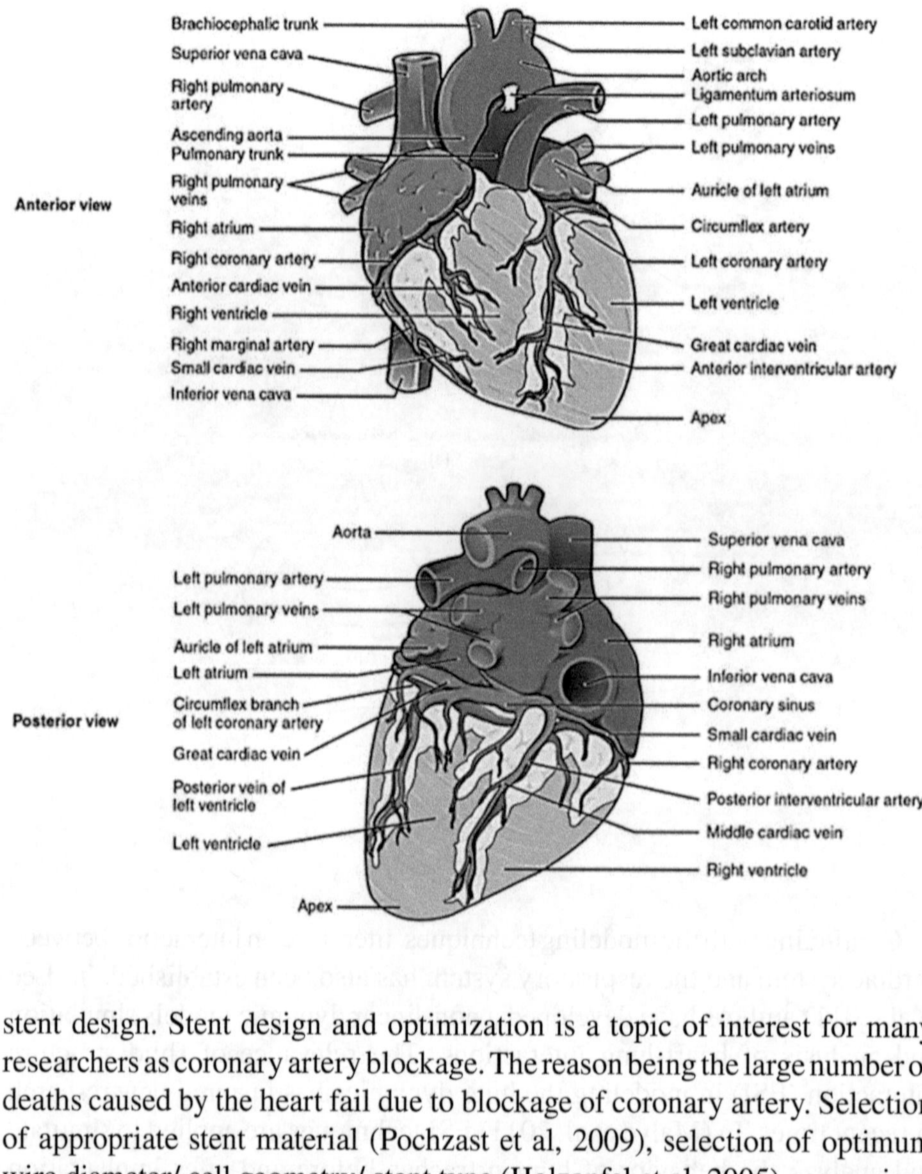

stent design. Stent design and optimization is a topic of interest for many researchers as coronary artery blockage. The reason being the large number of deaths caused by the heart fail due to blockage of coronary artery. Selection of appropriate stent material (Pochzast et al, 2009), selection of optimum wire diameter/ cell geometry/ stent type (Holzapfel et al, 2005) comparison of various models of stent according to arterial stress distribution considering stent-tissue friction and plaque properties (Gu et al, 2012), experimental investigation of real stents and comparison of mechanical behaviour (Tambaca et al, 2011), consideration of arterial stress/strain due to stenting (Zhao et al, 2012) are some of the many researches in this domain. In a recent paper

Figure 11. a) Heart anatomy (frontal half); b) heart valves
(OpenStax College, n.d.)

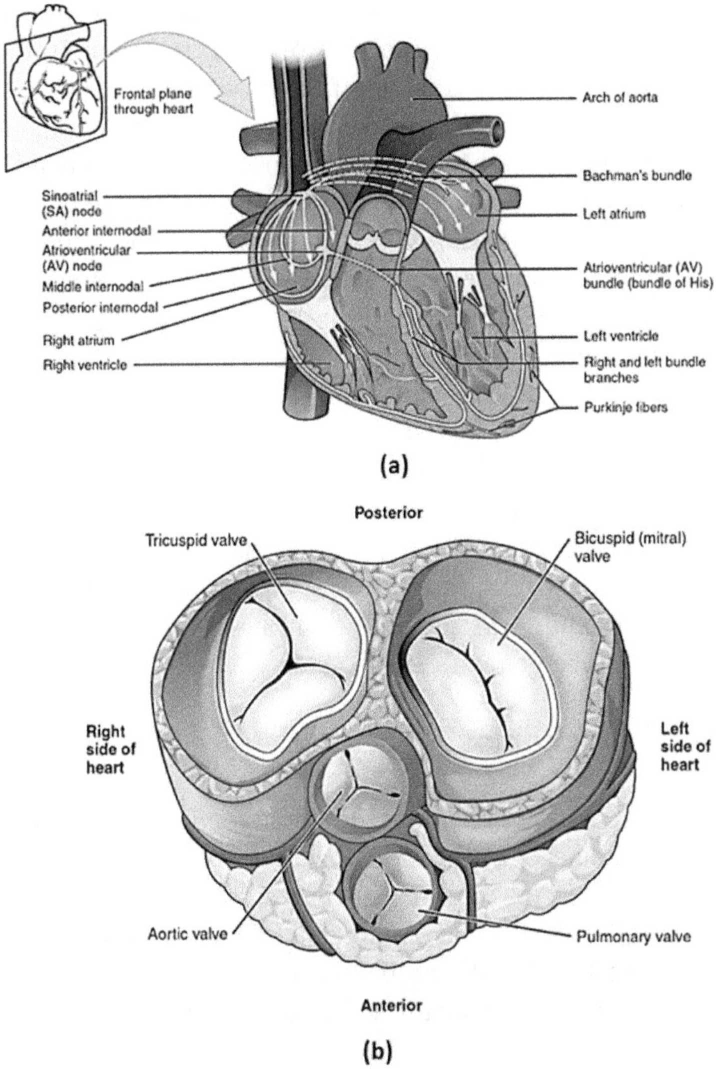

(Imani et al, 2013), Imani et al have analyzed the expansion characteristics of three different multi-link stents using FEA and taking into account all the parameters like stress distribution in stent and artery, amount of flattening in radial direction, changes in dimensions, deposition at the ends called dog boning etc., with and without considering the effect of plaque. It is significant to mention here that a number of publications on CFD/ FSI analysis of arteries and arterial environment are also available.

Biomechanical Analysis of Arteries and Veins

Arteries are flexible tubes that supply fresh oxygenated blood from heart to tissues and organs while the function of veins is to supply the impure blood back to heart. Arteries are classified in two types viz. One is elastic artery and other is muscular. Elastic arteries are larger in size and are in the vicinity of heart, and are highly elastic in nature. On the other hand muscular arteries show visco-elastic nature and function as distributing theblood to the organs (Holzapfel et al, 2004). Figure-13 depicts the cross-sectional details of an artery and veins thereby giving an idea of the different layers prenet in them. Valuable information regarding the basic mechanical aspects of arterial mechanics and properties required for modelling can be found in (Humphrey et al, 2003; Black et al, 1998). Excellent reviews on the arterial mechanics with comparison of various constitutive models can be found in (Humphrey, 1995; Holzapfel et al, 2000; Holzapfel et al, 2010). A common disease associated with arteries is atherosclerosis/ stenosis i.e.thickening and stiffening of intima, the innermost layer of artery. This results in alterations in both wall properties and flow of blood. A common treatment for stenosis is angioplasty and stenting. FE modelling and analysis of balloon angioplasty is reported in (Kleinberger et al, 1994).

MEMS in Biomechanics

Micro electro-mechanical systems are micron size devices with sensors and actuators have a number of applications e.g. Inkjet printers, digital projectors, automotive motion sensing etc. Such devices are used in the field of medical science also and BioMEMS is a rapidly emerging field. An overview of the various aspects of BioMEMS can be viewed in (Imani et al, 2013). From mechanical point of view (Lobontiu et al, 2005) gives good exposure towards the principles governing the mechanics of MEMS. Application of MEMS in cardiac surgery (Bonanomi et al, 2003), development of micro/nano knife (Chang et al, 2007), MEMS forceps (Bhisitkul et al, 2005) are some of the recent researches relevant in this area.

CONCLUSION

This report has been written to cover prominent researches that may help a beginner to have an overview of the realm of biomechanics. The present work has been selectively classified into seven sections so as to describe the terminologies and recent advances of biomechanics in a concise and comprehensive way for a researcher with non-medical background. Thus each subsection of the survey attempts to highlight a particular segment of biomechanical study by summarizing the pertinent fundamental ideas and published reports. The studies relevant to mechanics of human movement have been covered in the first part; such studies are especially needed for researches on prosthetic orthopedics, in sports, animations and many more. The next subsection summarizes the mechanical study of human skeleton i.e. the study of bones, their joints and their motion using muscles. In order to have a smooth working of human skeletal system a collective effort of these is an absolute necessity. However to simplify things, studies have been made specific to each functional element; hence bones, joints and muscles are separately studied and reported. Spine, a complex assembly of bones, muscles and fibers with prominent functional characteristics, has been covered in the next subsection. The mechanical studies pertinent to spine are covered separately due to its significant functional requirement in overall functioning of human body. A virtual model of spine and its simulation studies may be highly supportive in customized patient specific prosthetics. In the next subsection study of head, neck and shoulder has been covered. Modeling and analysis of brain injuries due to impact load is one of the prime research areas in this category; similar other reports have been summarized in this section. Shoulder joints are also prone areas of injury, more common amongst athletes and sportsperson. Studies pertinent to shoulder has also been covered and reported in this section. Another crucial area of research has been modeling, simulation and analysis of functioning of heart and its valves; and is reported in the next section. Various studies like reports on modeling and dynamics of heart valves, synthesis and analysis of stents; cardiac-respiratory interactions; modeling of lung and respiratory dynamics has been covered. The studies relevant to modeling and simulation of arteries and veins have been reported in the next section. Another emerging area in the field of biomechanical applications has been Bio-MEMS and it is felt that micro and nano-mechanical components aided with smart materials will be highly significant in biomechanics in particular. Although considerable

Figure 12. Major blood vessels (arteries) in human body
(OpenStax College, n.d.)

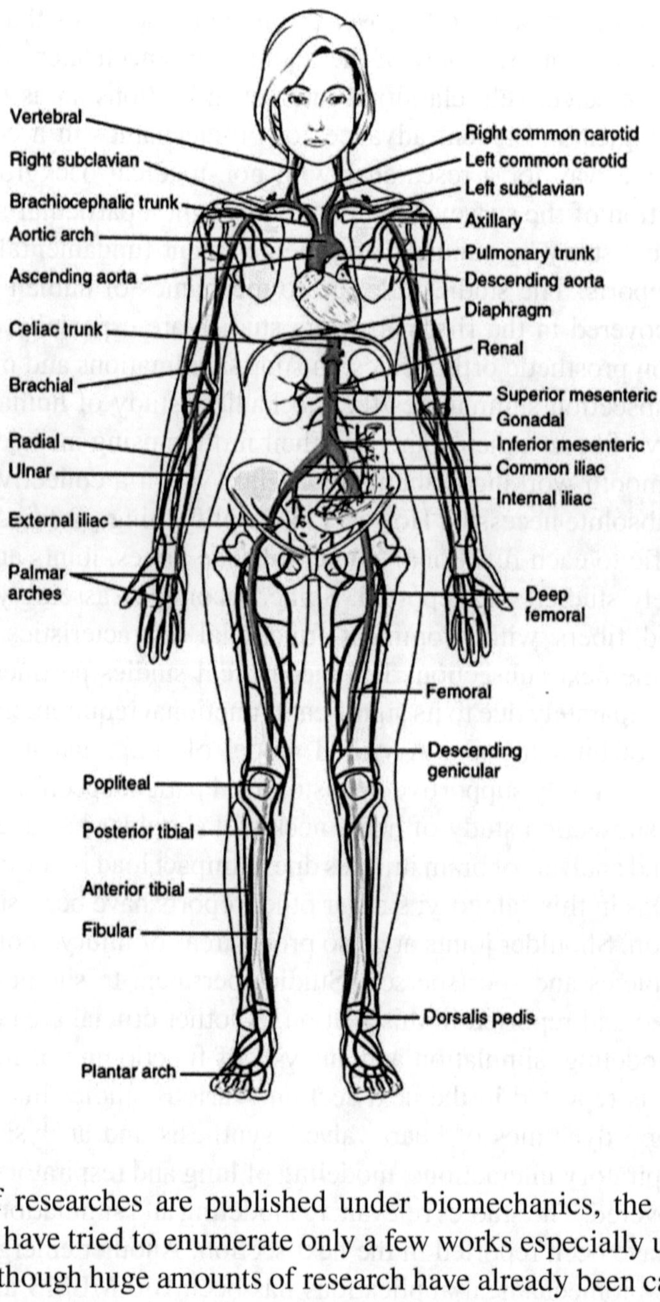

volumes of researches are published under biomechanics, the authors in this review have tried to enumerate only a few works especially useful for a layman. Although huge amounts of research have already been carried over in recent times in the area of bio-mechanical and bio-medical engineering, but eminent personalities predict that many prominent areas of biomechanical analysis areas are still untouched and can be explored in near future.

Figure 13. Section showing components of a healthy elastic artery and vein *(OpenStax College, n.d.)*

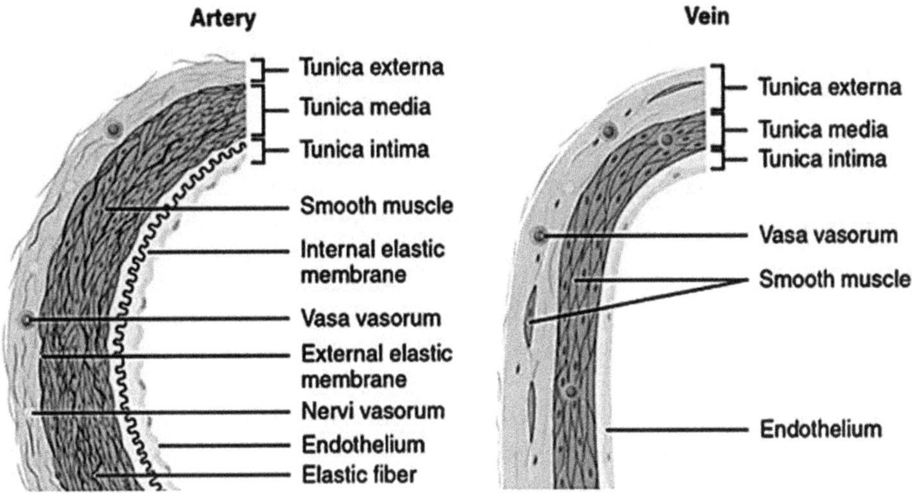

Figure 14. Balloon angioplasty and Stenting. (a) Positioning of balloon tipped catheter in the diseased area and placing of the stent near coronary narrowing, (b) Inflation of the balloon to expand the stent to press the arterial wall, the balloon is deflated, removed while stent remains permanently in place, helping to keep the artery open.

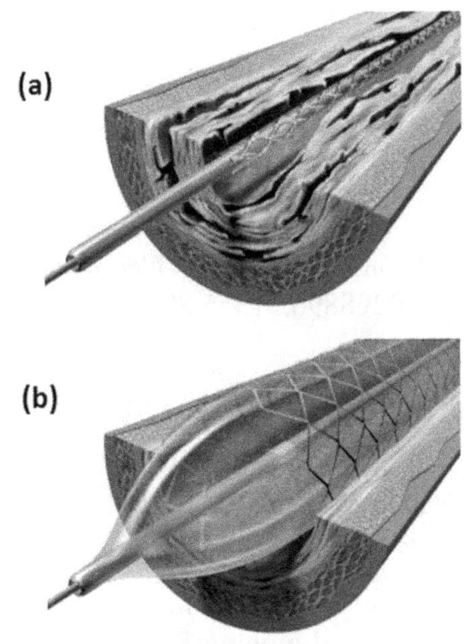

REFERENCES

Astorino, M., Gerbeau, J. F., Pantz, O., & Traor, K. F. (2008). Fluid-Structure Interaction and Multi-Body Contact Application to Aortic Valves. *8th. World Congress on Computational Mechanics (WCCM8).*

Auricchio, Ferrara, & Morganti. (2012). Comparison and critical analysis of invariant-based models with respect to their ability in fitting human aortic valve data. In *Annals of Solid and Structural Mechanics*. Springer.

Behrsin, J. F., & Briggs, C. A. (1988). Ligaments of the lumbar spine: A review. *Surgical and Radiologic Anatomy*, *10*(3), 211–219. doi:10.1007/BF02115239 PMID:3147534

Bhisitkul, R. B., & Keller, C. G. (2005). Development of Microelectromechanical Systems (MEMS) forceps for intraocular surgery. *Journal of Ophthalmology*, *89*, 1586–1588. PMID:16299136

Black, J., & Hastings, G. (1998). *Handbook of Biomaterial Properties*. Chapman & Hall. doi:10.1007/978-1-4615-5801-9

Bonanomi, G., Rebello, K., Lebouitz, K., Riviere, C., Di Martino, E., Vorp, D., & Zenati, M. A. (2003). Microelectromechanical systems for endoscopic cardiac surgery. *The Journal of Thoracic and Cardiovascular Surgery*, *126*(3), 851–852. doi:10.1016/S0022-5223(03)00393-3 PMID:14502165

Boyce, E. (2009). Simulating the Fluid Dynamics of Natural and Prosthetic Heart Valves using the Immersed Boundary Method. *International Journal of Applied Mechanics*, *1*(1), 137–177. doi:10.1142/S1758825109000113

Chang, W. C., Hawkes, E. A., Kliot, M., & Sretavan, D. W. (2007). In Vivo Use of aNanoknife for Axon Microsurgery. *Neurosurgery*, *61*(4), 683–692. doi:10.1227/01.NEU.0000298896.31355.80 PMID:17986929

Christina, A. (2004). Degenerative mechanics of the lumbar spine. *The Spine Journal*, *4*(6), 202–208. doi:10.1016/j.spinee.2004.07.013 PMID:15016399

Coombs, D. J., Laz, P. J., Rao, M., Smith, S. D., Bushelow, M., & Rullkoetter, P. J. (2012). Stepwise Validated Finite Element Model of the Human Lumbar Spine. *SIMULIA Customer Conference.*

De Hart. (2002). *Fluid-Structure Interaction in the Aortic Heart Valve-a three-dimensional computational analysis* (PhD thesis). Eindhoven University of Technology.

De Hart, J., Cacciola, G., Schreurs, P. J. G., & Peters, G. W. M. (1998). A three-dimensional analysis of a fibre-reinforced aortic valve prosthesis. *Journal of Biomechanics, 31*(7), 629–638. doi:10.1016/S0021-9290(98)00063-3 PMID:9796685

de Jager, M. (1993). Mathematical Modelling of the Human Cervical Spine: A Survey of the Literature. *Proceedings of the 1993 International IRCOBI Conference on the Biomechanics of Impact.*

Diniz Dos Santos, N. M. (2007). *Numerical methods for fluid-structure interaction problems with valves* (PhD thesis). University of Parie and Marie Curie.

Douglas, B. (2006). *Generation of 3-D parametric solid model of human spine using anthropomorphic parameters* (MS Thesis). Ohio University.

El Sayed, T., Mota, A., Fraternali, F., & Ortiz, M. (2008). Biomechanics of traumatic brain injury. *Computer Methods in Applied Mechanics and Engineering*, *197*(51-52), 4692–4701. doi:10.1016/j.cma.2008.06.006

Eli, J. (2010). On the multiscale modeling of heart valve biomechanics in health and disease. *Biomechanics and Modeling in Mechanobiology*, *9*(4), 373–387. doi:10.100710237-009-0181-2 PMID:20066464

Erdemir, A., McLean, S., Herzog, W., & van den Bogert, A. J. (2007). Model-based estimation of muscle forces exerted during movements. *Clinical Biomechanics (Bristol, Avon)*, *22*(2), 131–154. doi:10.1016/j.clinbiomech.2006.09.005 PMID:17070969

Freivalds. (2004). *Biomechanics of the upper limbs- Mechanics, modeling and musculoskeletal injuries*. CRC Press.

Gasser & Holzapfel. (2007). Finite element modeling of balloon angioplasty by considering overstretch of remnant non-diseased tissues in lesions. *Computational Mechanics, 40*, 47–60.

Gu, Zhao, & Froemming. (2012). Arterial Wall Mechanics and Clinical Implications after Coronary Stenting: Comparisons of Three Stent Designs. *International Journal of Applied Mechanics*, *4*(2), 1–12.

Guise, Mezghani, Aissaoui, & Hagemeister. (2011). New comprehensive methods for the biomechanical analysis of knee osteoarthritis. Understanding Osteoarthritis from Bench to Bedside, 85-102.

Hall, S. J. (2011). *Basic Biomechanics* (6th ed.). McGraw Hill.

Holzapfel, G. A., Gasser, T. C., & Ogden, R. W. (2000). A New Constitutive Framework for Arterial Wall Mechanics and a Comparative Study of Material Models. *Journal of Elasticity*, *61*(1/3), 1–48. doi:10.1023/A:1010835316564

Holzapfel, G. A., & Ogden, R. W. (2010). Constitutive modeling of arteries. *Proceedings of Royal Society*, *466*(2118), 1551–1597. doi:10.1098/rspa.2010.0058

Holzapfel, G. A., Stadler, M., & Gasser, T. C. (2005). Changes in the Mechanical Environment of Stenotic Arteries during interaction with Stents: Computational Assessment of Parametric Stent Designs. *Transactions of the ASME*, 127, 167-180. 10.1115/1.1835362

Holzapfel. (2004). Computational Biomechanics of Soft Biological Tissue. In Encyclopedia of Computational Mechanics. John Wiley & Sons.

Horgan, T. J., & Gilchrist, M. D. (2003). The creation of three-dimensional finite element models for simulating head impact biomechanics. *International Journal of Crash*, *8*(4), 353–366. doi:10.1533/ijcr.2003.0243

Hou, S.-M., Hsu, C.-C., Wang, J.-L., Chao, C.-K., & Lin, J. (2004). Mechanical tests and finite element models for bone holding power of tibial locking screws. *Clinical Biomechanics (Bristol, Avon)*, *19*(7), 738–745. doi:10.1016/j.clinbiomech.2004.04.012 PMID:15288461

Huelke, D. F., & Nusholtz, G. S. (1986). Cervical Spine Biomechanics: A Review of the Literature. *Journal of Orthopedics Research*, *4*(2). PMID:3519910

Humphrey, J. D. (1995). Mechanics of arterial wall: Review and directions. *Critical Reviews in Biomedical Engineering*, *23*(1-2), 1–162. doi:10.1615/CritRevBiomedEng.v23.i1-2.10 PMID:8665806

Humphrey, J. D., & Delange, S. L. (2003). *An introduction to Biomechanics-Solids and Fluids, Analysis & Design*. Springer.

Jagadamma. (2010). *The biomechanical optimisation (tuning) of The Ankle Foot Orthosis - Footwear Combination (AFO-FC) of children with Cerebral Palsy - the effects on sagittal gait characteristics, muscle and joint characteristics and quality of life* (PhD Thesis). Queen Margret University.

Jang, T. H., & Ekwaro-Osire, S. (2010). *Stochastic Finite Element Approach in Low Cervical Spine For Increasing Analysis Reliability*. Society for Design and Process Science.

Jones, D. B., Broeckmann, E., Pohl, T., & Smith, E. L. (2003). Development of a Mechanical Testing and Loading System for Trabecular Bone Studies for Long Term Culture. *European Cells & Materials*, *5*, 48–60. doi:10.22203/eCM.v005a05 PMID:14562272

Joshi, Mehta, Vresilovic, Karduna, & Marcolongo. (2005). Nucleus Implant Parameters Significantly Change the Compressive Stiffness of the Human Lumbar Intervertebral Disc. *Transactions of the ASME,* 127.

Joshi, A. (2006). *Functional compressive mechanics of a PVA/PVP nucleus pulposus replacement* (Vol. 27). Biomaterials.

Karadogan & Williams. (2012). Three-Dimensional Static Modeling of the Lumbar Spine. *Journal of Biomechanical Engineering*, *134*. PMID:22938364

Khatib, O., & Demircan, E. (2005). *Robotics-based Synthesis of Human Motion*. Academic Press.

Kiousis, D. E. (2008). *Biomechanical and Computational Modeling of Atherosclerotic Arteries-Insights into Plaque Vulnerability and Vascular Stenting* (Vol. 4). Computation in Engineering and Science.

Kleiven. (2002). *Finite Element Modeling of the Human Head* (PhD thesis). Royal Institute of Technology.

Knudson, D. (2007). *Fundamentals of Biomechanics* (2nd ed.). Springer.

Kuo, Hu, Lin, Huang, Lin, Zhong, & Hsei. (2010). Bio-mechanical analysis of the lumbar spine on facet joint force and intra-discal pressure - a Finite element study. *BMC Musculoskeletal Disorders*.

Kurutz & Fornet. (2006). Experimental And Numerical Biomechanical Analysis of the Human Lumbar Spine. *Journal of Computational and Applied Mechanics*, *7*(1), 23–39.

Lee. (2008). *Biomechanical Modeling and Control of the Human Body for Computer Animation* (PhD Thesis). University of California, Los Angeles, CA.

Lee. (2009). Comprehensive Biomechanical Modeling and Simulation of the Upper Body. Academic Press.

Lee, R.-M., & Chiu, H.-L. (2011). Mathematical Model of Interactive Respiration/Cardiovascular Composite System. *International Conference on Trends in Mechanical and Industrial Engineering (ICTMIE'2011)*, 136-139.

Lester. (2009). *The Biomechanical Analysis Of The Hand In Rheumatoid Arthritis Patients with McpArthroplasty* (PhD Thesis). University of Birmingham.

Lobontiu & Garcia. (2005). Mechanics of Microelectromechanical Systems. Kluwer Academic Publishers.

Lori, A. (2003). Anatomical and biomechanical mechanisms of subacromial impingement syndrome. *Clinical Biomechanics (Bristol, Avon)*, *18*(5), 369–379. doi:10.1016/S0268-0033(03)00047-0 PMID:12763431

Malve, M., Pe'rez del Palomar, A., Chandra, S., Lo'pez-Villalobos, J. L., & Finol, E. A. (2011). FSI Analysis of a Human Trachea Before and After Prosthesis Implantation. *Journal of Biomechanical Engineering*, *133*(7), 071003–1, 12. doi:10.1115/1.4004315 PMID:21823742

Malve, M., Pe'rez del Palomar, A., Chandra, S., Lo'pez-Villalobos, J. L., Finol A. Mena, E. A., Ginel, A., & Doblaré, M. (2011). FSI Analysis of a Healthy and a Stenotic Human Trachea Under Impedance-Based BoundaryConditions. *Journal of Biomechanical Engineering*, *133*(2), 021001–1, 12. doi:10.1115/1.4003130 PMID:21280873

Manal, K. T., & Buchanan, T. S. (2004). *Biomechanics of Human Movement*. McGraw Hill.

Martijn, D., & Horsman, K. (2007). *The Twente Lower Extremity Model, Consistent Dynamic Simulation of the Human Locomotor Apparatus* (PhD Thesis). University of Twente.

Michaels, A. D., & Chatterjee, K. (2002). Angioplasty Versus Bypass Surgery for Coronary Artery Disease. *Circulation*, *106*(23), e187–e190. doi:10.1161/01.CIR.0000044747.37349.64 PMID:12460885

Misagh Imani, A.M., Goudarzi, M.H., & Hojjati. (2013). Finite Element Analysis of Mechanical Behaviors of Multi-Link Stent in a Coronary Artery with Plaque. *World Applied Sciences Journal*, *21*(11), 1597–1602.

van den Bogert, Samorezov, Davis, & Smith. (2012). Modeling and Optimal Control of an Energy-Storing Prosthetic Knee. *Journal of Biomechanical Engineering*, *134*. PMID:22757495

Namjoshi, D. R., Good, C., Wai, H. C., Panenka, W., Richards, D., Cripton, P. A., & Wellington, C. L. (2013). Towards clinical management of traumatic brain injury: A review of models and mechanisms from a biomechanical perspective. *Disease Models & Mechanisms*, *6*(6), 1325–1338. doi:10.1242/dmm.011320 PMID:24046354

Nareliya & Kumar. (2011). Biomechanical Analysis of Human Femur Bone. *International Journal of Engineering Science and Technology*, *3*(4).

Nigg, B., & Herzog, W. (1999). *Biomechanics of the Musculoskeletal System* (2nd ed.). John Wiley & Sons.

Nobili, M., Morbiducci, U., Ponzini, R., Del Gaudio, C., Balducci, A., Grigioni, M., ... Redaelli, A. (2008). Numerical simulation of the dynamics of a bileaflet prosthetic heartvalve using a fluid–structure interaction approach. *Journal of Biomechanics*, *41*(11), 2539–2550. doi:10.1016/j.jbiomech.2008.05.004 PMID:18579146

Oh, S., Kleinberger, M., & McElhaney, J. H. (1994). Finite Element analysis of balloon angioplasty. *Medical & Biological Engineering & Computing*, *32*(S1), S108–S114. doi:10.1007/BF02523336 PMID:7967823

Ommaya, A. K., Goldsmith, W., & Thibault, L. (2002). Biomechanics and neuropathology of adult and paediatric head injury. *British Journal of Neurosurgery*, *16*(3), 220–242. doi:10.1080/02688690220148824 PMID:12201393

OpenStax College. (n.d.). *Anatomy and Physiology*. OpenStax CNX. Retrieved from http://cnx.org/contents/14fb4ad7-39a1-4eee-ab6e-3ef2482e3e22@12.8

Peterson, D. R., & Bronzino, J. D. (2008). *Biomechanics- Principles and Applications*. CRC Press.

Pierce, M. C., Bertocci, G. E., Vogeley, E., & Moreland, M. S. (2004). Evaluating long bone fractures in children: A biomechanical approach with illustrative cases. *Child Abuse & Neglect*, *28*(5), 505–524. doi:10.1016/j.chiabu.2003.01.001 PMID:15206413

Pinnoji, P. K., & Mahajan, P. (2007). Finite element modeling of helmeted head impact under frontal loading. *Sadhana*, *32*(4), 445–458. doi:10.100712046-007-0034-6

Pochrząst, M., Walke, W., & Kaczmarek, M. (2009). Biomechanical characterization of the balloon-expandable slotted tube stents. *Journal of Achievements in Materials and Manufacturing Engineering*, *3*(2), 340–347.

Prot. (2008). *Modelling and numerical analysis of the porcine and human mitral apparatus* (PhD thesis). Norwegian University of Science and Technology.

Quarteroni & Formagga. (2002). Mathematical modeling and numerical simulation of the cardiovascular system. In Modeling of living systems: Handbook of numerical analysis series. Elsevier.

Rebello, K. J. (2004). Applications of MEMS in Surgery. *Proceedings of the IEEE*, *92*(1), 43–55. doi:10.1109/JPROC.2003.820536

Samaka & Tarlochan. (2013). Finite Element (FE) Human Head Models / Literature Review. *International Journal of Scientific & Technology Research*, *2*(7).

Stijnen. (2004). *Interaction between the mitral and aortic heart valve- an experimental and computational study* (PhD thesis). Eindhoven University of Technology.

Tambaca, Canic, Kosor, Fish, & Paniagua. (2011). Mechanical Behavior of Fully Expanded Commercially Available Endovascular Coronary Stents. Texas Heart Institute Journal, 491-501.

Reilly, D. T. & Cleveland, A. H. B. (1974). The Mechanical Properties of Cortical Bone. *The Journal of Bone and Joint Surgery*, *56a*(5). PMID:4603167

Torii, R., Oshima, M., Kobayashi, T., Takagi, K., & Tezduyar, T. E. (2004). Computation of Cardiovascular Fluid-Structure Interactions with the DSD/SST Method. *Proceedings of the 6th World Congress on Computational Mechanics*.

Tözeren, A. (2000). *Human Body Dynamics Classical Mechanics and Human Movement*. Springer.

Tyndyk, M. A., Barron, V., Mchugh, P. E., & O'mahoney, D. (2007). Generation of a finite element model of the thoracolumbar spine. *Acta of Bioengineering and Biomechanics*, *9*(1). PMID:17933103

Van De Vosse, F. N., De Hart, J., Van Oijen, C. H. G. A., Bessems, D., Gunther, T. W. M., Segal, A., ... Baaijens, F. P. T. (2003). Finite-element-based computational methods for cardiovascular fluid-structure interaction. *Journal of Engineering Mathematics*, *47*(3/4), 335–368. doi:10.1023/B:ENGI.0000007985.17625.43

van Loon, R. (2005). *A 3D method for modeling the fluid-structure interaction of heart valves* (PhD thesis). Eindhoven University of Technology.

van Loon, R., Anderso, P. D., & van de Vosse, F. N. (2006). A fluid–structure interaction method with solid-rigid contact for heart valve dynamics. *Journal of Computational Physics*, *217*(2), 806–823. doi:10.1016/j.jcp.2006.01.032

van Loon, R., Anderson, P. D., de Hart, J., & Baaijens, F. P. T. (2004). A combined fictitious domain /adaptive meshing method for fluid–structure interaction in heart valves. *International Journal for Numerical Methods in Fluids*, *46*(5), 533–544. doi:10.1002/fld.775

Vena, P., Franzoso, G., Gastaldi, D., Contro, R., & Dallolio, V. (2005). A finite Element Model of the L4-L5 spinal motion segment: Biomechanical compatibility of an inter-spinous device. *Computer Methods in Biomechanics and Biomedical Engineering*, *8*(1), 7–16. doi:10.1080/10255840500062914 PMID:16154865

Wahab. (2009). *Design and Implementation of MEMS Biomechanical Sensors for Real-Life Measurements of Gait Parameters* (PhD Thesis). Victoria University, Australia.

Weiss, J. A., & Gardiner, J. C. (2001). Computational Modeling of Ligament Mechanics. *Critical Reviews in Biomedical Engineering*, *29*(4), 1–70. PMID:11730098

Zahedmanesh, H., & Lally, C. (2009). Determination of the influence of stent strut thickness using the finite element method: Implications for vascular injury and in-stent restenosis. *Medical & Biological Engineering & Computing*, *47*(4), 385–393. doi:10.100711517-009-0432-5 PMID:19189146

Zhao, S., Gu, L., & Froemming, S. R. (2012). Effects of Arterial Strain and Stress in the Prediction of Restenosis Risk: Computer Modeling of Stent Trials. *Biomedical Engineering Letters*, *2*(3), 158–163. doi:10.100713534-012-0067-6

APPENDIX

Description of Terminologies/ Important Terms

1. Biomechanics of Human Motion

Abduction: Motions that move a structure away from or towards the centre of the body.

Adduction: Motions that move a structure towards the centre of the body.

Anterior: Refers to the "front"(ventral) of the individual other than in the head.

Extension: Describes movements that increase the angle between two parts of the body.

Flexion: Describes a bending movement that decreases the angle between two parts of the body.

Frontal Plane: Is any vertical plane that divides the body into ventral (front) and dorsal (back) sections. It is one of the planes of the body used to describe the location of body parts in relation to each other.

Kinesiology: The science dealing with the Interrelationship of the physiological processes and anatomy of the human body with respect to movement. It includes measures from motion tracking systems, electrophysiology of muscle and brain activity, various methods for monitoring physiological functions, and other behavioral and cognitive research techniques.

Musculoskeletal System: The complete muscular and skeletal system made up of bones muscles, joints, tendons, ligaments that supports and binds the tissues and organs together. Its functions include supporting the body, allowing motion, and protecting vital organs.

Posterior: Refers to the "back" (dorsal) of the individual other than in the head.

Rotation: Rotation towards (internal) or away(external) from the center of the body.

Saggital Plane: Is a vertical plane which passes from ventral (front) to dorsal (rear) dividing the body into right and left halves.

2. Biomechanics of Bone, Joint and Muscle

Actin: Is a globular multi-functional protein that forms microfilaments in muscles. Its functions include muscle contraction, cell motility, cell division cell signalling, and the establishment and maintenance of cell junctions and cell shape.

Arthritis: A form of joint disorder that involves inflammation of one or more joints.

Arthroplasty: Is an orthopedic surgery where the articular surface of a musculoskeletal joint is replaced, remodeled, or realigned to relieve pain and restore function to the joint after damage by arthritis or some other type of trauma.

Carpus: Is the anatomical assembly connecting the hand to forearm. In human anatomy, the main role of the carpus is to facilitate effective positioning of the hand and powerful use of the extensors and flexors of the forearm, but the mobility of individual carpal bones increase the freedom of movements at the wrist.

Clavicle: Is a long bone lying horizontally below neck and it serves as a strut between the scapula and the sternum. It makes up part of the shoulder and the pectoral girdle

Collagen: Is the main structural protein of the various connective tissues in animals and is mostly found in fibrous tissues such as tendons, ligaments and skin, and is also abundant in corneas, cartilage, bones, blood vessels, the gut, and inter-vertebral discs.

Fascia: Is a structure of connective tissue that surrounds muscles, groups of muscles, blood vessels, and nerves, binding some structures together, while permitting others to slide smoothly over each other.

Femur: Is a bone in the human leg extending from the pelvis to the knee and is the longest, largest, and strongest in the body; also called thighbone.

Fibula: Also called calf bone is a leg bone located on the lateral side of the tibia, with which it is connected above and below.

Humerus: Is the long bone in the arm of humans extending from the shoulder to the elbow.

Ligaments: Is the fibrous tissue that connects bones to other bones

Metacarpus: Is the intermediate part of the hand skeleton that is located between the phalanges (bones of the fingers) and the carpus which forms the connection to the forearm

Metatarsus: The intermediate part of the foot skeleton that is located between the phalanges (bones of the toes) and the tarsus

Myofibril: Also known as a muscle fibril is a basic rod-like unit of a muscle. Muscles are composed of tubular cells called myocytes, also known as muscle fibers, and these cells in turn contain many chains of myofibrils.

Myosin: Comprise of a family of ATP-dependent motor proteins and are best known for their role in muscle contraction and their involvement in a wide range of other eukaryotic motility processes

Patella: Also known as the kneecap is a thick, circular-triangular bone which articulates with the femur (thigh bone) and covers and protects the anterior/ articular surface of the knee joint.

Phalanges: Are bones that exist on each finger and toe. There are 56 phalanges in the human body, with fourteen phalanges on each hand and foot. Three phalanges are present on each finger and toe, with the exception of the thumb and large toe, which possess only two.

Prosthesis: Is an artificial device that replaces a missing body part lost through trauma, disease, or congenital conditions.

Scapula: Is flat, triangular bone, forming the back part of a shoulder in humans; it is also called shoulder blade.

Tarsus: Is a cluster of seven articulating bones in each foot situated between the lower end of tibia and fibula of the lower leg and the metatarsus.

Tendon: A tendon (or sinew) is a tough band of fibrous connective tissue that usually connects muscle to bone and is capable of withstanding tension. Tendons are similar to ligaments and fasciae; all three are made of collagen. Ligaments join one bone to another bone; fasciae connect muscles to other muscles. Tendons and muscles work together to move bones.

Tibia: Also known as the shinbone, is the larger and stronger of the two bones in the leg below the knee in vertebrates (the other being the fibula), and it connects the knee with the ankle bones.

Ulna: Is the bone of the forearm on the side opposite to the thumb.

3. Biomechanics of Spine

Cervical Spine: Comprises of seven bony segments lying near the neck, typically referred to as C-1 to C-7 with cartilaginous discs between each vertebral body.

Coccygeal: Also known as the tailbone, is the final segment of the spine in tailless primates comprising three to five separate or fused vertebrae.

Lumbar Spine: Are the five vertebrae between the rib cage and the pelvis. They are the largest segments of the vertebral column.

Sacrum: Is a large, triangular bone at the base of the spine and at the upper and back part of the pelvic cavity, where it is inserted like a wedge between the two hip bones. Its upper part connects with the last lumbar vertebra, and bottom part with the coccyx (tailbone).

Thoracic Spine: Composes the middle segment of the spine between the cervical and the lumbar and are 12 in number in humans.

4. Biomechanics of Head, Neck and Shoulder

Acromioclavicular Joint: The acromioclavicular joint, or AC joint, is a joint at the top of the shoulder. It is the junction between the acromion (part of the scapula that forms the highest point of the shoulder) and the clavicle. It is a plane synovial joint.

Acromion: Is a bony process on the scapula (shoulder blade).

Glenohumeral Joint: Is a multiaxialsynovial ball and socket joint and involves articulation between the glenoid fossa of the scapula (shoulder blade) and the head of the humerus (upper arm bone). Due to the very limited interface of the humerus and scapula, it is the most mobile joint of the human body.

Rotator cuff Impingement Syndrome/ Subacromial Impingement Syndrome/ Shoulder Impingement Syndrome: Is a clinical syndrome which occurs when the tendons of the rotator cuff muscles become irritated and inflamed as they pass through the subacromial space, the passage beneath the acromion. This can result in pain, weakness and loss of movement at the shoulder.

Scapulothoracic Joint: Is a physiological joint formed by an articulation of the anterior scapula and the posterior thoracic rib cage. It is musculotendinous in nature and is formed predominantly by the trapezius, rhomboids and serratus anterior muscles.

Sternoclavicular Joint: Is structurally classed as a synovial double-plane joint and functionally classed as a diarthrotic joint. It is composed of two portions separated by an articular disc which is made from fibrocartilage.

Trapezius: Is a large superficial muscle that extends longitudinally from the occipital bone to the lower thoracic vertebrae and laterally to the spine of the scapula (shoulder blade). Its functions are to move the scapulae and support the arm.

5. Biomechanical Analysis of Heart and Lungs

Aortic Valve: Lies between the left ventricle and the aorta.

Cardiovascular: THE essential components of the human cardiovascular system are the heart, blood, and blood vessels.

Coronary Circulation: Is the circulation of blood in the blood vessels of the heart muscle (myocardium). The vessels that deliver oxygen-rich blood to the myocardium are known as coronary arteries.

Mitral Valve: Also known as the bicuspid valve is a dual-flap valve in the heart that lies between the left atrium (LA) and the left ventricle (LV).

Pulmonary Circulation: Is the portion of the cardiovascular system which carries deoxygenated blood away from the heart, to the lungs, and returns oxygenated (oxygen-rich) blood back to the heart.

Pulmonary Valve: Is the semi lunar valve of the heart that lies between the right ventricle and the pulmonary artery and has three cusps.

Systemic Circulation: Refers to the part of the circulatory system in which the blood leaves the heart through the left ventricle to the aorta then to smaller arteries, arterioles, and finally capillaries, services the body's cells, and then re-enters the heart.

Tricuspid Valve: Is on the right dorsal side of the heart, between the right atrium and the right ventricle. The function of the valve is to prevent back flow of blood into the right atrium.

6. Biomechanical Analysis of Arteries and Veins

Adventitia: Or tunica is the outermost tunica (layer) of a blood vessel, surrounding the tunica media. It is mainly composed of collagen and, in arteries, is supported by external elastic lamina. The collagen serves to anchor the blood vessel to nearby organs, giving it stability.

Angioplasty: Is the technique of mechanically widening narrowed or obstructed arteries by passing a balloon catheter into the narrowed locations and then inflated to a fixed size.

Arteries: Are blood vessels that carry blood away from the heart.

Balloon Catheter: Is a type of "soft" catheter with an inflatable "balloon" at its tip which is used during a catheterization procedure to enlarge a narrow opening or passage within the body. The deflated balloon catheter is positioned, then inflated to perform the necessary procedure, and deflated again in order to be removed.

Carotid Arteries: Are arteries that supply the head and neck with oxygenated blood

Intima: Or tunica intima is the innermost tunica (layer) of an artery or vein. It is made up of one layer of endothelial cells and is supported by an internal elastic lamina. The endothelial cells are in direct contact with the blood flow.

Media: Or tunica media is the middle tunica (layer) of an artery or vein. It lies between the tunica intima on the inside and the tunica externa on the outside.

Stenosis: Is an abnormal narrowing in a blood vessel or other tubular organ or structure.

Stent: Is a mesh 'tube' inserted into a natural passage/conduit in the body to prevent or counteract a disease-induced, localized flow constriction. The term may also refer to a tube used to temporarily hold such a natural conduit open to allow access for surgery.

Veins: Carry deoxygenated blood from the tissues back to the heart.

Chapter 2
A Brief History of Prosthetics and Orthotics of the Lower Body and Their Types

Dheeman Bhuyan
https://orcid.org/0000-0001-9772-0028
Girijananda Chowdhury Institute of Management and Technology, India

Kaushik Kumar
Birla Institute of Technology, India

ABSTRACT

Prosthetics and orthotics are items taken for granted in today's day and age. However, this has not always been the case. The history of these everyday items is long and very colorful. In this chapter, the authors shed light on the history and development of prosthetics and orthotics of the lower body in order to better understand the current state of the art in the fields. A historical perspective is provided followed by enumeration of the types of devices and techniques available without going into the form and function of individual products.

INTRODUCTION

With advances in science and technology, the efforts to replicate natures work have been bolstered over the years. There are numerous techniques and technologies available today. The replacement of ailing organs and lost limbs is now a reality. Prosthetics and orthotics are today playing an important

DOI: 10.4018/978-1-5225-8235-9.ch002

and ever more effective role in improving the quality of life of people who otherwise would not have been able to lead a normal, healthy life.

The words prosthetics and orthotics bring to the mind visualizations of plastic legs and arms without any form of articulation. Some even think of the wooden stump which would be used by seafarers as prosthetic legs and the hooks used in place of lost arms. While the history of prosthetics does include these, today prosthetics could not be further from these popular images. This is a growing field, with new developments and advances being made almost every day.

Advances in the fields of medicine and engineering have today given the world a new breed of prosthetics and orthotics which not just look and feel like the physiological part but also resemble them strongly in function.

This chapter is aimed at providing coverage of the history and current state of the art in the fields of prosthetics and orthotics. Starting from the mechanics of the physiological parts, performances of various prosthetics are discussed.

PROSTHETICS

Historical Perspective

An effective prosthesis delivers renewed functionality and is cosmetically pleasing, but it also serves to complete the wearer's sense of wholeness. A prosthesis then, is as much medical device as it is an emotional comfort, and so the history of prosthetics is not only a scientific history, but the story of human beings since the dawn of civilization who by birth, wound, or accident were left with something missing.

The evolution of prosthetics is a long and storied history, from its primitive beginnings to its sophisticated present, to the exciting visions of the future. As in the development of any other field, some ideas and inventions have worked and been expanded upon, such as the fixed-position foot, while others have fallen by the wayside or become obsolete, such as the use of iron in a prosthesis. The long and winding road to today's technology began about 1500 B.C. and has been evolving ever since. There have been many refinements to the first peg legs and hand hooks that have led to the highly individualized fitting and casting of today's devices.

One entry in the Rig Veda, dating to around 3500 BC – 1800 BC, stated that during a battle with a neighboring territory Queen Vishpala, received a blow that amputated one of her legs. After a time, having healed, she was fitted with an iron leg in order to be able to return to the battle field in defense of her kingdom once more (Rig Veda, 1.112, 116, 117, 118 & 10.39). While there is written record of the limb, there has been no discovery of the iron leg used by Queen Vishpala, or one like it.

The evidence of usage of prosthetics dates back to as early as the ancient Egyptians. In one case, it was found that a mummy's big toe had been amputated during its life and supplanted with a carefully crafted wooden toe, which attached by a series of wooden plates and leather strings (Vanderwerker, 1976). A big toe, belonging to a noblewoman, was found in Egypt and dated to between 950-710 B.C.E.

An artificial leg dating to about 300 B.C. was unearthed at Capua, Italy, in 1858. It was made of bronze and iron, with a wooden core, apparently for a below-knee amputee. The prosthesis was destroyed during an air raid on London in 1941 (Vanderwerker, 1976). Ancient literature contains references to prosthetic limbs in stories and poems, but some of the earliest historical accounts of prosthetic limb use were recorded in Greek and Roman times. For instance, there's the historical account of Marcus Sergius, a Roman general who lost his right hand while battling in the second Punic War. Famously, he had a replacement hand fashioned out of iron for the purpose of holding his shield and was able to return to battle and continue fighting (Dellon & Matsouka, 2007).

The Dark Ages saw little advancement in prosthetics other than the hand hook and peg leg. Most famously attributed to seafaring pirates, peg legs with wooden cores and metal hands shaped into hooks have actually been the prosthetic standard throughout much of history. While Hollywood has exaggerated their use of hooks and peg legs, pirates did sometimes rely on these types of prostheses. The required materials for these devices could be scavenged from a common pirate ship.

Most prostheses of this time were made to hide deformities or injuries sustained in battle (Clements, 2008). A knight would be fitted with a prosthesis that was designed only to hold a shield or for a leg to appear in the stirrups. Little attention was paid to functionality. Outside of battle, only the wealthy were lucky enough to be fitted with a peg leg or hand hook for daily function (Marshall, 2015).

It was common for tradesmen, including armourers, to design and create artificial limbs. People of all trades often contributed to making the devices;

watchmakers were particularly instrumental in adding intricate internal functions with springs and gears (Marshall, 2015).

In 1508, German mercenary Gotz von Berlichingen had a pair of technologically advanced iron hands made after he lost his right arm in the Battle of Landshut. The hands could be manipulated by setting them with the natural hand and moved by relaxing a series of releases and springs while being suspended with leather straps (Marshall, 2015).

Around 1512, an Italian surgeon travelling in Asia recorded observations of a bilateral upper extremity amputee who was able to remove his hat, open his purse, and sign his name (Marshall, 2015). Another story surfaced about a silver arm that was made for Admiral Barbarossa, who fought the Spaniards in Bougie, Algeria, for a Turkish sultan.

French Army barber/surgeon Ambroise Paré is considered by many to be the father of modern amputation surgery and prosthetic design. In the early part of the 16th century Paré, contributed some of the first major advances in prosthetics seen for many years. Paré invented a hinged mechanical hand as well as prosthetic legs that featured advances such as locking knees and specialized attachment harnesses (Clements, 2008). A colleague of Paré's, Lorrain, a French locksmith, offered one of the most important contributions to the field when he used leather, paper and glue in place of heavy iron in making a prosthesis.

Around 1690, a Dutch surgeon, Pieter Verduyn, later developed a lower leg prosthesis with specialized hinges and a leather cuff for improved attachment to the body (Norton, 2007).

In 1800, a Londoner, James Potts, designed a prosthesis made of a wooden shank and socket, a steel knee joint and an articulated foot that was controlled by catgut tendons from the knee to the ankle. It would become known as the "Anglesey Leg" after the Marquis of Anglesey, who lost his leg in the Battle of Waterloo and wore the leg. William Selpho would later bring the leg to the U.S. in 1839 where it became known as the "Selpho Leg." In 1846, Benjamin Palmer saw no reason for leg amputees to have unsightly gaps between various components and improved upon the Selpho leg by adding an anterior spring, smooth appearance, and concealed tendons to simulate natural-looking movement (Vanderwerker, 1976; Marshall, 2005 & Norton, 2007).

Douglas Bly invented and patented the Doctor Bly's anatomical leg in 1858, which he referred to as "the most complete and successful invention ever attained in artificial limbs."

Figure 1. Artificial leg invented by Ambroise Pare (middle sixteenth century)
Source: Malgaigne (1841)

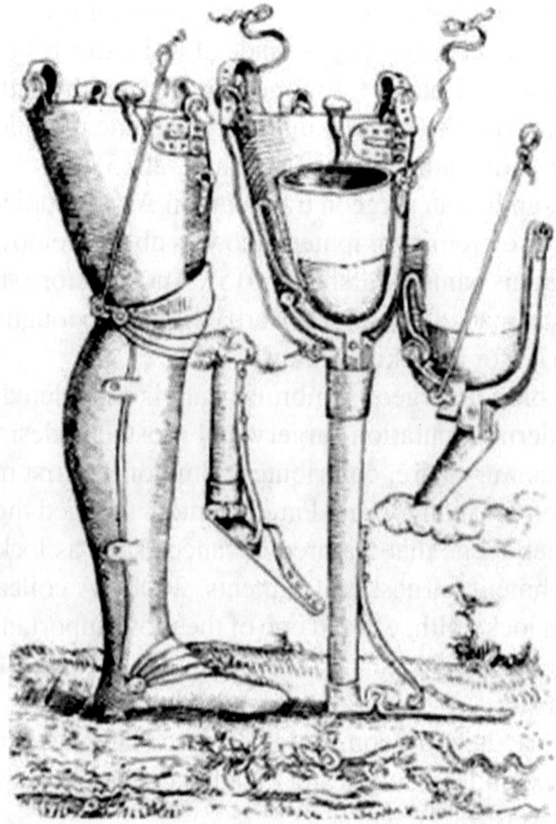

In 1863, Dubois Parmlee invented an advanced prosthesis with a suction socket, polycentric knee and multi-articulated foot. Later, Gustav Hermann suggested in 1868 the use of aluminium instead of steel to make artificial limbs lighter and more functional. However, the lighter device would have to wait until 1912, when Marcel Desoutter, a famous English aviator, lost his leg in an airplane accident, and made the first aluminium prosthesis with the help of his brother Charles, an engineer.

The American Civil War hastened the development of prosthetic limbs. The drastic rise in the number of amputees forced the development of new prosthetics such as the Hanger Limb. The next watershed events that hastened the development of prosthetics were the World Wars, followed by the Vietnam conflict. Unlike the Civil War, World War I did not foster much advancement in the field. Following World War II, veterans were dissatisfied with the lack of technology in their devices and demanded improvement. This paved the way to the development and production of modern prostheses. Today's devices are much lighter, made of plastic, aluminum and composite materials to provide amputees with the most functional devices.

Prostheses of the Lower Body

Transtibial Prosthetics

A person who has undergone a transtibial amputation retains the knee joint. This is a major advantage as a healthy knee not only provides the power to lift and lower, it also helps in maintaining overall balance. A surgeon will want to preserve a viable, healthy knee joint because it provides a transtibial amputee with many functional advantages, not available to those who have undergone a trans-femoral amputation or a knee disarticulation (amputation through the knee joint). The knee is very important in transfers, such as on and off the toilet, in and out of bed, and up and down stairs, and it also gives greater ability to push forward, slow down, and walk on slopes and stairs.

For the transtibial amputee, the major challenge is replacing the foot and ankle. The major roles of the ankle are accommodation, shock absorption and motion. However, the general perception about it is that it pushes down and pulls up. The physiologic foot adjusts to different and uneven surfaces. Movements from concrete to gravel or between other surfaces is smooth and the person is still able stand or walk steadily. The foot perceives when there's a change in the surface and responds rapidly to nerve signals to accommodate it. This ability of the foot to feel position and surface, the sensation of the foot's relation to the ground, whether the ground slopes up or down, and whether it's hard or soft, slippery or dry, rough or smooth is called proprioception. Without a foot and ankle, proprioception is lost along with the sense of positioning and shock absorption. The partial foot amputation preserves a small bit of this ability, but with a transtibial amputation, all of it is lost.

Prosthetic feet generally can be designed to be firm and spring like or soft and accommodating, but not both. A prosthetic foot that's soft and accommodating usually remains that way and is not suitable for dynamic use, while a prosthetic foot that's made to provide the firmer foundation needed for push off and the spring like propulsion of stored energy is often described as too "stiff" for less vigorous uses.

Hence, the construction of a prosthesis depends largely on is function. Prosthetic legs serve as substitutes for a major structural part of the patient's body and bear their entire weight. Typically, a strong and durable but lightweight material such as carbon fiber, covered with foam padding (for comfort) or flesh-colored plastic is preferred for the construction of a prosthetic. The weight of prosthetic limbs also, is another very important factor. Given that the legs amount to 30–40 percent of a person's total body weight while the arms amount to only about 10 percent, it is amply clear why prosthetic limbs need to be much lighter: the energy expenditure of the patient would be much higher in moving prosthetic limbs that weighed as much as natural ones.

The effectiveness and comfort of a prosthesis largely depends by how well it fits onto the portion of the patient's physiologic limb left after amputation, called the residual limb or informally the "stump". The interfacing between the prosthetic and the residual limb is done by what is called the socket and it is custom molded around a plaster cast of the residual limb. The fit of a socket has to be precise or the new prosthetic may damage the residual limb resulting in increased discomfort and/or tissue damage and in extreme cases, making it impossible to wear the pros-thesis for an extended time. A patient's residual limb matures and changes in its shape and size occur over months and years, necessitating the fitting of new sock-ets from time to time. 3D scans of a patient's residual limb, combined with modern techniques such as 3D printing are now being used to give the patient better and more closely fitting sockets. These tend to be more comfortable and eliminate the need for the patient to wait for a precise fit, which otherwise takes multiple attempts and can be quite cumbersome.

A number of designs for artificial feet are commercially available, each having its own advantages and disadvantages. Currently available prosthetic foot designs can be divided into two classes

- Articulated i.e. those with moving joints
- Non – articulated.

Articulated joints generally require more maintenance and are heavier than most of the non-articulated kind. Articulated feet may have one or more joints.

Transfemoral Prosthetics

The above-knee amputee faces considerable challenges since he/she has lost both the knee and ankle joints. The loss of the knee poses a major challenge in re-habilitation of the amputee. Problems with stumbling and falling increase, and much greater concentration is needed for walking. Also, the power provided by the knee during transfers i.e. moving from one position to another is lost (Hofstad et al., 2004). In children, it results in the loss of the growth plate located at the end of the femur. As such, what was initially a long residual limb in the juvenile amputee ends as a short stump, post maturity.

The above knee prosthesis consists of:

- Foot-ankle assembly
- Shank
- Knee unit
- Socket
- Suspension device

For the above-knee or transfemoral amputee, the prosthetic knee joint is one of the most critical components of the prosthesis. Replacing the complex human knee is an ongoing challenge, one yet to be fully addressed, since the beginning of modern prosthetics. A prosthetic knee is tasked with mimicking the function of the normal knee while providing safety and stability at a reasonable weight and cost (Dupes, n.d.).

The type of knee used in an above knee prosthesis is dependent on a number of factors including, but not limited to, the patient's activity level, weight, strength and ability to control the knee, residual limb length, funding, and patient preference. Foot-ankle assembly and shank are same as those that are used with BK prostheses.

Friction is used in order to control the knee joint during walking. How far and how fast the knee bends and straightens during gait is controlled by friction. Some knees utilize mechanical friction while others employ hydraulic resistance. Computerized, microprocessor mounted knees are also available that control the knee speed based on the person's gait. Computerized and hydraulic knees change the knee speed depending on how fast the person is walking whereas mechanical knees provide constant friction.

Prosthetic knees can be classified into two distinct types based on the mode of control of the swing and/or stance phases of gait:

- Non-microprocessor: those that use mechanical control of the knee joint
- Microprocessor those that use some form of computer chips

Figure 2. Human gait cycle
Source: Schaffer, Kort, and Kreuter (2008)

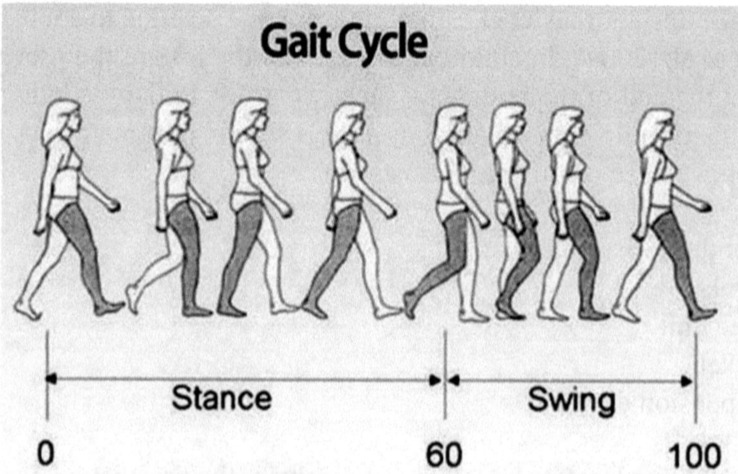

There exist many designs of non-microprocessor knees which are commercially available worldwide. All of them use a mechanical hinge, the speed and ease of the swing, of which, is controlled by one of the following mechanisms (Dupes, n.d.):

- Free swing
- Manual lock
- Constant friction
- Weight-activated friction
- Geometrical locking
- Hydraulics.

Muscular and mechanical control need to be exerted by mechanical-knee users to alter speed and step length and provide stability in the weight-bearing phase of gait. Some mechanical knee joints can manually be adjusted to set the controls based on the patient's needs in the swing and stance phases by the prosthetist or the user. These adjustments however, can only be made when the person is in a static (still) position.

In microprocessor controlled knees, the speed and ease with which the knee swings throughout the swing phase are controlled by the microprocessor. It also controls the degree of stability of the knee joint maintained during stance phase. Microprocessor controlled prosthetic knees continuously detect the position of the knee during the stance and swing phases of gait through fitted sensors. The input from these sensors goes to the microprocessor so that the knee "knows" which gait phase it's in and can adapt accordingly. This allows it to change performance characteristics in relation to different walking speeds, terrain and environmental conditions as the user walks n order to provide a semblance of proprioception. In addition to these features, a microprocessor knee senses that the user is not walking and thus resists collapsing of the knee. As such, it has been shown to improve the stability in the stance phase of gait because it. This feature adds an improved safety layer when standing and more confidence when walking. The ability to control the swing phase during walking and to provide resistance in the stance phase allows for the user of such knees to enjoy a reduction in the amount of energy it takes to walk and provides additional safety for walking.

Commercial units are described according to 4 features:

1. Axis
2. Friction mechanism
3. Extension aid
4. Mechanical stabilizer

The thigh piece can be connected to the shank by either a single-axis hinge which permits flexion and extension at a point correlating to the anatomic axis of the knee or by a polycentric linkage, where the mechanism that permits the momentary axis of knee flexion to change through the arc of motion. Polycentric linkage is more stable.

The friction mechanism changes the knee swing by modifying the speed of knee motion during the various parts of swing phase and adjusts knee swing ac-cording to cadence. The friction mechanism may be such that it is a constant friction mechanism that applies uniform resistance throughout the swing phase or variable friction mechanism in which greater friction is applied at early and late swing.

The medium through which the resistance is applied influences performance. Several types of media are used of which the most common is sliding friction which consists of solid structures that resist motion by moving up against each other. Another popular medium is fluid friction. It consists of a cylinder (hydraulic is oil-filled, pneumatic is air-filled) in which a piston connected to the knee hinge moves up and down. These units automatically compensate for changes in walking speed.

Hip and Transpelvic Prosthetics

Hip disarticulation and transpelvic amputation, also known as the hemipelvectomy, are the rarest of all the lower limb amputations. In fact, only 2% of all amputations are at the hip disarticulation level (Stark, 2001). These are cases when amputations are performed at the hip or pelvic level and the entire leg is removed. These amputations are the ones in which the patient does not retain a residual limb. Instead, the patient has an incision line and padding in the hip or pelvic area (Smith, March/April 2005).

A transtibial amputee has the advantage of being able to use the thigh, the knee, and part of the lower leg for control and positioning. The transfemoral amputees can use their hip strength and buttock muscles to flex and extend the hip to control the prosthesis and for stabilization. At any of these amputation levels, if the amputee feels the leg buckling, he or she can move the hip and residual limb to stabilize the knee and keep from falling. But none of these motion segments are available for control and balance to an individual with a hip or pelvic level amputation and control of the prosthetic limb must come from the pelvis and lower back.

Transpelvic amputations mean the loss of three weight bearing joints – the hip, the knee and the ankle. Although there's no way to predict the recovery from any amputation with any degree of certainty, people who have these high level amputations generally face greater challenges (Smith, January/ February 2005).

The hip functions as a lever, bringing the thigh forward and directing where the foot will go during walking. It allows the thigh to be brought back, stabilizing the knee during standing. The hip abductor and extensor musculature – the gluteus and buttock muscles – provide strength so that the leg supports the body weight and does not buckle. While a portion of these muscles might remain after a hip disarticulation, they're no longer connected to the part of the leg that makes them work (Smith, March/April 2005).

One of the major problems in surgical reconstruction at the hip or at the pelvic level is where to place the new hip joint. For lower level amputations, the ankle or knee prosthesis can be located relatively close to where the physiological location of ankle or knee. However, that is not possible in the case of higher level amputations. After the amputation, the original location is usually covered by soft tissue padding. Once the thickness of the socket and the connector to attach the hip to the socket is added, the hip joint will be located 3 to 4 inches away from its original center, either to the outside, down below the anatomic location, to the front, or to the back.

Although the anatomic differences between hip disarticulation and transpelvic (hemipelvectomy) amputations are considerable, prosthetic component selection and alignment for both levels are almost the same (van der Waarde & Michael, 2002).

Myoelectric Prosthetics

This is included as a separate subheading as this is considered to be the cutting edge of prosthetics technology. Once just Sci-Fi, this technology is inching closer to achieving what was previously thought to be impossible. With the advent of myoelectrics, full function of the amputated part is now being made possible.

The primary purpose of any prosthetic is to mimic the appearance and replace the function of a missing limb. While a single prosthetic that achieves both a natural appearance and functionality similar to the physiologic part would be ideal, in most artificial limbs that exist today a tradeoff has to happen. As such the designs sacrifice some degree of one for the other. Hence, there is a wide spectrum of specialized prosthetics that range from those that are purely cosmetic, which are inert to the primarily functional models whose appearance is obviously mechanical. Myoelectric prosthetics are an attempt to bridge the gap and serve both purposes of an artificial limb equally, without sacrificing either appearance or functionality.

Myoelectric controlled prostheses offer the ultimate combination of function and natural appearance to amputees. Designed to mimic human anatomy and motion, these electronic components have come the closest to mimicking the physiological limb. These have become the best replacement to an anatomical limb lost due to any circumstance.

"Myoelectric" is the term used to describe electric properties of muscles. A myoelectric controlled prosthesis is an externally powered artificial limb that the amputee can control with the electrical signals generated naturally by the muscles.

Myoelectric components for the hand, wrist and elbow are available today. With amputations above the elbow, a "hybrid prosthesis" may combine myoelectric components with body powered ones to control shoulder and/or elbow function. A skin like glove covers the prosthesis for a natural appearance.

A myoelectric prosthesis uses the existing muscles in the residual limb to control its functions. Sensors fabricated into the prosthetic socket receive electrical signals when specific muscles in the residual limb are activated. The sensors relay information to a controller, which translates the data into commands for the electric motors to move the joints. If muscle signals cannot be used to control the prosthesis, switches with a rocker or pull – push mechanisms or a touch pad may be used.

The strength and speed of movements can be controlled by varying muscle intensity. For those with damage to nerves or muscles in the residual limb or for people with bilateral amputation, muscles in the chest or back can be used to direct movements of a myoelectric prosthesis.

When a myoelectric prosthesis has several joints, each joint might need to be controlled by the same muscle. Sequential control allows positioning of one joint at a time. For example, a muscle contraction may be used to signal the elbow to bend, and then another contraction to signal the hand to close.

Although a myoelectric prosthesis is controlled by electricity generated by the own muscles, the system needs a battery to power motors and electronics. Some batteries need to be removed from the prosthesis for charging while for others, a cord from a charging unit can be plugged into the prosthesis.

A myoelectric prosthesis is connected to the residual limb via a custom fabricated suction socket. The user ‘pulls in’ to the socket with a donning sock, which creates suction and helps suspend the socket. A hybrid prosthesis, which combines both myoelectric and body powered components, is another option. A hybrid prosthesis may include a myoelectric hand and wrist controlled along with an elbow that is controlled by a harness and cables worn on the torso and controlled by shoulder movements. Compared to a traditional body powered prosthesis, a myoelectric arm provides greater comfort, more range of motion, a larger functional area and a more natural appearance. It may, however, cost and weigh more.

Targeted muscle reinnervation (TMR) is a technique in which motor nerves which would control muscles on an amputated limb, are surgically rerouted to reinnervate a small region of a large, intact muscle, such as the pectoralis major (Childress, 1985). As a result, when a patient thinks about moving the thumb of his missing hand, a small area of muscle on his chest will contract instead. These contractions can be made to control movement of an appropriate part of the robotic prosthesis by placing sensors over the reinnervated muscle.

ORTHOTICS

Historical Perspective

The word "Orthotics" comes from the Greek: Ορθός (orthos) which means "to straighten" or "align". It is a specialty within the medical field concerned with the design, manufacture and application of orthoses. An orthosis (plural: orthoses) can be defined as "an externally applied device used to modify the structural and functional characteristics of the neuromuscular and skeletal system" (ISO 8549-1:1989).

The general functions of orthoses span:

- Control, guide, limit and/or immobilize an extremity, joint or body seg-ment for a particular reason
- Restriction of movement in a given direction
- Assisting of movement generally
- Reduction weight bearing forces for a particular purpose
- Aiding rehabilitation from fractures after the removal of a cast
- The correction the shape and/or function of the body, to provide easier movement capability or reduce pain

Orthotics combines knowledge of anatomy and physiology, pathophysiology, biomechanics and engineering. Orthoses are generally indicated for patients who may have a condition such as spina bifida or cerebral palsy, or have experienced a spinal cord injury or stroke. At the same time, orthoses also find prophylactic use in order to optimize performance in sports.

Tracing the origins of the discipline, a key development was a wrote a book called "*Orthopedie*", published in 1741, in which he demonstrated the theory of human anatomy, skeletal structure and gave methods to correct deformations of the bones. The author of the volume was Nicolas Andry de Bois-Regard, a French doctor and writer, who played a key role in parasitology and orthopaedics. This book was translated to English in 1743 as "*Orthopaedia*" and was designed more for parents then doctors.

The father of orthopaedic studies is considered to be the 18th century Swiss doctor, Jean Andre Venel. Venel specialized in the treatment of deformations in children In 1780 he set up the world's first ever orthopaedic clinic in Orbe where he offered orthopaedic, rehabilitation and prophylactic services. It was the first clinic where children with skeletal deformation received comprehensive treatment. In his institute, he pioneered the production of various orthotic devices to treat children.

In 19th century, Hugh Owen Thomas, a Welsh surgeon, considered the father of the orthopaedics in the UK, created the 'Thomas splint', 'Thomas collar', multiple lower limb and hip orthosis and developed the method of examination of deformation in a lying position.

At the beginning of the 20th century the first modern orthoses and orthopaedic splints were invented. These were the first solutions for body support.

The field of orthotics has transformed from a traditional craft-based industry into a modern professional clinical specialty. The modern era of lower limb orthotics can reasonably be considered as having begun during the early 1970s. Prior to then the design and construction of lower limb orthoses had not changed substantially since the beginning of the century. Orthoses, in general, were assembled from metal components – some prefabricated some customized – with their body contact areas padded with felt and covered in leather by skilled craftsmen (Condie, 2008).

The only significant change in practice in recent years had been the introduction of thermo-setting resins to produce plastic shells. Two revolutionary designs, the PTB Brace and the UCLA Long Leg Brace (Scott 1971) owed a lot more than their material features to the rapidly developing field of prosthetics. The pioneering developments of Engen in Houston, and Lehneis et al. in New York, both of whom had recognized the enormous potential and opportunities for the use of thermoplastic materials in orthotic construction can justifiably be described as revolutionary (Condie, 2008).

During this first phase of innovative activity a variety of materials were employed, including polyethylene, PVC, ABS and polycarbonate; however it was polypropylene which quickly emerged as most versatile and most easily applied within the comparatively unsophisticated environment of a typical orthotic work-shop.

A comparatively unknown general practitioner published a brief article in the year 1968 describing the use of polypropylene to fabricate below-knee braces for children with spina bifida after visiting Houston and suddenly every parent wanted 'plastic braces' for their child.

One of the consequences of the sudden emergence of a whole new range of orthotic designs was to highlight the very poor quality of the existing guidance on the prescription of orthotics. The jargon phrase to describe this process was 'patient/orthosis matching'. Virtually all the orthotic manuals and text books avail-able at the time tended to classify patients by reference to their medical diagnosis and routinely used terms such as 'drop foot brace' or 'hemiplegic brace' to de-scribe both the devices and their clinical applications. These practices had many pitfalls and a more logical approach to the description of both the orthosis user and their device was required if the goal of matching them was to be realized.

The key to the realization of the first of these objectives – a method for the description of the potential user of an orthotic device and their orthotic needs – was provided by Jacqueline Perry in 1975. Perry described a model of normal physical activity and identified the body tissues and systems which contributed to each element of it. Using this model as a basis she then proceeded to propose a classification of 'functional loss' which completely eliminated the need for diagnostic labels to describe the disorder needing treatment (Condie, 2008).

It was not until 2003 that the Prosthetics and Orthotics Technical Committee of the International Standards Organization (ISO) devised and published a standard (ISO 2003) which formalized the original 'Perry/AAOS' approach.

The basic objective of lower limb orthoses hasn't changed for more than 100 years. The leather straps were replaced by Velcro straps which are friendlier to the skin and leather orthopaedic shoes were replaced by dynamic ankle brace made of light carbon fibres. Nowadays, light splints are used instead of steel. In recent years the huge development of the orthopaedic devices is noticed. Modern orthopaedic braces are friendlier for patients thanks to materials and design.

Today orthoses are made from various types of materials including thermoplastics, carbon fibre, metals, elastomers, EVA, fabric or a combination of similar materials. Some designs may be purchased at a local retailer. Others are more specific and require a prescription from a physician, who will fit the orthosis according to the patient's requirements. Over the counter braces are basic and available in multiple sizes. They are generally slid on or strapped on with Velcro, and are held tightly in place.

Orthoses of the Lower Body

The Knee Ankle Foot Orthosis is an externally applied orthosis used for the control and bracing of the knee and ankle joints. It is beneficial for individuals with varus (bow legs), valgus (knock knees) or hyperextension deformities in combination with other neuromuscular problems in the lower legs. Patients afflicted by ailments such as spinal cord injuries, post polio etc. are usually pre-scribed KAFOs. These devices control the knee, ankle and foot so as to provide support during standing and walking for some patients, while others use them for stability during transfers, for example to and from wheel chairs.

When bracing of the ankle joint is necessitated because of various factors which prevent dorsiflexion, it is necessary to consider the foot not in isolation but in conjunction with the neighbouring joints, the other joints of the lower limb and even those of the trunk. Walking, running and jumping are highly complex and coordinated movements, and limitations on anyone joint may derange neighbouring joints and cause disorders in weight bearing.

Knee – ankle–foot orthosis are systems used for the restoration of human gait by providing stability during the stance phase of walking. They are prescribed as partial solutions for disorders caused by different pathologies resulting in muscle weakness, while providing stability and keeping joints at their functional positions.

In endeavouring to give the patient the full advantages of bracing, the aim should be to achieve stability without unduly restricting mobility. In concentrating on the function the difference in the mechanism of disability is often forgotten. The spring assistance which helps the polio patient will only aggravate hemiplegic spasticity.

Knee-Ankle-Foot Orthoses

There are two general designs of KAFOs. One utilizes metal and the other combines plastic along with metal (Scheck & Siress, n.d.). The metal design consists of a metallic structure shaped to conform to the limb and upholstered with leather at the points where the device makes contact with the patient's body. This is the more traditional of the two designs. The plastic and metal design is most frequently encountered today and usually comprises of a plastic device, custom moulded to the patient's body, with metal components in key structural areas only (Gravlee & Van Durme, 2007). The reason for the increased use of the plastic and metal design is reduction in the weight of the orthosis and that it is considered to be more cosmetic. The latest developments include stance control exoskeletons, which are externally powered exoskeletons.

It is of prime importance when selecting a brace to restrict only the unwanted motion and to ensure that no limitation is placed on other movements within the walking cycle. Adaptations should be considered to meet the needs of individual patients.

Ankle Braces

Ankle sprains are some of the most common musculoskeletal injuries (Gravlee & Van Durme, 2007). The treatment of lateral ankle sprains can be confusing because of the various designs of braces and splints that are available for this kind of injury.

Ankle braces can be classified broadly into two categories:

- Rigid
- Functional.

Rigid braces immobilize the entire ankle while functional braces, including semi rigid and soft braces, allow some flexion at the ankle while providing bracing to control inversion and eversion.

Semi rigid braces make use of thermoplastic contoured lateral stirrups lined with foam pads for support of the medial and lateral malleoli. Soft, lace-up braces are usually manufactured from canvas. Semi rigid stirrup braces have been seen to restrict ankle inversion and eversion comparatively more than lace up braces. Proprioception, an important component in the reduction of recurrent ankle sprains, has also been shown to improve with external ankle support (Gravlee & Van Durme, 2007).

Knee Braces

Knee braces are used to treat anterior knee pain, to immobilize the knee and to reduce the load on the medial compartment for patients with varus osteoarthritis. Many designs are available as over the counter models while others are custom fitted by an orthotist

Stance Control Knee-Ankle-Foot Orthoses

Persons with muscle weakness in the quadriceps are often prescribed KAFOs that lock the knee during both the stance and swing phases of gait in full extension resulting in abnormal gait patterns characterized by hip-hiking and circumduction of the leg during swing phase (Yakimovich, 2009). Stance Control Knee-Ankle-Foot Orthoses (SCKAFO) permit free knee motion during swing while resisting knee flexion during stance, thereby supporting the limb during weight bearing.

Hip and Pelvic Orthoses

The purpose of a pelvic or hip brace is to provide support and stabilization to the pelvic and/or hip joints by limiting the motion of the leg in relation to the body. The hip brace limits the bending of the leg forward, backward and across the body. It is designed to keep the leg out to the side of the body, holding the thigh bone in the hip socket and allowing for proper healing to take place (Ballert Orthopaedic, n.d.). Pelvic fractures might carry a significant risk of bleeding. Pelvic fractures have a mortality rate of 5% to 50% caused mainly in part by the significant hemorrhage that may occur in the pelvis with minimal external signs (Pyng Medical Corp, 2011). A wide variety of pelvic binders along with pelvic sheets is available to aid the initial management of poly-trauma patients with pelvic injuries. These devices are collectively referred to as pelvic circumferential compression devices (PCCDs) (Bakhshayesh et al., 2016).

Though the survival rate after pelvic fractures has greatly improved during the recent years, the overall high mortality rate has been shown to have resulted pri-marily from injuries sustained from high-energy trauma rather than isolated pelvic fractures (SPS Co., n.d.). Historically, attempts have been made to develop a treatment that will rapidly reduce and stabilize the disrupted pelvic ring in order to provide improved hemodynamic stability (Bakhshayesh et al., 2016).

Until recently initial pelvic stabilization was achieved through invasive surger-ies such as the application of an external fixator or a pelvic C-clamp (Bakhshayesh et al., 2016). These approaches were inadvertently associated with a time delay owing to the need for an operating theatre environment. Non – invasive external compression devices, have rapidly gained popularity since their introduction (Bakhshayesh et al., 2016). Factors such as speed, safety, ease of application and their biomechanical capability to reduce a disrupted pelvic ring and pelvic volume have contributed to this rise in popularity (DeAngelis et al., 2008).

CONCLUSION

While progress has been made by leaps and bounds in the fields of prosthetics and orthotics, the state of the art is far from perfect. Continuous evolution and growth is happening daily and devices are inching closer to the optimal solution i.e. total replication of physiological function in case of prosthetics and complete restoration of natural form and function in the case of orthotics. Whatever, the development, it can safely be said that the future holds a lot of promise.

REFERENCES

Bakhshayesh, P., Boutefnouchet, T., & Tötterman, A. (2016). Effectiveness of non invasive external pelvic compression: A systematic review of the literature. *Scandinavian Journal of Trauma, Resuscitation and Emergency Medicine*, *1824*(1), 73. doi:10.118613049-016-0259-7 PMID:27193135

Childress, D. S. (1985). Historical Aspects of Powered Limb Prostheses. *Clinical Prosthetics & Orthotics*, *9*(1), 2–13.

Clements, I. P. (2008). *How Prosthetic Limbs Work*. Retrieved 16 April 2016 from http://science.howstuffworks.com/prosthetic-limb.htm

Condie, D. N. (2008). The modern era of orthotics. *Prosthetics and Orthotics International*, *32*(3), 313–323. doi:10.1080/03093640802113006 PMID:18825575

DeAngelis, N. A., Wixted, J. J., Drew, J., Eskander, M. S., Eskander, J. P., & French, B. G. (2008). Use of the trauma pelvic orthotic device (TPOD) for provisional stabilisation of anterior–posterior compression type pelvic fractures: A cadaveric study. *Injury*, *39*(8), 903–906. doi:10.1016/j.injury.2007.12.008 PMID:18586248

Dellon, B., & Matsuoka, Y. (2007, March). Prosthetics, Exoskeletons, and Rehabilitation: Now and for the Future. *IEEE Robotics & Automation Magazine*, 30–34. doi:10.1109/MRA.2007.339622

Dupes, B. (n.d.). *Prosthetic Knee Systems*. Retrieved 19 April 2016 from http://www.amputee-coalition.org/military-instep/knees.html

Gravlee, J. R., & Van Durme, D. J. (2007). Braces and Splints for Musculoskeletal Conditions. *American Family Physician*, *75*, 342–348. PMID:17304865

Hofstad C.J., van der Linde H., van Limbeek J. & Postema, K. (2004). Prescription of Prosthetic Ankle-Foot Mechanisms after Lower Limb Amputation. *Cochrane Database of Systematic Reviews, 1*.

Marshall, J. (2015). *The History of Prosthetics*. Retrieved 16 April 2016 from http://unyq.com/the-history-of-prosthetics/

Norton, K. M. (2007). A Brief History of Prosthetics. *inMotion, 17*(7), 11-13.

Orthopaedic, B. (n.d.). *Hip Abduction Brace*. Retrieved 26 July 2016 from http://www.ballert.com/pdf/HipAbductionOrthosis.pdf

Pyng Medical Corp. (2011). *T-POD® Pelvic Stabilization Device Training Session*. Retrieved 25 July 2016 from www.pyng.com/wp/wp-content/uploads/2011/02/PM-088a T-POD Training PowerPoint Presentation.pdf

Schaffer, E., Kort, C. & Kreuter P. (2008). The Prosthetic Knee Microprocessor and Non-Microprocessor Knee Joints. *inMotion, 18*(7), 34-36.

Scheck & Siress. (n.d.). *KAFO (Knee-Ankle-Foot Orthosis)*. Retrieved 1 July 2016 from www.scheckandsiress.com

Smith, D. G. (2005a). Higher Challenges: The Hip Disarticulation and Transpelvic Amputation Levels. *inMotion, 15*(1).

Smith, D. G. (2005b). Higher Challenges: Amputations at the Hip and Pelvis, Part 2. *inMotion, 15*(2).

SPS Co. (n.d.). *Orthotic catalogue section 7: Hip orthoses*. Retrieved from http://www.spsco.com/education/downloadable-resources/orthotic/

Stark, G. (2001). Overview of Hip Disarticulation Prostheses. *JPO, 13*(2), 50.

van der Waarde, T., & Michael, J. W. (2002). Hip Disarticulation and Transpelvic Amputation: Prosthetic Management. In Atlas of Limb Prosthetics: Surgical, Prosthetic, and Rehabilitation Principles. Academic Press.

Vanderwerker, E. E. Jr. (1976). A Brief Review of the History of Amputations and Prostheses. *Inter-Clinic Information Bulletin., 15*(5), 15–16.

Yakimovich, T., Lemaire, E. D., & Kofman, J. (2009). Engineering design review of stance control knee – ankle – foot orthoses. *Journal of Rehabilitation Research and Development, 46*(2), 257–268. doi:10.1682/JRRD.2008.02.0024 PMID:19533539

Chapter 3
Bioresorbable Composites and Implant

Divya Zindani
National Institute of Technology Silchar, India

ABSTRACT

Different biomaterials in the form of ceramics, metal alloys, composites, glasses, polymers, etc. have gained wide-range acceptance in the realm of medical sciences. Bioimplants from such biomaterials have been constructed and used widely for different clinical applications. With the continual progress, biomaterials that may be resorbed inside the body have been developed. These have done away with the major challenge of removal of an implant after it has served its intended function. Important factors are taken into consideration in design and development of implants from such biomaterials are mechanical properties, degradation rate, surface modification, rate of corrosion, biocompatibility, and non-toxicity. Given the importance of such materials in clinical applications, the chapter presents an overview of the bioresorable composites and their implants. The related properties and the functions served have been outlined briefly. Further, the challenges associated and the remedies to overcome them have also been delineated.

DOI: 10.4018/978-1-5225-8235-9.ch003

INTRODUCTION

Progressive research and advancements in medical sciences have resulted in the development of implants for human body. The implants that replaces or assists in functioning of a human organ are referred to as bioimplants (Soler-Botija et al., 2014). Various bioimplants such as cosmetic implants (Yahyavi-Firouz-Abadi et al., 2015), dental implants (Klein et al., 2014), subcutaneous implants (Guo et al., 2015), organ stimulation implants (Oka et al., 2015), sensory implants (Huang et al., 2015), neural implants (Takmakov et al., 2015), spinal implants (Bagga et al., 2017) and other structural implants such as braces, hip prosthesis etc. have been widely applied in the medical milieu to suit different applications. Given the quantum of road accidents as well as the trauma injuries, an upsurge in the usage of bioimplants can be predicted.

Biomaterials for bioimplants can be categorised into: single crystals, polycrystals, polymers, composites, bioceramics and glass-ceramics (Shackelford, 1999). The inherent nature of a biomaterial is dominant in deciding the type and mechanism of their interaction with the adjacent tissue surface. An implant may be biotoxic if the surrounding tissue dies, bioactive and nontoxic, bioinert and nontoxic and bioresorable in which case it dissolves to replace the surrounding tissue. Resorable bioceramics (Shikinami and Okuno, 1999) degrade with time and therefore replace the existing surrounding tissue. Major challenges associated with bioresorable bioceramics is that of maintenance of strength and stability throughout their lifetime. Some of the important characteristics desired to be possessed by a bioactive and nontoxic bioceramics are biocompatibility, osteoinductivity, osteoconductivity, biodegradability and the flexibility to acquire different shapes. A very well-known class of material that is used predominantly in the tissue engineering applications are calcium phosphates bioceramics having similar mineral content to that of bone.

Continual advancements in the development of bioresorable implants have led to their wider acceptability than the metallic biomaterials in sports related traumas and injuries (Weiler et al., 2000). Disadvantages such as inflammatory reactions, distortion of metallic screws and other postoperative complications are associated with metallic biomaterials. Polymeric materials are used as bioresorable materials for drug delivery devices and bone implants (Vert, 2009).

Bioresorable materials in the form of metallic alloys have also been considered for medical strength owing to them having higher stiffness and mechanical strength in comparison to the polymeric bioresorable materials. Iron (Schinhammer et al., 2010) and Magnesium (Chen et al., 2014) are the major explored bioresorable metallic alloys that have been observed to degrade as per the human body metabolism. Porous metallic implants are desired to have the following major characteristics: porosity, pore interconnectivity, pore size in accordance with the tissues they would be replacing and assist the natural organs to serve their intended function. Porosity Angiogenesis results with a higher porosity.

The objective of the present work is to brief the readers with the progress and development of bioresorable composites and their implants. Various applications and associated challenges have been illuminated in the work. Future developments have been highlighted towards the end of the work.

BIORESORBABLE COMPOSITES AND THEIR IMPLANTS

Biodegradable Polymers

Natural as well as synthethic polymeric materials (Chiellini and Solaro, 2014; Gunatillake and Adhikari, 2003) are the preferred polymeric material choices possessing biodegradability. Covalently bonded monomers are the building blocks of polymeric materials. Polymeric materials can be classified into copolymers as well as homopolymers depending on the number of repeating monomers that may belong to the same or different molecules. Chitosan, starch, collagen, silk and derivatives of hyalunoric acid are some of the examples of known nature-based polymers. However, natural polymers possesses lower mechanical strength, higher physiological activity, repellence and unknown degradation rate and therefore restricts their application. Synthetic polymers have been largely investigated to overcome the challenges associated with the natural polymers. The degradation rate of polymeric material can be altered on the basis of chain arrangement and the degree of crystallinity. Polymers are required to be made biodegradable above normal body temperature owing to their higher flexibility and glass transition temperature (Lodge and McLeish, 2000). Poly-ε-caprolactone, poly (lactic acid-co-glycolic acid), poly-β-hydroxybutyrate, polyglycolic acid and polylactic acid are some of the commonly used polymeric materials that inhibit biodegradability (Hollinger and Battistone, 1985). Polylactic acid is synthesized from corns and starch and has been used for degradable sutures (Middleton and Tipton,

2000). Resistance to hydrolysis is more for crystalline polylactic acid than the amorphous form of polylactic acid (Karst and Yang, 2006). Low solubility, higher rate of degradation and higher crystallinity is possessed by polyglycolic acid. The higher degradation rate of polyglycolic acid is responsible for its decreased mechanical strength over years when implanted in human body (Sung et al., 2004). Poly-β-hydroxybutyrate is another type of biodegradable polymer that possesses higher crystallinity. However, its practical application is restricted because of higher brittleness and is therefore blended with other available and biodegradable polymers. Another commonly used biodegradable polymer is poly-para-dioxanone (Pezzin et al., 2003) and is known for its good biodegradability, biocompatibility, flexibility and resorbability. This polymer is used in varied forms viz-a-viz coatings, films and foams and has been prominently used for fixation of internal fractures. Disintegration phenomenon with the poly-para-dioxanone implants have been observed within six months of its implantation. The rate of disintegration could be controlled by varying molecular weight, melting temperature and crystallinity (Tan et al., 2003). Poly-ε-caprolactone is an aliphatic polymer that has wider acceptability for medical implants. It possesses excellent permeability and crystallinity. Furthermore, it renders higher level of flexibility and therefore can be shaped as required. These characteristics allow it to be used for drug delivery systems as well in addition to being used for long term implants. However, it is very difficult to control its degradation rate. Polylactic acid is yet another biodegradable polymer and can be classified into poly (D-lactide) acid (PDLA) and poly (L-lactide) acid (PDLA) on the bais of their stereoisomers (Maurus and Kaeding, 2003). The characteristics of polylactic acid are determined by the constituting polymeric chain.

Hydrolysis of ester bond is mainly responsible for the degradation phenomenon in polymers. The microorganism when attracted by the polymers, secret enzymes that results in conversion of macromolecular to tiny particles and finally these get converted to H_2O and CO_2. As a result, biodegradable process occurs that results in ultimately the formation of oligomer debris. The oligomer debris are formed because of the ensuing hydrolysis process. It is worth noting that the mechanism of biodegradation for different polymers differ and therefore has been one of the prominent research topics amongst the researchers (David et al., 1994; Premraj and Doble, 2005; Shtilman et al., 2015).

Higher mechanical strength is required for load bearing implants and that used for bone repairing. Therefore ceramics and metals are preferred over their polymeric counterparts. Further, with degradation over time, mechanical strength also tends to decrease for the polymeric materials. Also, these materials are transparent to X-rays and it is also difficult to analyse the foreign body interactions. Although they have mechanical strength but some adverse effects such as corrosion (Witte et al., 2008), loss of bone (Cappiello et al., 2008) and inflammation are also observed (Broggini et al., 2006). Therefore, polymers are generally considered for repairing of bones (Sheikh et al., 2015).

Another polymeric material that renders itself as an instant adhesive in surgery are cyanoacrylates (Almeida et al., 2013). The biodegradation of cyanoacrylates involves unzipping of base-catalysts from the chain terminus. As a result of the biodegradation process, the adhesiveness decreases and also reduced resistance to water is observed (Robello et al., 1999). Polymers as implants is still a topic of great interest amongst the researchers.

Bioceramics

The properties possessed by biomaterials such as osteoconduction, osteoinduction, mechanical strength and inflammatory properties are similar to that of a native bone. Biomaterials in the form of bioceramics results in reduced disease transmission risk as well as immunogenicity. On implantation, bioceramics tends to experience humid conditions. The application domain of bioceramics include dental, spinal discs, otolarynhgology, periodontal and so on (LeGeros et al., 2003). Alumina (Al_2O_3) (Wittenbrink et al., 2015) and Zirconia (ZrO_2) (Lohbauer et al., 2008) were the initial bioinert bioceramics. These initial construction materials were used in the fabrication of femoral heads for hip prosthesis. Bioactive bioceramics have recently gained widespread popularity because of their potential ability to form bone bonding without ensuing inflammation. Varied studies have been conducted on various types of calcium phosphates (Bohner, 2000) such as that based on tricalcium phosphate, dicalcium phosphate dehydrate and hydroxyapatite for bone replacements. Resorbability of tricalcium phosphate is relatively higher to that of tricalcium phosphate. The resorbable bioceramics although have lesser mechanical strength in comparison to their non-resorbable counterpart (de Groot, 1993). The biological response of a specific bioceramics is determined by their physical and chemical compositions. Bioactive ceramics promotes osteoconduction i.e., production of proteins and also adhesibility with the cells. This can be attributed to the presence of inorganic phase.

Major inorganic component in a bone tissue is that of calcium phosphate. Calcium, phosphate and water are the main ingredients of Dicalcium phosphate (Gbureck et al., 2007), which is a biodegradable bioceramics. Dicalcium phosphate is generally known to change the physical properties for the bone tissues. Brushite is one of the form of Dicalcium Phosphate that has calcium and phosphate in equal ratio. It is basically dehydrated form of Dicalcium phosphate. Conversion of Dicalcium phosphate into hydroxyapatite takes place under physiological conditions or in vivo environment. This fact is solely responsible for restricting the resorbability as well as degradation rate of Brushite. Fractures in tibial plates are mainly addressed using Brushite.

Hydroxyapatite is another such bioceramics that possesses similar calcium and phosphate contents. When in either amorphous or crystalline state, hydroxyapatite is both bioactive as well as resorbable. Reactivity of either natural or synthetic hydroxyapatite depends on the method of preparation. Further, the crystallinity of hydroxyapatite is higher when prepared at high temperatures. Hydroxyapatite possesses very slow resorbability. Loss of bones or fractures in vertebra, calcaneus and tibia or any other bone related small defects are taken care off by the hydroxyapatite bioceramics. However, hydroxyapatite are not recommended for load-bearing applications owing to their poor mechanical properties. Research is ongoing with major objective of improving mechanical and biological properties of hydroxyapatite. Mechanical and biological properties have been revealed to be enhanced for hydroxyapatite using metal ions such as silicon, magnesium and strontium (Boanini et al., 2010). Quicker resorption mechanism have been reported with doping of hydroxyapatite with zinc (Thian et al., 2013) and manganese (Mayer et al., 2003). Better osteogenecity as well as osteoconductivity have also been reported for hydroxyapatite which has further strengthened its prospect for load bearing tissue engineering applications.

Tricalcium phosphate (Knaack et al., 1998) also has chemical composition similar to that of a bone tissue. α-TCP and β-TCP are the two main variants of Tricalcium phosphate. Good resorbability as well as bioactivity are possessed by Tricalcium phosphate. Tricalcium phosphate also possesses higher biodegradability rate in comparison to hydroxyapatite (Teramoto et al., 2005). Due to the excellent resorption properties as well as osteoconductivity. Tricalcium phosphate has been used widely for bone graft applications. Applications such as orthopaedic, dental and maxillofacial are addressed by Tricalcium phosphate. Bone grafts made using Tricalcium phosphate have revealed to have a slow resorbability when observed for a period ranging two years.

Other prominent bioceramics that has been reported for bone regeneration and augmentation applications is that of Monetite ($CaHPO_4$) (Tamimi et al., 2012). Monetite has also been used for orthopaedic and dental applications.

Magnesium Alloys

Magnesium alloys find applications in tissue engineering, cardiovascular cases and in orthopaedics. As such their suitability with respect to mechanical properties as well as biodegradability is of utmost importance and should be checked before their intended application. Many research studies have been reported on the magnesium alloys and their applications in medical domain. A study on novel magnesium alloys for biomedical applications was reported by Li and Zheng (2013). Corrosion of different types of magnesium alloys under in vivo conditions was reported by Witte et al. (2006). They reported that better osteointegration was exhibited by magnesium alloys owing to the accumulation of calcium phosphate and other minerals. Better mechanical properties were reported for magnesium alloys when alloyed with rare earth elements and aluminium (Tang et al., 2008). However, the aluminium alloyed magnesium alloys can't be used for biomedical applications because of neurotoxicity because of accumulation of aluminium (Taïr et al., 2016). Further, due to accumulation of rare earth elements, hepatoxicity results and therefore restricting their biomedical applications too (Wang et al., 2017). These disadvantages supersedes the better mechanical properties of the aluminium and rare earth elements alloyed magnesium alloys.

Extensive research has been carried out to develop magnesium alloys that are non-toxic or possesses low toxicity (Gu and Zheng, 2010). Various researchers have conducted investigations on magnesium alloys such as that based on rare earth alloy, Strontium, Silicon, Calcium (Li et al., 2008) and Zinc (Gao and Nie, 2007) used in biomedical applications. Magnesium alloys however have higher rate of corrosion (Song and Atrens, 2003) which can be reduced to a large extent by enhancing the purity through the process of purification. Iron, copper and nickel are the prominent impurity particles in magnesium. Addition of calcium results in refinement of granular particles of magnesium (Suthar and Patel, 2018). Fine grains have been reported with rapid rate of solidification of calcium based magnesium alloys (He et al., 2017). Improved cell activity as well as corrosion resistance was also reported in the same study. In another study on degradation behaviour of calcium based magnesium alloys (Lee et al., 2016), degradation was observed for period ranging three months. Improved mechanical properties could be achieved with zinc based magnesium alloys (Zhang et al., 2010). Other than the binary formation, zinc based magnesium alloys with ternary and quaternary configurations have also been achieved (Wang et al., 2015). An investigation on one of the binary zinc based magnesium alloy configurations i.e., Mg-6Zn (Wang et al., 2012) was carried out for their biocompatibility and galvanic corrosion. A good resistance to galvanic corrosion as well as good biocompatibility was reported. The biodegradability properties were obtained both for the in vitro as well as in vivo conditions. The bio corrosion for in vitro conditions were lower than that for the in vivo condition (He et al., 2009). When employed as a rods in rabbit femur, the rate of biodegradation was reported to be around 2 mm/year. The corrosion rate was revealed to be reduced with addition of Y in the binary zinc based magnesium alloy configuration. The addition of zirconium to the binary zinc based magnesium alloy resulted in refinement of grains and also enhanced the osteointegration properties of the binary alloy configuration. Addition of manganese to the zinc based magnesium binary alloy configuration led to their enhanced corrosion resistance and also removal of iron. The percentage of the constituting elements in the manganese alloyed binary zinc based magnesium alloy dictates their degradation behaviour. Further, the calcium doped binary zinc based magnesium alloys showcased higher mechanical as well as corrosion resistance properties under the in vivo conditions (Hofstetter et al., 2014; Hofstetter et al., 2009). Rare earth metals have also been added as a dopant to the magnesium alloys, however owing to their toxicity these can be employed for implant applications.

Various fabrication processes (Xu et al., 2011) have been employed for the development and fabrication of magnesium alloys. Some of the prominent ones are spin melting, metal casting and powder metallurgy. However still there is a wider scope on the investigation of magnesium alloys for orthopaedic and cardiovascular applications. As for instance research could be directed towards biodegradation rate and its control. Formation of hydrogen is one of the major challenges associated with magnesium based alloys. Alternative to the crystalline alloy is that of magnesium glasses, wherein the hydrogen formation can be avoided or reduced (Yang et al., 2016).

Orthodontic Wire

Wires and braces made from different metal alloys are used for dental applications. There has been continuous investigations to develop archwires that minimizes the human discomfort (Yap et al., 2014). The currently used materials are stainless steel, copper, titanium alloys in beta form or based on nickel. Orthodontic wires with surfaces of various shapes such as square, rectangular etc. have been used by the medical community (Bellini et al., 2016). Investigators have also worked significantly to minimize friction between the bracket and the archwires. Dentists have considered Nickel Titanium wires (Scattina et al., 2015) encompassing enhanced resilience, however, permanent distortions with overstressing is one of the major disadvantages associated with the Nickel titanium orthodontic wires. Surface coatings on nickel titanium wires have been employed in order to reduce the wire surface friction. The orthodontic wires from beta titanium possesses properties that are intermediary to that made from stainless steel and nickel titanium. These beta titanium wires have flexibility twice that of stainless steels. Nickel titanium wires with copper as one of the dopants has been reported to have more resistance to permanent distortion in comparison to the other variants of nickel titanium wires (Ravi Shantharaj et al., 2014). Cobalt-chromium is another material that has been used in the fabrication of orthodontic wires.

Metals for Knee Replacement

Various metallic have been employed for knee replacement applications. Metal such as steel possesses are stiffer in comparison to the cortical bone (Daniels et al., 1990). However, a much stiffer material weakens the normal bone because of stress shielding effect. Therefore in order to decrease the shielding effect, bone cement is employed as an interfacial substance (Nagels et al., 2003). The steel variants employed in medical implants are much cheaper than their other counterparts. Iron alloyed with Molybdenum, Nickel and Chromium have been used commonly for medical applications. However, the release of these metallic ions in the body results in allergy and other related symptoms. Investigations have been carried out by the research community to minimize the effect of releasing metal ions into the body. Stainless steel implants if used are mainly for short-term or as used with some coatings to avoid any aforementioned inconveniences to the patient. The coating material used commonly is that of hydroxyapatite. A success rate of 80-90% have been reported for steel implants (Zimmerli, 2014). Cobalt-chrome alloys have been used for implants and radiographic loosening has been reported in such cases. The osteointegration potential is one of the governing factors for surface finish for cementless cobalt-chromium alloys.

Titanium Alloys

Low density is one of the major reasons for titanium alloys being an attractive option for biomedical applications. Other important characteristic properties are their biocompatibility (Kopova et al., 2016), lower modulus (Mohammed et al., 2014) and corrosion resistance (Wang et al., 2014). Deforming processes or alloying with other elements aids in strengthening of titanium alloy (Kwasniak et al., 2016). Investigations have been ongoing on metastable β titanium alloys and also on (α+ β) Titanium alloys (Barriobero-Vila et al., 2017). Transformation of β to α titanium alloy takes place at a temperature of around 900 °C. Presence of elements such as oxygen, nitrogen, carbon, boron and hydrogen effects the transformation temperature. Further, the interstitial elements also have effect on the microstructural as well as mechanical properties of titanium alloys (Li et al., 2014). β phase of titanium alloys can be stabilized with the addition of substitutional elements such as Vanadium, Copper, Iron, Silicon, Molybdenum, Tungsten etc. in comparison to other alloys, titanium alloys possess superior biocompatibility as well as corrosion resistance. β phase of titanium alloy have modulus in proximity to that of the bone and are considered to be safe. The fatigue strength of (α+ β) titanium alloy is however poor. Inclusion of ZrO_2, SiO_2 etc. results in enhanced fatigue strength for the (α+ β) titanium alloys. Titanium alloys find a wider range of applications such as that in pacemakers, drug delivery pumps, dental implants, craniofacial implants and ventricular devices. However, the risks associated with titanium based alloys is much higher owing to the releasing of aluminium and vanadium. This results in complicated neurological conditions. Investigations have been carried out to develop titanium alloys free from vanadium (Gepreel, and Niinomi, 2013) and their applicability has been evidenced in fracture plates, wires, screws, rods, nails and femoral prosthesis stems. Another disadvantage associated with the titanium alloy implants is that of reduced wear resistance and bending strength in comparison to other alloys. Titanium alloys based on Molybdenum, Zirconium and Iron have been used for total hip replacement hip prosthesis. Addition of refractory materials to titanium alloys have reported to enhance their wear resistance properties (Mohammed et al, 2014b). However, poor mechanical strength of titanium alloys restricts their applicability for implant applications.

CONCLUSION

Implants made from ceramics and bioresorable composites have been used increasingly owing to their ability to provide for the required mechanical functions as desired for the tissue engineering mainly reconstruction and other intended functions in the body. Degradation of the bioresorable materials is controllable and therefore the rate of degradation can be optimized as is desired by the function it serves in the body. However, a number of challenges are associated with the bioresorable implants. The implants from magnesium based alloys have got a faster rate of degradation of mechanical properties when employed for tissue engineering applications. Surface coatings have been recommended for achieving magnesium based alloys with consistency in their mechanical strength throughout their intended functions. Research community has been active on carrying out research activities for magnesium and iron based alloys. Their main focus has been to determine and enhance the mechanical properties as well as the degradation kinetics. The types of bioresorable and ceramics implants are dictated by various parameters such as physical conditions, age, type of fracture and the risks associated with the infections. Polymers have also been used for various medical applications such as for fixation plates, screws, sutures and so on. However, it is very difficult to control their degradation rate. Further, the do not provide for the required mechanical strength and also ensues in inflammations when implanted in human body. There are some metallic polymeric composite materials that demonstrates properties similar to that of cancellous bones and possess excellent cytocompatability.

REFERENCES

Almeida, J. I., Javier, J. J., Mackay, E., Bautista, C., & Proebstle, T. M. (2013). First human use of cyanoacrylate adhesive for treatment of saphenous vein incompetence. *Journal of Vascular Surgery. Venous and Lymphatic Disorders*, *1*(2), 174–180. doi:10.1016/j.jvsv.2012.09.010 PMID:26992340

Bagga, C. S., Erbe, E. M., Murphy, J. P., Freid, J. M., & Pomrink, G. J. (2017). *U.S. Patent No. 9,629,728*. Washington, DC: U.S. Patent and Trademark Office.

Barriobero-Vila, P., Gussone, J., Haubrich, J., Sandlöbes, S., Da Silva, J. C., Cloetens, P., ... Requena, G. (2017). Inducing stable α+ β microstructures during selective laser melting of Ti-6Al-4V using intensified intrinsic heat treatments. *Materials (Basel)*, *10*(3), 268. doi:10.3390/ma10030268 PMID:28772630

Bellini, H., Moyano, J., Gil, J., & Puigdollers, A. (2016). Comparison of the superelasticity of different nickel–titanium orthodontic archwires and the loss of their properties by heat treatment. *Journal of Materials Science. Materials in Medicine*, *27*(10), 158. doi:10.100710856-016-5767-5 PMID:27623709

Boanini, E., Gazzano, M., & Bigi, A. (2010). Ionic substitutions in calcium phosphates synthesized at low temperature. *Acta Biomaterialia*, *6*(6), 1882–1894. doi:10.1016/j.actbio.2009.12.041 PMID:20040384

Bohner, M. (2000). Calcium orthophosphates in medicine: From ceramics to calcium phosphate cements. *Injury*, *31*, D37–D47. doi:10.1016/S0020-1383(00)80022-4 PMID:11270080

Broggini, N., McManus, L. M., Hermann, J. S., Medina, R., Schenk, R. K., Buser, D., & Cochran, D. L. (2006). Peri-implant inflammation defined by the implant-abutment interface. *Journal of Dental Research*, *85*(5), 473–478. doi:10.1177/154405910608500515 PMID:16632764

Cappiello, M., Luongo, R., Di Iorio, D., Bugea, C., Cocchetto, R., & Celletti, R. (2008). Evaluation of peri-implant bone loss around platform-switched implants. *International Journal of Periodontics & Restorative Dentistry*, *28*(4). PMID:18717373

Chen, Y., Xu, Z., Smith, C., & Sankar, J. (2014). Recent advances on the development of magnesium alloys for biodegradable implants. *Acta Biomaterialia*, *10*(11), 4561–4573. doi:10.1016/j.actbio.2014.07.005 PMID:25034646

Chiellini, E., & Solaro, R. (1996). Biodegradable polymeric materials. *Advanced Materials*, *8*(4), 305–313. doi:10.1002/adma.19960080406

Daniels, A. U., Chang, M. K., Andriano, K. P., & Heller, J. (1990). Mechanical properties of biodegradable polymers and composites proposed for internal fixation of bone. *Journal of Applied Biomaterials*, *1*(1), 57–78. doi:10.1002/jab.770010109 PMID:10148987

David, C., De Kesel, C., Lefebvre, F., & Weiland, M. (1994). The biodegradation of polymers: Recent results. *Die Angewandte Makromolekulare Chemie: Applied Macromolecular Chemistry and Physics, 216*(1), 21–35. doi:10.1002/apmc.1994.052160102

de Groot, K. (1993). Clinical applications of calcium phosphate biomaterials: A review. *Ceramics International, 19*(5), 363–366. doi:10.1016/0272-8842(93)90050-2

Gao, X., & Nie, J. F. (2007). Characterization of strengthening precipitate phases in a Mg–Zn alloy. *Scripta Materialia, 56*(8), 645–648. doi:10.1016/j.scriptamat.2007.01.006

Gbureck, U., Hölzel, T., Klammert, U., Würzler, K., Müller, F. A., & Barralet, J. E. (2007). Resorbable dicalcium phosphate bone substitutes prepared by 3D powder printing. *Advanced Functional Materials, 17*(18), 3940–3945. doi:10.1002/adfm.200700019

Gepreel, M. A. H., & Niinomi, M. (2013). Biocompatibility of Ti-alloys for long-term implantation. *Journal of the Mechanical Behavior of Biomedical Materials, 20*, 407–415. doi:10.1016/j.jmbbm.2012.11.014 PMID:23507261

Gu, X. N., & Zheng, Y. F. (2010). A review on magnesium alloys as biodegradable materials. *Frontiers of Materials Science in China, 4*(2), 111–115. doi:10.100711706-010-0024-1

Gunatillake, P. A., & Adhikari, R. (2003). Biodegradable synthetic polymers for tissue engineering. *European Cells & Materials, 5*(1), 1–16. doi:10.22203/eCM.v005a01 PMID:14562275

Guo, R., Merkel, A. R., Sterling, J. A., Davidson, J. M., & Guelcher, S. A. (2015). Substrate modulus of 3D-printed scaffolds regulates the regenerative response in subcutaneous implants through the macrophage phenotype and Wnt signaling. *Biomaterials, 73*, 85–95. doi:10.1016/j.biomaterials.2015.09.005 PMID:26406449

He, C., Bin, S., Wu, P., Gao, C., Feng, P., Yang, Y., ... Shuai, C. (2017). Microstructure evolution and biodegradation behavior of laser rapid solidified Mg–Al–Zn alloy. *Metals, 7*(3), 105. doi:10.3390/met7030105

He, Y., Tao, H., Zhang, Y., Jiang, Y., Zhang, S., Zhao, C., ... Zhang, X. (2009). Biocompatibility of bio-Mg-Zn alloy within bone with heart, liver, kidney and spleen. *Chinese Science Bulletin, 54*(3), 484–491.

Hofstetter, J., Becker, M., Martinelli, E., Weinberg, A. M., Mingler, B., Kilian, H., ... Löffler, J. F. (2014). High-strength low-alloy (HSLA) Mg–Zn–Ca alloys with excellent biodegradation performance. *JOM*, *66*(4), 566–572. doi:10.100711837-014-0875-5

Hofstetter, J., Martinelli, E., Weinberg, A. M., Becker, M., Mingler, B., Uggowitzer, P. J., & Löffler, J. F. (2015). Assessing the degradation performance of ultrahigh-purity magnesium in vitro and in vivo. *Corrosion Science*, *91*, 29–36. doi:10.1016/j.corsci.2014.09.008

Hollinger, J. O., & Battistone, G. C. (1985). *Biodegradable bone repair materials: synthetic polymers and ceramics*. Army Inst of Dental Research.

Huang, Y., Van Dessel, J., Martens, W., Lambrichts, I., Zhong, W. J., Ma, G. W., ... Jacobs, R. (2015). Sensory innervation around immediately vs. delayed loaded implants: A pilot study. *International Journal of Oral Science*, *7*(1), 49–55. doi:10.1038/ijos.2014.53 PMID:25214361

Karst, D., & Yang, Y. (2006). Molecular modeling study of the resistance of PLA to hydrolysis based on the blending of PLLA and PDLA. *Polymer*, *47*(13), 4845–4850. doi:10.1016/j.polymer.2006.05.002

Klein, M. O., Schiegnitz, E., & Al-Nawas, B. (2014). Systematic review on success of narrow-diameter dental implants. *International Journal of Oral & Maxillofacial Implants*, 29. PMID:24660189

Knaack, D., Goad, M. E. P., Aiolova, M., Rey, C., Tofighi, A., Chakravarthy, P., & Lee, D. D. (1998). Resorbable calcium phosphate bone substitute. *Journal of Biomedical Materials Research*, *43*(4), 399–409. doi:10.1002/(SICI)1097-4636(199824)43:4<399::AID-JBM7>3.0.CO;2-J PMID:9855198

Kopova, I., Stráský, J., Harcuba, P., Landa, M., Janeček, M., & Bačáková, L. (2016). Newly developed Ti–Nb–Zr–Ta–Si–Fe biomedical beta titanium alloys with increased strength and enhanced biocompatibility. *Materials Science and Engineering C*, *60*, 230–238. doi:10.1016/j.msec.2015.11.043 PMID:26706526

Kwasniak, P., Garbacz, H., & Kurzydlowski, K. J. (2016). Solid solution strengthening of hexagonal titanium alloys: Restoring forces and stacking faults calculated from first principles. *Acta Materialia*, *102*, 304–314. doi:10.1016/j.actamat.2015.09.041

Lee, J. W., Han, H. S., Han, K. J., Park, J., Jeon, H., Ok, M. R., ... Yang, S. J. (2016). Long-term clinical study and multiscale analysis of in vivo biodegradation mechanism of Mg alloy. *Proceedings of the National Academy of Sciences of the United States of America, 113*(3), 716–721. doi:10.1073/pnas.1518238113 PMID:26729859

LeGeros, R. Z., Lin, S., Rohanizadeh, R., Mijares, D., & LeGeros, J. P. (2003). Biphasic calcium phosphate bioceramics: Preparation, properties and applications. *Journal of Materials Science. Materials in Medicine, 14*(3), 201–209. doi:10.1023/A:1022872421333 PMID:15348465

Li, N., & Zheng, Y. (2013). Novel magnesium alloys developed for biomedical application: A review. *Journal of Materials Science and Technology, 29*(6), 489–502. doi:10.1016/j.jmst.2013.02.005

Li, Y., Yang, C., Zhao, H., Qu, S., Li, X., & Li, Y. (2014). New developments of Ti-based alloys for biomedical applications. *Materials (Basel), 7*(3), 1709–1800. doi:10.3390/ma7031709 PMID:28788539

Li, Z., Gu, X., Lou, S., & Zheng, Y. (2008). The development of binary Mg–Ca alloys for use as biodegradable materials within bone. *Biomaterials, 29*(10), 1329–1344. doi:10.1016/j.biomaterials.2007.12.021 PMID:18191191

Lodge, T. P., & McLeish, T. C. (2000). Self-concentrations and effective glass transition temperatures in polymer blends. *Macromolecules, 33*(14), 5278–5284. doi:10.1021/ma9921706

Lohbauer, U., Zipperle, M., Rischka, K., Petschelt, A., & Müller, F. A. (2008). Hydroxylation of dental zirconia surfaces: Characterization and bonding potential. *Journal of Biomedical Materials Research Part B: Applied Biomaterials, 87*(2), 461–467. PMID:18506815

Maurus, P. B., & Kaeding, C. C. (2004). Bioabsorbable implant material review. *Operative Techniques in Sports Medicine, 12*(3), 158–160. doi:10.1053/j.otsm.2004.07.015

Mayer, I., Jacobsohn, O., Niazov, T., Werckmann, J., Iliescu, M., Richard-Plouet, M., ... Reinen, D. (2003). Manganese in precipitated hydroxyapatites. *European Journal of Inorganic Chemistry, 2003*(7), 1445–1451. doi:10.1002/ejic.200390188

Middleton, J. C., & Tipton, A. J. (2000). Synthetic biodegradable polymers as orthopedic devices. *Biomaterials*, *21*(23), 2335–2346. doi:10.1016/S0142-9612(00)00101-0 PMID:11055281

Mohammed, M. T., Khan, Z. A., & Siddiquee, A. N. (2014a). Beta titanium alloys: the lowest elastic modulus for biomedical applications: a review. *Int. J. Chem. Mol. Nucl. Mater. Metall. Eng*, *8*(8).

Mohammed, M. T., Khan, Z. A., & Siddiquee, A. N. (2014b). Surface modifications of titanium materials for developing corrosion behavior in human body environment: A review. *Procedia Materials Science*, *6*, 1610-1618.

Nagels, J., Stokdijk, M., & Rozing, P. M. (2003). Stress shielding and bone resorption in shoulder arthroplasty. *Journal of Shoulder and Elbow Surgery*, *12*(1), 35–39. doi:10.1067/mse.2003.22 PMID:12610484

Oka, Y., Ye, M., & Zuker, C. S. (2015). Thirst driving and suppressing signals encoded by distinct neural populations in the brain. *Nature*, *520*(7547), 349–352. doi:10.1038/nature14108 PMID:25624099

Pezzin, A. P. T., Van Ekenstein, G. A., Zavaglia, C. A. C., Ten Brinke, G., & Duek, E. A. R. (2003). Poly (para-dioxanone) and poly (L-lactic acid) blends: Thermal, mechanical, and morphological properties. *Journal of Applied Polymer Science*, *88*(12), 2744–2755. doi:10.1002/app.11984

Premraj, R., & Doble, M. (2005). Biodegradation of polymers. *Indian Journal of Biotechnology*, *4*(2), 186–193.

Ravi Shantharaj, M. D. S., Panchali Batra, M. D. S., Pradeep Subbiah, M. D. S., & Lakshmi, B. (2014). Total Recall: An Update On Orthodontic Wires. *IJO*, *25*(3).

Robello, D. R., Eldridge, T. D., & Swanson, M. T. (1999). Degradation and stabilization of polycyanoacrylates. *Journal of Polymer Science. Part A, Polymer Chemistry*, *37*(24), 4570–4581. doi:10.1002/(SICI)1099-0518(19991215)37:24<4570::AID-POLA14>3.0.CO;2-#

Scattina, A., Alovisi, M., Paolino, D. S., Pasqualini, D., Scotti, N., Chiandussi, G., & Berutti, E. (2015). Prediction of Cyclic Fatigue Life of Nickel-Titanium Rotary Files by Virtual Modeling and Finite Elements Analysis. *Journal of Endodontics*, *41*(11), 1867–1870. doi:10.1016/j.joen.2015.07.010 PMID:26361644

Schinhammer, M., Hänzi, A. C., Löffler, J. F., & Uggowitzer, P. J. (2010). Design strategy for biodegradable Fe-based alloys for medical applications. *Acta Biomaterialia, 6*(5), 1705–1713. doi:10.1016/j.actbio.2009.07.039 PMID:19654056

Shackelford, J. F. (1999). Bioceramics-current status and future trends. *Materials Science Forum, 293*, 99. doi:10.4028/www.scientific.net/MSF.293.99

Sheikh, Z., Najeeb, S., Khurshid, Z., Verma, V., Rashid, H., & Glogauer, M. (2015). Biodegradable materials for bone repair and tissue engineering applications. *Materials (Basel), 8*(9), 5744–5794. doi:10.3390/ma8095273 PMID:28793533

Shikinami, Y., & Okuno, M. (1999). Bioresorbable devices made of forged composites of hydroxyapatite (HA) particles and poly-L-lactide (PLLA): Part I. Basic characteristics. *Biomaterials, 20*(9), 859–877. doi:10.1016/S0142-9612(98)00241-5 PMID:10226712

Shtilman, M. I. (2015). Biodegradation of Polymers. Journal of Siberian Federal University. *Biology (Basel), 8*(2), 113.

Soler-Botija, C., Bagó, J. R., Llucià-Valldeperas, A., Vallés-Lluch, A., Castells-Sala, C., Martínez-Ramos, C., ... Bayes-Genis, A. (2014). Engineered 3D bioimplants using elastomeric scaffold, self-assembling peptide hydrogel, and adipose tissue-derived progenitor cells for cardiac regeneration. *American Journal of Translational Research, 6*(3), 291. PMID:24936221

Song, G., & Atrens, A. (2003). Understanding magnesium corrosion—a framework for improved alloy performance. *Advanced Engineering Materials, 5*(12), 837–858. doi:10.1002/adem.200310405

Sung, H. J., Meredith, C., Johnson, C., & Galis, Z. S. (2004). The effect of scaffold degradation rate on three-dimensional cell growth and angiogenesis. *Biomaterials, 25*(26), 5735–5742. doi:10.1016/j.biomaterials.2004.01.066 PMID:15147819

Suthar, J., & Patel, K. M. (2018). Processing issues, machining, and applications of aluminum metal matrix composites. *Materials and Manufacturing Processes, 33*(5), 499–527. doi:10.1080/10426914.2017.1401713

Taïr, K., Kharoubi, O., Taïr, O. A., Hellal, N., Benyettou, I., & Aoues, A. (2016). Aluminium-induced acute neurotoxicity in rats: Treatment with aqueous extract of Arthrophytum (Hammada scoparia). *Journal of Acute Disease*, *5*(6), 470–482. doi:10.1016/j.joad.2016.08.028

Takmakov, P., Ruda, K., Phillips, K. S., Isayeva, I. S., Krauthamer, V., & Welle, C. G. (2015). Rapid evaluation of the durability of cortical neural implants using accelerated aging with reactive oxygen species. *Journal of Neural Engineering*, *12*(2), 026003. doi:10.1088/1741-2560/12/2/026003 PMID:25627426

Tamimi, F., Le Nihouannen, D., Eimar, H., Sheikh, Z., Komarova, S., & Barralet, J. (2012). The effect of autoclaving on the physical and biological properties of dicalcium phosphate dihydrate bioceramics: Brushite vs. monetite. *Acta Biomaterialia*, *8*(8), 3161–3169. doi:10.1016/j.actbio.2012.04.025 PMID:22522010

Tan, L., Yu, X., Wan, P., & Yang, K. (2013). Biodegradable materials for bone repairs: A review. *Journal of Materials Science and Technology*, *29*(6), 503–513. doi:10.1016/j.jmst.2013.03.002

Tang, A., Pan, F., Yang, M., & Cheng, R. (2008). Mechanical properties and microstructure of magnesium-aluminum based alloys containing strontium. *Materials Transactions*, *49*(6), 1203–1211. doi:10.2320/matertrans.MOV2007315

Teramoto, H., Kawai, A., Sugihara, S., Yoshida, A., & Inoue, H. (2005). Resorption of apatite-wollastonite containing glass-ceramic and beta-tricalcium phosphate in vivo. *Acta Medica Okayama*, *59*(5), 201. PMID:16286959

Thian, E. S., Konishi, T., Kawanobe, Y., Lim, P. N., Choong, C., Ho, B., & Aizawa, M. (2013). Zinc-substituted hydroxyapatite: A biomaterial with enhanced bioactivity and antibacterial properties. *Journal of Materials Science. Materials in Medicine*, *24*(2), 437–445. doi:10.100710856-012-4817-x PMID:23160913

Vert, M. (2009). Degradable and bioresorbable polymers in surgery and in pharmacology: Beliefs and facts. *Journal of Materials Science. Materials in Medicine*, *20*(2), 437–446. doi:10.100710856-008-3581-4 PMID:18815731

Wang, J., Tang, J., Zhang, P., Li, Y., Wang, J., Lai, Y., & Qin, L. (2012). Surface modification of magnesium alloys developed for bioabsorbable orthopedic implants: A general review. *Journal of Biomedical Materials Research. Part B, Applied Biomaterials*, *100*(6), 1691–1701. doi:10.1002/jbm.b.32707 PMID:22566412

Wang, J., Zhang, J., Zong, X., Xu, C., You, Z., & Nie, K. (2015). Effects of Ca on the formation of LPSO phase and mechanical properties of Mg-Zn-Y-Mn alloy. *Materials Science and Engineering A*, *648*, 37–40. doi:10.1016/j.msea.2015.09.046

Wang, S., Liu, Y., Zhang, C., Liao, Z., & Liu, W. (2014). The improvement of wettability, biotribological behavior and corrosion resistance of titanium alloy pretreated by thermal oxidation. *Tribology International*, *79*, 174–182. doi:10.1016/j.triboint.2014.06.008

Wang, X. H., Ni, J. S., Cao, N. L., Yu, S., Chen, Y. G., Zhang, S. X., ... Yan, J. (2017). In vivo evaluation of Mg–6Zn and titanium alloys on collagen metabolism in the healing of intestinal anastomosis. *Scientific Reports*, *7*(1), 44919. doi:10.1038rep44919 PMID:28317926

Weiler, A., Hoffmann, R. F., Stähelin, A. C., Helling, H. J., & Südkamp, N. P. (2000). Biodegradable implants in sports medicine: The biological base. *Arthroscopy*, *16*(3), 305–321. doi:10.1016/S0749-8063(00)90055-0 PMID:10750011

Witte, F., Fischer, J., Nellesen, J., Crostack, H. A., Kaese, V., Pisch, A., ... Windhagen, H. (2006). In vitro and in vivo corrosion measurements of magnesium alloys. *Biomaterials*, *27*(7), 1013–1018. doi:10.1016/j.biomaterials.2005.07.037 PMID:16122786

Witte, F., Hort, N., Vogt, C., Cohen, S., Kainer, K. U., Willumeit, R., & Feyerabend, F. (2008). Degradable biomaterials based on magnesium corrosion. *Current Opinion in Solid State and Materials Science*, *12*(5-6), 63–72. doi:10.1016/j.cossms.2009.04.001

Wittenbrink, I., Hausmann, A., Schickle, K., Lauria, I., Davtalab, R., Foss, M., ... Fischer, H. (2015). Low-aspect ratio nanopatterns on bioinert alumina influence the response and morphology of osteoblast-like cells. *Biomaterials*, *62*, 58–65. doi:10.1016/j.biomaterials.2015.05.026 PMID:26022980

Xu, Z., Smith, C., Chen, S., & Sankar, J. (2011). Development and microstructural characterizations of Mg–Zn–Ca alloys for biomedical applications. *Materials Science and Engineering B*, *176*(20), 1660–1665. doi:10.1016/j.mseb.2011.06.008

Yahyavi-Firouz-Abadi, N., Menias, C. O., Bhalla, S., Siegel, C., Gayer, G., & Katz, D. S. (2015). Imaging of cosmetic plastic procedures and implants in the body and their potential complications. *AJR. American Journal of Roentgenology*, *204*(4), 707–715. doi:10.2214/AJR.14.13516 PMID:25794060

Yang, Y., Scenini, F., & Curioni, M. (2016). A study on magnesium corrosion by real-time imaging and electrochemical methods: Relationship between local processes and hydrogen evolution. *Electrochimica Acta*, *198*, 174–184. doi:10.1016/j.electacta.2016.03.043

Yap, J., Walsh, L. J., Naser-ud Din, S., Ngo, H., & Manton, D. J. (2014). Evaluation of a novel approach in the prevention of white spot lesions around orthodontic brackets. *Australian Dental Journal*, *59*(1), 70–80. doi:10.1111/adj.12142 PMID:24528001

Zhang, S., Zhang, X., Zhao, C., Li, J., Song, Y., Xie, C., ... Bian, Y. (2010). Research on an Mg–Zn alloy as a degradable biomaterial. *Acta Biomaterialia*, *6*(2), 626–640. doi:10.1016/j.actbio.2009.06.028 PMID:19545650

Zimmerli, W. (2014). Clinical presentation and treatment of orthopaedic implant-associated infection. *Journal of Internal Medicine*, *276*(2), 111–119. doi:10.1111/joim.12233 PMID:24605880

Section 2

Scaffolds and Tissue Engineering

Chapter 4
Scaffolds and Tissue Engineering Applications by 3D Bio-Printing Process:
A New Approach

Ranjit Barua
Om Dayal Group of Institutions, India

Sudipto Datta
Indian Institute of Engineering Science and Technology Shibpur, India

Pallab Datta
Indian Institute of Engineering Science and Technology Shibpur, India

Amit Roy Chowdhury
Indian Institute of Engineering Science and Technology Shibpur, India

ABSTRACT

3D bio-printing is a revolutionary manufacturing process that is widely used in medical fields especially in preparing bone scaffolds and tissue engineering. With the help of new biocompatible material like polymers, bio-gels, ceramics, this technology has created a new site in advanced tissue engineering and scaffolds manufacturing area. Another important thing is that, with the use of CAD file software, any complex design can be prepared (i.e., this technology does not have any limited sites). But here it is very much essential to study and analyze machine printability characteristics, cross-linking time and biocompatibility of printing objects as well as bio-ink. However, mechanical properties like shear thinning, mechanical elasticity are also required. In this chapter, different types of scaffold-preparing methods and the bio-printing process are discussed, which are used in scaffold and tissue engineering.

DOI: 10.4018/978-1-5225-8235-9.ch004

INTRODUCTION

Three dimensional printing is growing up innovatively in medical application especially in scaffolds preparing and tissue engineering are. 3D printing is nothing but a process of additive manufacturing process. As per ASTM-F42 Committee, Additive manufacturing is manufacturing method of joining materials to make an objects from 3D model data, normally layer upon layer, contradictory of traditional manufacturing process [ASTM F2792–10]. Basically the objects are made by different types of materials like metal, polymers, powders, ceramics, in case of bio-printing process, biocompatible materials like bioink even also living cells are also used for making scaffolds [Banks.,2013, Sun et al., 2005, Hornbeck,1997]. Bio-printing technique initially starts from collecting the image data from any patients' body through Magnetic Resonance Imaging (MRI) or Computed Tomography (CT) process [Mertz et al.,2013]. After collecting the image data, all data are converting the Computer Aided Design (CAD) file [Yandell,2013] through Digital Imaging and Communication Medicine (DICOM) directory [Science and society,2013]. A uniform process is exists for preparing the essential Standard Triangulation Language (STL) format of implants [Cheah et al., 2003]. After all this process, final objects is printed. Table 1 shows the time wise evolutionary list of 3D printing technology. On the increase bioactive three-dimensional (3D) scaffolds to hold up bone regeneration has consequently develop into a solution part of spotlight inside tissue engineering specially bone tissue. Three dimensional scaffolds that have effectively linked bone defects even as vigorously reminding bone regeneration will be emphasized. Most significant things is that the fast advances have been stimulated by the novel bio-printing manufacturing process, innovative features of bio-printers, printable biomaterials like bioinks and exhilarating applications for transplantable tissues or invitro models.

IDEAL SCAFFOLD CHARACTERISTICS

Basically, the idyllic three dimensional scaffold is compiled with biodegradable and biocompatible material, which have similar mechanical properties of tissue. Normally scaffold is not a planed to be constant position in implants, it will preferably assist the host cells for depositing in extracellular matrix (ECM)

Table 1. The time wise evolutionary list of 3D printing technology

Year	Details
1984	3D printing technology invented by Charles Hull named stereo-lithography.
1991	First fused deposition modelling (FDM) created by stratasys where 3D model are made by polymers like PLA, ABS materials.
1992	Selective laser sintering process (SLS) made by DTM applying powder materials with laser to print the object.
2000	Inkjet 3D printer and multi-colour printer manufactured. Next year, desktop based 3D printer launched.
2009	Commercial 3D printer machine existing to the marketplace.

and after then the scaffold structure will replace. Three dimensional scaffold architecturally must has to be porous with an interrelated structure to permit cell and also nutrient relocation. Scaffold surface always to be optimized for facilitating cell addition, differentiation and proliferation. Form a medical surgical position; it is also an advantageous for the scaffold material to be effortlessly operated into a various shapes and sizes for allowing *in-situ* medical treatment for individual problem of patient bone defects [Sun et al.,2005, Hutmacher, 2010, Albrektsson et al.,2001, Bose et al., 2102, Young et al., 2003]. It is necessary that scaffold materials must have to be biocompatiable, does not any toxicity reaction with cell, also can easily removed from the body, to obtain small immune reaction through their existence [O'Keefe et al., 2011, Brydone et al., 2010, Lloyd, 2001, Vaccaro, 2002]. One more things is that, controlling the biodegradability is also a vital characteristic for a scaffold to complete; if a scaffold degrades so rapidly then mechanical failure could happens . This is mostly applicable in bone tissue engineering (BTE), where an implanted scaffold is expected to endure load-bearing and it could fracture, if there have not present mechanical support at the same time as new bone is forming. On the other hand, if a scaffold does not able to degrade properly then an inflammatory reaction could be generated to the foreign material of the scaffold, damaging the tissue regeneration [Mountziaris et al.,2008, Brydone, 2010]. Growth is also an important factor to cooperate in successful bone tissue engineering scaffolds. The developments of new bone formation and extracellular matrix deposition are controlled by a variety of growth factors and also biomolecules. For developing bone and cartilage, Bone morphogenic proteins (BMP) play a serious function, it have the facility to activate proliferation as well as differentiation of osteo-progenitor cells

[Cao, 2010]. There are numerous examples of scaffolds which have fruitfully integrated BMPs ensuing in developed bone formation. Still, there have a threat of bone formation inside soft tissues, heterotopic ossification, is also related with use of BMPs [Leblanc et al., 2011, Li et al., 2006, Nie et al., 2007, Shi et al., 2009, Cipitria et al., 2015]. Now a day in scaffold, Vascular endothelial growth factor (VEGF) are used frequently for adding the ability to increase bone and blood vessel formation in-vivo [Schantz et al., 2007, Kaigler et al., 2006, Wernike et al., 2010]. In bone and cartilage tissue engineering [Dimitriou et al.,2005, Salgado et al., 2004] different kind of growth factors are applied like insulin-like growth-factor 1 (IGF-1),Transforming growth factor b (TGF b), fibroblast growth factors (FGFs) and platelet-derived growth factor (PDGF). For cell viability and development tissue in growth, micro-architecture of scaffolds is necessary. Interconnected pore structure helps to supply nutrients and oxygen in scaffold and also exits the waste product from it without any blood supply. Porosity can help cell migration and it also advances existing surface area for binding cell scaffold for interacting with adjacent tissues [Hing et al., 2004, Zhang et al., 2006, Barrere et al., 2008]. Scaffold pore size and density are considerably impact on cellular attachment and growth [O'Brien et al. 2005, Zeltinger et al., 2001]. Surface area of the scaffold will be increased when pore size will be decreased. Though, due to small pore size, it will difficult to cell migration in scaffold structure. That's why scaffolds must be accurately fabricated with approving parameters. Scaffolds implanted in vivo system with 300 mm pore sizes which supports osteogenesis for higher permeability and good for vascularisation, while smaller pore sizes like 100mm more suitable for chondrogenesis [Walthers et al., 2014, Kuboki et al., 2001]. With increasing of macroporosity of scaffold which can help to progress of angiogenesis invivo system [Tsuruga et al., 1997], at the same time as a degree of microporosity also improves cell-scaffold contacts [Ashman et al., 2013, Rosa et al., 2003, Habibovic et al., 2005, Boccaccio et al., 2011]. Over and above porosity and pore size, mechanoregulatory effect plays a vital role for influencing bone cellular differentiation and tissue growth in vivo system [Kelly et al.,2006]. It is required same mechanical stiffness of scaffold materials and native bone [Sandino et al., 2011, Chen et al., 2015, Breuls et al., 2008]. Though, mechanical stiffness of scaffold and porosity are straightly differing with physical properties, if scaffold porosity is increased then the mechanical strength will reduce. Mechanical properties of scaffold such as Young's modulus fatigue strength and compressive strength are also very important[Howk et al., 2006, Corrales et al., 2014]. An ideal scaffold have Young's modulus ike to cortical bone is almost 7 to 30 GPa and compressive strength is around 100-230 MPa and range of tensile strength is 50-151 MPa [Hutmacher et al., 2007, Kokubo et al., 2003, Amaral et al., 2002, Chen et al., 2012].

Scaffold Fabrication Process

A large variety of methods have been employed for fabrication 3D scaffold. Normally, it is not easy to make difficult scaffold micro-architectures with exact control by traditional technique process. Though, the incorporation into BTE of three dimensional printing with computer-aided design (CAD) modeling has significantly augmented with scaffold manufacture accuracy and interchangeability, with possible to control scaffold macro and micro-

Table 2. Different types of scaffold fabrication processes with advantage and disadvantage

Sl. No.	Fabrication Process	Advantages	Limitations
1	Solvent casting-particle leaching process	It is simple technique which can allow for creating of scaffolds with standard porosity, also controlled pore size and composition.	Restricted thickness of structures also mechanical properties achievable.
2	Freeze-drying	Solid porogens are not required.	Organic solvents must be needed and require small pore size.
3	Gas foaming	Reduces utilize of chemical solvents	To control pore sizes is very complicated and also can not ensure interconnectivity.
4	Electro-spinning	Generates scaffold with wide surface area for cell addition.	It have limited mechanical properties and Organic solvents may be needed, which causes harmful to cells.
5	Phase Separation	Removes leaching step of porogen, it be joined with another techniques effortlessly.	Require long processing time.
6	3D Printing	i. Difficult 3D shapes can be fabricated with high resolution, controlled internal structures, morphology and pore size. ii. With the help of this technique, cells may be incorporated in high concentration directly in scaffold materials	Arrangement costs are expensive for machinery.

porosity. Table 2 shows different types of scaffold manufacturing processes and also advantages and disadvantages.

Traditional Method of Scaffold Fabrication Process

Different types of traditional scaffolds fabrication processes are available like solvent casting- particle leaching process, freeze- drying, gas foaming, electro-spinning and phase separation [Puppi et al., 2010]. All processes are described below.

Solvent Casting-Particle Leaching Process

Solvent casting is a traditional method of scaffold manufacturing process which starts with a polymer dissolution in an organic solvent. Figure 1 describes the solvent casting-particle leaching technique, in this technique porogens is used, which can be scattered into a moulded structure and consequently closed once the structure has place, producing in the formation of pores. Normally, porogens are mixed with polymer solution to prepare a polymer-porogen network. Then the polymer is consequently hardened as evaporating of solvent, through water then inured to break up the porogen which is frequently a salt like as sodium chloride. A hardedged polymer scaffold with a porous network is made, though it is not easy to control pore shape and interconnectivity of scaffolds formed by this process [Liao, et al., 2002].

Figure 1. Solvent casting-particle leaching process

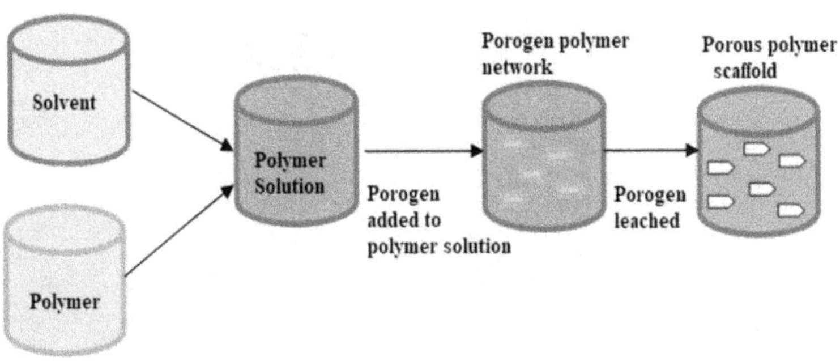

Freeze-Drying Process

This process starts with freezing of a polymer solution (Figure 2), making in the arrangement of solvent ice crystals encircled by polymer aggregates. The contiguous pressure is then decreased through a vacuum, to a level less than the frozen solvent equilibrium vapor pressure. Therefore the solvent is generated to endure sublimation straightly into gas. After the solvent is totally sublimated, interconnected porous structure of dry polymer scaffold relics. In primary scaffold fabrication process an emulsification freeze drying is used, and the process commences by dissolving polymers or ceramics into the solvent and adding with water for obtaining an emulsion. Then the mixture is poured into the mould and after frozen then two phases can detach. After that the frozen emulsion is freeze-dried for removing the solvent and detached water for making pores into a solidified scaffold [Whang et al., 1995].

Gas Foaming

In this process removes the applications of solvents positioned in solvent casting technique (Figure 3). This process makes a porous structure during the nucleation, development of gas bubbles scattered all over a polymer. Compression moulding process was first used for making solid discs of a scaffold material, for example poly(lactic-co-glycolic acid). Subsequent this, the discs are drenched with carbon dioxide by revelation to high pressure CO_2 gas of 5.5 MPa for 72 hrs at room temperature, previous to solubility of the

Figure 2. Freeze-drying process

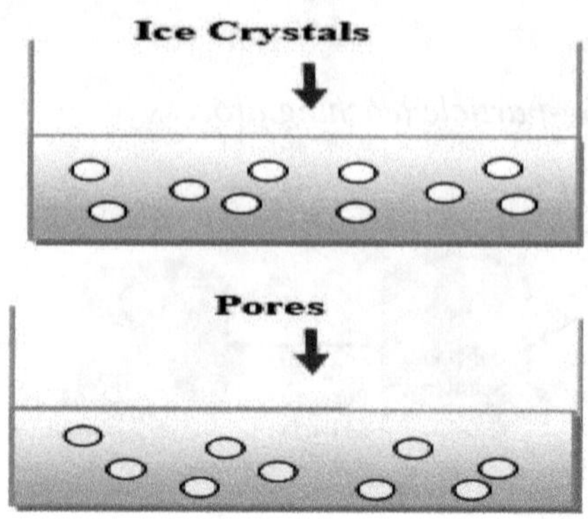

Figure 3. Gas forming process

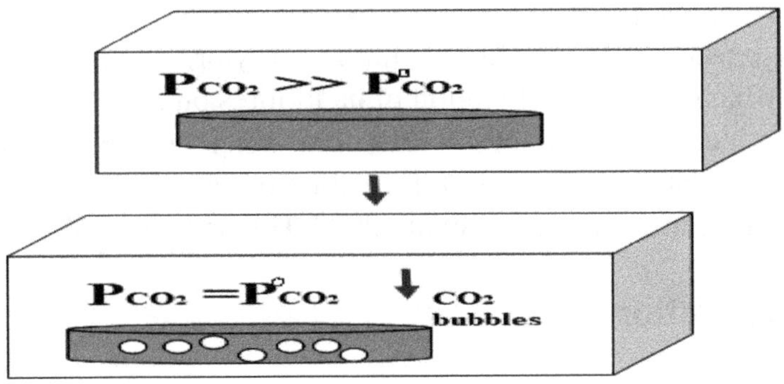

gas in the polymer is quickly declined by dipping CO_2 pressure to atmospheric levels (P^0CO_2). This sources the CO_2 gas to tuft mutually and making pores. Here pore sizes and porosities up to 100 mm 93% can be gained by using this process. Though, pore connectivity is not easy to control and also creates pore sizes by gas foaming [Hollister; 2005, Manke et al., 2013, Mooney et al., 1996, Whang et al., 1995, Dehghani et al., 2011].

Electro-Spinning

Another technique of scaffold fabrication process is Electrospinning which have the facility to make nano fibrous with interconnected porous in scaffolds

Figure 4. Electro-Spinning process

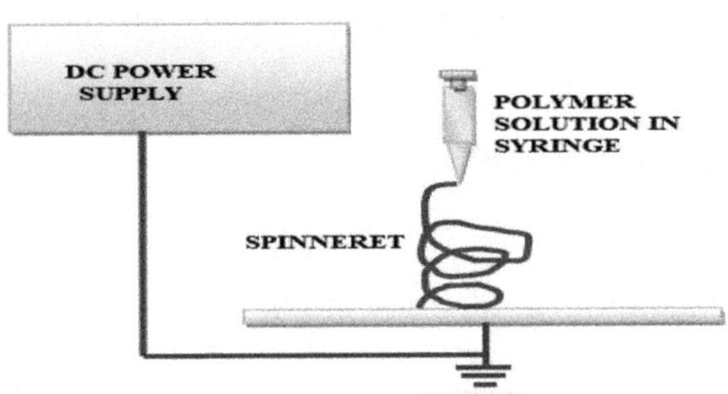

(Figure 4). An externally DC high voltage is applied on the anode syringe needle in which the polymer is present. When the external voltage exceeds the surface tension of the polymer solution a Taylor cone is formed on the needle tip which result in production of nanofibres on the collector plate of cathode. Various fibres diameter from micro to nano ranges are created on the deposition plate which result in formation of various types of scaffolds for tissue engineering[Matthews et al., 2002, Huang et al., 2003].

Phase Separation

This process relies on thermal energy for de-mixing the homogenous polymer. Polymer like as PLLA is mixed with solvent, basically it is unstable at a low temperature and impulsively split into a a solvent-rich phase and polymer rich phase. This scaffold manufacture obtains advantage and in high boiling polymer becomes dissolute. At an elevated temperature, low molecular weight obtains. Homogenous met-blend obtain normally around the of polymer melting point. After that the solution can cast in desired shape of scaffold (Figure 5). The solvent of solvent-rich phase is removed during extraction, sublimation and evaporation. This process makes a porous scaffold, in the polymer matrix pores are left behind after solvent removal.

Three Dimensional Printing Process

Conventional scaffold fabrication process is limited in geometry of shape, scaffolds' interconnectivity and pore size. Three dimensional printing is a revolutionary manufacturing process which can help to overcome all this difficulties. This manufacturing process also called additive manufacturing

Figure 5. Phase separation process

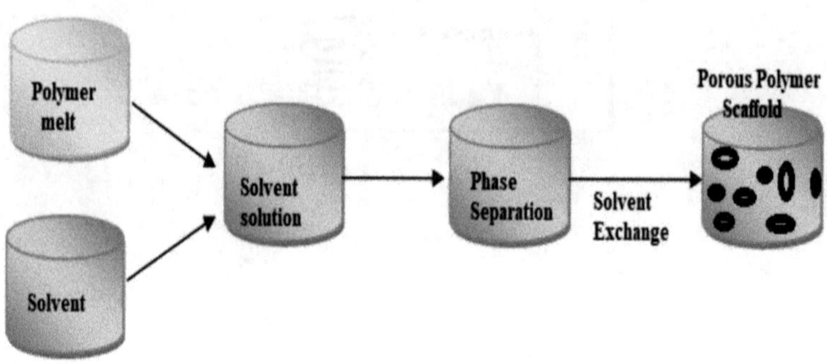

process because in this process the final object is fabricated by depositing printable material on collecting plate surface layer by another layer. 3D printing process offers to make any complex design, normally a model is drawn by design software like computer aided design (CAD) then the model is converted into .stl format. After forming the .stl file, this file is converted to G-code format and uploaded into the 3D printer for printing the desired model. By using different kind of medical imaging data like computed tomography (CT), magnetic resonance imaging (MRI), X-rays can be converted to CAD models which can helps to print the imaging reports into 3D model. 3D printing technology is also applied in bone tissue engineering (BTE), the first three dimensional object is made by stereolithography (SLA) process where UV light was applied on liquid photo polymer to solidify for making 3D substance and remaining area was liquid form. SLA technique is very expansive method and also limited materials can be printed [Kim et al., 2010]. Another process named Fused deposition modelling (FDM) are also available, thermoplastic polymer like PLA, ABS are used as base material for printing the objects. In this process an hot extruder involves to melt the thermoplastic material, after melting the material, through printer head the liquid material deposits on the print bed and forming the objects. This process has been effectively modified into bone tissue engineering (BTE) as synthetic scaffolds are made by this technique, even though the high temperatures engaged limit the addition of hydrogels and biomolecules [Zein et al., 2002, Do, et al., 2015]. Various achievement with this technique has been established, during the production of composite and bioactive scaffold with comparable mechanical properties of trabecular bone [Williams et al., 2005, Xia et al., 2013].

Bio-Printing Process of Scaffold Fabrication

Conventional scaffold fabrication process is limited in geometry of shape, scaffolds' interconnectivity and pore size. Three dimensional printing is a revolutionary manufacturing process which can help to overcome all these difficulties. This manufacturing process also called additive manufacturing process because in this process the final object is fabricated by depositing printable material on collecting plate surface layer by another layer.3D printing process offers to make any complex design, normally a model is drawn by design software like computer aided design (CAD) then the model is converted into .stl format. After forming the .stl file, this file is converted to G-code format and uploaded into the 3D printer for printing the desired model. By using different kind of medical imaging data like computed tomography (CT), magnetic resonance imaging (MRI), X-rays can be converted to CAD models which can helps to print the imaging reports into 3D model.3D printing technology is also applied in bone tissue engineering (BTE), the first three dimensional object is made by stereolithography (SLA) process where UV light was applied on liquid photo polymer to solidify for making 3D substance and remaining area was liquid form. SLA technique is very expansive method and also limited materials can be printed [Shafiee et al., 2016].Another process named Fused deposition modeling (FDM) are also available, thermoplastic polymer like PLA, ABS are used as base material for printing the objects. In this process a hot extruder involves to melt the thermoplastic material, after melting the material, through printer head the liquid material deposits on the print bed and forming the objects. This process has been effectively modified into bone tissue engineering (BTE) as synthetic scaffolds are made by this technique, even though the high temperatures engaged limit the addition of hydrogels and biomolecules [Murphy et al., 2014, Fennema, et al., 2013].Various achievement with this technique has been established, during the production of composite and bioactive scaffold with comparable mechanical properties of trabecular bone [Handschel et al., 2007, Ventola, 2014].

DIFFICULTIES OF SCAFFOLD FABRICATION

Current challenges faced by the scaffold fabrications are choosing of the proper scaffold design and cell contain [Saunders et al., 2014, Cui et al., 2012] in bone tissue engineering scaffold. The most efficient cell for BTE still now remain unclear but cell inclusion in cartilage and bone regenerative therapies is clear positively. In clinical and experimental usages Mesenchymal stem cell are used mainly because of its varying and high degree of success depending on the delivery type. Though, the morbidity rate of this cells are high because they are taken from bone marrow and capacity of regeneration reduces with age of patients [Keriquel et al., 2017, Alan et al., 2015]. Induced-pluripotent stem cells (iPSCs) and Embryonic (ESCs) are also considered, without any lab treatment this cell are not basically engaged for repairing adult tissue, also have some limitation like ethical consideration and treatment trauma risk [Jones et al., 2013, Gurkan et al., 2014]. In case of scaffold vascularisation process [Yu et al., 2016, Ozbolat et al., 2016, Hunter et al., 2005, Robey, 2011] there also a big challenge to create interconnected vascular network, with out vascular network, cells cannot survive for further procedure [Colnot, 2011]. In case of large vessel fabrication, to print capillaries and micro vessel is very challenging, without any proper accuracy cell viability may decrease. Sometimes, microvessels infiltration creates big problem for bone cell viability in bone tissue engineering process[Stolzing et al., 2008, Muschler et al., 2001]. Consideration of mechanical properties [Kahle et al., 2010, Illich et al., 2011, Ting et al., 2017] for scaffold fabrication is very important, Sudipto et al, [Datta et al., 2017] has worked on alginate honey bioinks and studied there mechanical and cell viability, with increasing the concentration of honey in same concenyration of alginate solution the mechanical strength decrease but the cell viability increased. Analysis the mechanical properties like tensile, compressive strength, fatigue resistance, elasticity, young modulus also help to stimulate osteogenesis [Jakus et al., 2016]. Another difficulty of this technique is very costly, that why this technique has limited boundary in huge medical practice area. In vivo process, there have a risk factor to replace bio-printed cell in to the patient's body. Biocompatibility, biomaterial degradation, and tissue integration [Kolesky, et al., 2016] are most essential considerations.

FUTURE SCOPE OF SCAFFOLD FABRICATION

There are number of ways on which the cost effectiveness of the three dimensional bio-printing can be increased by using osteogenic differentiation which reduce the reliance on differentiating media. For an example, in Glasgow Dalby et al, reported a nano-scale vibration which was transferred through a bioreactor of nanovibrational type for differentiating MSCs culturing mineralised tissue with collagen gels by three dimensional bio-printing. By this technology they came to a conclusion that this technology is more readily and efficient as compared to 3D scaffold fabrication and also the maintenance is easier irrespected to rotary or perfusion chamber type bioreactors [Tsimbouri et al., 201794]. The modification 3D printed constructs can be modified by using smart hydrogels having properties like degradation rate, bioa activity and mechanical stiffness etc [Byambaa, et al., 2017]. The biomimetic construct can be produced easily from the 2d clinical images taken from X-ray, MRI or CT scan also from mathematical modeling like FEM. There is also important role of surface modification for bio materials developments and scaffold of tissue engineering for the repair of cartilage and bone regeneration.

CONCLUSION

One of the most vital challenges in tissue engineering is to repair complicated bone defects, even though considerable and novel research involves. Present challenges among many patients are improving structural biomimicry, tailoring scaffold degradation, incorporating sufficient vascularisation of scaffold manufacture to manage huge scale defects. Day by day composite materials are involved in scaffold preparation due to enhancing bioactivity like good mechanical, cell affable properties which makes a great role in tissue engineering. A number of examples have in there, where bioactive polymers and ceramics are using in bone tissue engineering (BTE) specially bone as well as cartilage creates. Three dimensional bio-printing processes presents rapidly accurate control for making scaffolds' microarchitecture. With the help of 3D bio-printing all the factors like growth factor, material bioactive properties, and bio-mimetic scaffold designs can precisely combined together with in a same platform which will help to make critical BTE applications. This technology also makes a hope for facing critical challenges in medico treatment like serious bone defects, osteoporosis and osteonecorosis. This technology gradually develops day by day, many researchers are involving to make this procedure as much as increase efficiency, cost effective and mimicable in such a way which can takes a revolutionary role in medical treatments area.

REFERENCES

Alan, F.J. (2015). Bioprinting of human pluripotent stem cells and their directed differentiation into hepatocyte-like cells for the generation of minilivers in 3D. *Biofabrication*, *7*(4), 044102.

Albrektsson, T., & Johansson, C. (2001). Osteoinduction, osteoconduction and osseointegration. *European Spine Journal*, *10*(Suppl 2), S96–S101. doi:10.1007005860100282 PMID:11716023

Amaral, M., Lopes, M. A., Silva, R. F., & Santos, J. D. (2002). Densification route and mechanical properties of Si3N4-bioglass biocomposites. *Biomaterials*, *23*(3), 857–862. doi:10.1016/S0142-9612(01)00194-6 PMID:11771704

Ashman, O., & Phillips, A. M. (2013). Treatment of non-unions with bone defects: Which option and why? *Injury*, *44*(1), 43–45. doi:10.1016/S0020-1383(13)70010-X PMID:23351870

ASTM F2792–10 Standard Terminology for Additive Manufacturing Technologies.

Banks, J. (2013). Adding value in additive manufacturing: Researchers in the United Kingdom and Europe look to 3D printing for customization. *IEEE Pulse*, *4*(6), 22–26. doi:10.1109/MPUL.2013.2279617 PMID:24233187

Barrere, F., Mahmood, T. A., de Groot, K., & van Blitterswijk, C. A. (2008). Advanced biomaterials for skeletal tissue regeneration: Instructive and smart functions, Mater. Sci. Eng. *R Rep.*, *59*(1), 38–71. doi:10.1016/j.mser.2007.12.001

Boccaccio, A., Ballini, A., Pappalettere, C., Tullo, D., Cantore, S., & Desiate, A. (2011). Finite element method (FEM), mechanobiology and biomimetic scaffolds in bone tissue engineering. *International Journal of Biological Sciences*, *7*(1), 112–132. doi:10.7150/ijbs.7.112 PMID:21278921

Bose, S., Roy, M., & Bandyopadhyay, A. (2012). Recent advances in bone tissue engineering scaffolds. *Trends in Biotechnology*, *30*(10), 546–554. doi:10.1016/j.tibtech.2012.07.005 PMID:22939815

Breuls, R. G. M., Jiya, T. U., & Smit, T. H. (2008). Scaffold stiffness influences cell behavior: Opportunities for skeletal tissue engineering. *The Open Orthopaedics Journal*, *2*(2), 103–109. doi:10.2174/1874325000802010103 PMID:19478934

Brydone, A. S., Meek, D., & Maclaine, S. (2010). Bone grafting, orthopaedic biomaterials, and the clinical need for bone engineering. *Proceedings of the Institution of Mechanical Engineers. Part H, Journal of Engineering in Medicine*, *224*(12), 1329–1343. doi:10.1243/09544119JEIM770 PMID:21287823

Byambaa, B., Annabi, N., Yue, K., Trujillo-de Santiago, G., Alvarez, M. M., Jia, W., ... Khademhosseini, A. (2017). Bioprinted osteogenic and vasculogenic patterns for engineering 3D bone tissue. *Advanced Healthcare Materials*, *6*(16), 1700015. doi:10.1002/adhm.201700015 PMID:28524375

Cao, X., & Chen, D. (2005). The BMP signaling and in vivo bone formation. *Gene*, *357*(1), 1–8. doi:10.1016/j.gene.2005.06.017 PMID:16125875

Cheah, C.M., Chua, C.K., Tan, K.H., & Teo, C.K. (2003). Integration of laser surface digitizing with CAD/CAM techniques for developing facial prostheses. Part 1: Design and fabrication of prosthesis replicas. *Int J Prosthodont Jul 1, 16*(4).

Chen, G., Dong, C., Yang, L., & Lv, Y. (2015). 3D scaffolds with different stiffness but the same microstructure for bone tissue engineering. *ACS Applied Materials & Interfaces*, *7*(29), 15790–15802. doi:10.1021/acsami.5b02662 PMID:26151287

Chen, Q., Zhu, C., & Thouas, G. A. (2012). Progress and challenges in biomaterials used for bone tissue engineering: Bioactive glasses and elastomeric composites. *Prog. Biomater.*, *1*(1), 2. doi:10.1186/2194-0517-1-2 PMID:29470743

Colnot, C. (2011). Cell sources for bone tissue engineering: Insights from basic science. *Tissue Engineering. Part B, Reviews*, *17*(6), 449–457. doi:10.1089/ten.teb.2011.0243 PMID:21902612

Cui, X., & ... . (2012). Thermal inkjet printing in tissue engineering and regenerative medicine, Recent Pat. drug Deliv. *Formulation*, *6*(2), 149–155. PMID:22436025

Datta, S., Sarkar, R., Vyas, V., Bhutoria, S., Barui, A., Roy Chowdhury, A., & Datta, P. (2018). Alginate-honey bioinks with improved cell responses for applicationsas bioprinted tissue engineered constructs. *Journal of Materials Research*, 1–11.

Dehghani, F. N., & Annabi, N. (2011). Engineering porous scaffolds using gas-based techniques. *Current Opinion in Biotechnology*, *22*(5), 661–666. doi:10.1016/j.copbio.2011.04.005 PMID:21546240

Dimitriou, R., Tsiridis, E., & Giannoudis, P. V. (2005). Current concepts of molecular aspects of bone healing. *Injury*, *36*(12), 1392–1404. doi:10.1016/j.injury.2005.07.019 PMID:16102764

Do, A. V., Khorsand, B., Geary, S. M., & Salem, A. K. (2015). 3D printing of scaffolds for tissue regeneration applications. *Advanced Healthcare Materials*, *4*(12), 1742–1762. doi:10.1002/adhm.201500168 PMID:26097108

Faulkner-Jones, A., Greenhough, S., A King, J., Gardner, J., Courtney, A., & Shu, W. (2013). Development of a valve-based cell printer for the bformation of human embryonic stem cell spheroid aggregates. *Biofabrication*, *5*(1), 15–13. doi:10.1088/1758-5082/5/1/015013 PMID:23380571

Fennema, E., Rivron, N., Rouwkema, J., van Blitterswijk, C., & de Boer, J. (2013). Spheroid culture as a tool for creating 3D complex tissues. *Trends in Biotechnology*, *31*(2), 108–115. doi:10.1016/j.tibtech.2012.12.003 PMID:23336996

Gurkan, U. A., El Assal, R., Yildiz, S. E., Sung, Y., Trachtenberg, A. J., Kuo, W. P., & Demirci, U. (2014). Engineering anisotropic biomimetic fibrocartilage microenvironment by bioprinting mesenchymal stem cells in nanoliter gel droplets. *Molecular Pharmaceutics*, *11*(7), 2151–2159. doi:10.1021/mp400573g PMID:24495169

Habibovic, P., Yuan, H., van der Valk, C. M., Meijer, G., van Blitterswijk, C. A., & de Groot, K. (2005). 3D microenvironment as essential element for osteoinduction by biomaterials. *Biomaterials*, *26*(17), 3565–3575. doi:10.1016/j.biomaterials.2004.09.056 PMID:15621247

Handschel, J. G. K. (2007). Prospects of micromass culture technology in tissue engineering. *Head & Face Medicine*, 3. PMID:17212823

Hing, K. A., Best, S. M., Tanner, K. E., Bonfield, W., & Revell, P. A. (2004). Mediation of bone ingrowth in porous hydroxyapatite bone graft substitutes. *Journal of Biomedical Materials Research. Part A*, *68*(1), 187–200. doi:10.1002/jbm.a.10050 PMID:14661264

Hollister, S. J. (2005). Porous scaffold design for tissue engineering. *Nature Materials*, *4*(7), 518–524. doi:10.1038/nmat1421 PMID:16003400

Hornbeck, L. J. (1997). Digital light processing for high-brightnesshigh-resolution applications. In *Proceedings of Electronic Imaging '97*. International Society for Optics and Photonics.

Howk, D., & Chu, T. M. (2006). Design variables for mechanical properties of bone tissue scaffolds. *Biomedical Sciences Instrumentation*, *42*, 278–283. PMID:16817621

Huang, Z. M., Zhang, Y.-Z., Kotaki, M., & Ramakrishna, S. (2003). A review on polymer nanofibers by electrospinning and their applications in nanocomposites. *Composites Science and Technology*, *63*(15), 2223–2253. doi:10.1016/S0266-3538(03)00178-7

Hunter, G. (2005). *Creation of Oxidized Zirconium Orthopaedic Implants*. Academic Press.

Hutmacher, D. W. (2000). Scaffolds in tissue engineering bone and cartilage. *Biomaterials*, *21*(24), 2. doi:10.1016/S0142-9612(00)00121-6 PMID:11071603

Hutmacher, D. W., Schantz, J. T., Lam, C. X. F., Tan, K. C., & Lim, T. C. (2007). State of the art and future directions of scaffoldbased bone engineering from a biomaterials perspective. *Journal of Tissue Engineering and Regenerative Medicine*, *1*(4), 245–260. doi:10.1002/term.24 PMID:18038415

Illich, D. J., Demir, N., Stojković, M., Scheer, M., Rothamel, D., Neugebauer, J., ... Zöller, J. E. (2011). Concise review: induced pluripotent stem cells and lineage reprogramming: prospects for bone regeneration. *Stem Cells (Dayton, Ohio)*, *29*(4), 555–563. doi:10.1002tem.611 PMID:21308867

Jakus, A.E. (2016). Hyperelastic "bone": A highly versatile, growth factorefree, osteoregenerative, scalable, and surgically friendly biomaterial. *Sci. Transl. Med., 8*(358).

Kahle, M. (2010). Embryonic stem cells induce ectopic bone formation in rats. *Bio-Medical Materials and Engineering*, *20*(6), 371–380. PMID:21263183

Kaigler, D., Wang, Z., Horger, K., Mooney, D. J., & Krebsbach, P. H. (2006). VEGF scaffolds enhance angiogenesis and bone regeneration in irradiated osseous defects. *Journal of Bone and Mineral Research*, *21*(5), 735–744. doi:10.1359/jbmr.060120 PMID:16734388

Kelly, D. J., & Prendergast, P. J. (2006). Prediction of the optimal mechanical properties for a scaffold used in osteochondral defect repair. *Tissue Engineering*, *12*(9), 2509–2519. doi:10.1089/ten.2006.12.2509 PMID:16995784

Keriquel, V., Oliveira, H., Rémy, M., Ziane, S., Delmond, S., Rousseau, B., ... Fricain, J.-C. (2017). In situ printing of mesenchymal stromal cells, by laserassisted bioprinting, for in vivo bone regeneration applications. *Scientific Reports*, *7*(1), 1778. doi:10.103841598-017-01914-x PMID:28496103

Kim, K., Yeatts, A., Dean, D., & Fisher, J. P. (2010). Stereolithographic bone scaffold design parameters: Osteogenic differentiation and signal expression. *Tissue Engineering. Part B, Reviews, 16*(5), 523–539. doi:10.1089/ten.teb.2010.0171 PMID:20504065

Kokubo, T., Kim, H. M., & Kawashita, M. (2003). Novel bioactive materials with different mechanical properties. *Biomaterials, 24*(13), 2161–2175. doi:10.1016/S0142-9612(03)00044-9 PMID:12699652

Kolesky, D. B., Homan, K. A., Skylar-Scott, M. A., & Lewis, J. A. (2016). Three-dimensional bioprinting of thick vascularized tissues. *Proceedings of the National Academy of Sciences of the United States of America, 113*(12), 3179–3184. doi:10.1073/pnas.1521342113 PMID:26951646

Kuboki, Y., Jin, Q., & Takita, H. (2001). Geometry of carriers controlling phenotypic expression in BMP-induced osteogenesis and chondrogenesis. *J. Bone Jt. Surg. Am., 83-A*(2), 105–115. PMID:11314788

Leblanc, E., Trensz, F., Haroun, S., Drouin, G., Bergeron, É., Penton, C. M., ... Grenier, G. (2011). BMP-9-induced muscle heterotopic ossification require changes to the skeletal muscle microenvironment. *Journal of Bone and Mineral Research, 26*(6), 1166–1177. doi:10.1002/jbmr.311 PMID:21611960

Li, C., Vepari, C., Jin, H.-J., Kim, H. J., & Kaplan, D. L. (2006). Electrospun silk-BMP-2 scaffolds for bone tissue engineering. *Biomaterials, 27*(16), 3115–3124. doi:10.1016/j.biomaterials.2006.01.022 PMID:16458961

Liao, C. J., Chen, C.-F., Chen, J.-H., Chiang, S.-F., Lin, Y.-J., & Chang, K.-Y. (2002). Fabrication of porous biodegradable polymer scaffolds using a solvent merging/particulate leaching method. *Journal of Biomedical Materials Research, 59*(4), 676–681. doi:10.1002/jbm.10030 PMID:11774329

Lloyd, A. W. (2001). Interfacial bioengineering to enhance surface biocompatibility. *Medical Device Technology, 13*(1), 18–21. PMID:11921776

Manke, A., Wang, L., & Rojanasakul, Y. (2013). Mechanisms of nanoparticle-induced oxidative stress and toxicity. *BioMed Research International, 2013*, 15. doi:10.1155/2013/942916 PMID:24027766

Matthews, J.A. (2002). Electrospinning of collagen nanofibers. *Biomacromolecules, 3*(2), 232-238.

Mertz, L. (2013). Dream it, design it, print it in 3-D: What can 3-D printing do for you? *IEEE Pulse*, *4*(6), 15–21. doi:10.1109/MPUL.2013.2279616 PMID:24233186

Mooney, D. J., Baldwin, D. F., Suh, N. P., Vacanti, J. P., & Langer, R. (1996). Novel approach to fabricate porous sponges of poly(d,llactic- co-glycolic acid) without the use of organic solvents. *Biomaterials*, *17*(14), 1417–1422. doi:10.1016/0142-9612(96)87284-X PMID:8830969

Mountziaris, P. M., & Mikos, A. G. (2008). Modulation of the inflammatory response for enhanced bone tissue regeneration. *Tissue Engineering. Part B, Reviews*, *14*(2), 179–186. doi:10.1089/ten.teb.2008.0038 PMID:18544015

Murphy, S.V., & Atala, A. (2014). 3D bioprinting of tissues and organs. *Nat. Biotechnol.*, *32*(8), 773-785.

Muschler, G. F., Nitto, H., Boehm, C. A., & Easley, K. A. (2001). Age- and gender-related changes in the cellularity of human bone marrow and the prevalence of osteoblastic progenitors. *Journal of Orthopaedic Research*, *19*(1), 117–125. doi:10.1016/S0736-0266(00)00010-3 PMID:11332607

Nie, H., & Wang, C. H. (2007). Fabrication and characterization of PLGA/HAp composite scaffolds for delivery of BMP-2 plasmid DNA. *Journal of Controlled Release*, *120*(1-2), 111–121. doi:10.1016/j.jconrel.2007.03.018 PMID:17512077

O'Brien, F. J., Harley, B. A., Yannas, I. V., & Gibson, L. J. (2005). The effect of pore size on cell adhesion in collagen-GAG scaffolds. *Biomaterials*, *26*(4), 433–441. doi:10.1016/j.biomaterials.2004.02.052 PMID:15275817

O'Keefe, R. J., & Mao, J. (2011). Bone tissue engineering and regeneration: From discovery to the clinicean overview. *Tissue Engineering. Part B, Reviews*, *17*(6), 389–392. doi:10.1089/ten.teb.2011.0475 PMID:21902614

Ozbolat, I. T., & Hospodiuk, M. (2016). Current advances and future perspectives in extrusion-based bioprinting. *Biomaterials*, *76*, 321–343. doi:10.1016/j.biomaterials.2015.10.076 PMID:26561931

Polo-Corrales, L., Latorre-Esteves, M., & Ramirez-Vick, J. E. (2014). Scaffold design for bone regeneration. *Journal of Nanoscience and Nanotechnology*, *14*(1), 15–56. doi:10.1166/jnn.2014.9127 PMID:24730250

PrimaryL. J. (2017). *3D Printing Processes*. Retrieved from https://www.printspace3d.com/3d-printing-processes/

Puppi, D., Chiellini, F., Piras, A. M., & Chiellini, E. (2010). Polymeric materials for bone and cartilage repair. *Progress in Polymer Science*, *35*(4), 403–440. doi:10.1016/j.progpolymsci.2010.01.006

Robey, P. G. (2011). Cell sources for bone regeneration: The good, the bad, and the ugly (but promising). *Tissue Engineering. Part B, Reviews*, *17*(6), 423–430. doi:10.1089/ten.teb.2011.0199 PMID:21797663

Rosa, A. L., Beloti, M. M., & van Noort, R. (2003). Osteoblastic differentiation of cultured rat bone marrow cells on hydroxyapatite with different surface topography. *Dental Materials*, *19*(8), 768–772. doi:10.1016/S0109-5641(03)00024-1 PMID:14511735

Salgado, A. J., Coutinho, O. P., & Reis, R. L. (2004). Bone tissue engineering: State of the art and future trends. *Macromolecular Bioscience*, *4*(8), 743–765. doi:10.1002/mabi.200400026 PMID:15468269

Sandino, C., & Lacroix, D. (2011). A dynamical study of the mechanical stimuli and tissue differentiation within a CaP scaffold based on micro-CT finite element models. *Biomechanics and Modeling in Mechanobiology*, *10*(4), 565–576. doi:10.100710237-010-0256-0 PMID:20865437

Saunders, R. E., & Derby, B. (2014). Inkjet printing biomaterials for tissue engineering: Bioprinting. *International Materials Reviews*, *59*(8), 430–448. doi:10.1179/1743280414Y.0000000040

Schantz, J. T., Chim, H., & Whiteman, M. (2007). Cell guidance in tissue engineering: SDF- 1 mediates site-directed homing of mesenchymal stem cells within threedimensional polycaprolactone scaffolds. *Tissue Engineering*, *13*(11), 2615–2624. doi:10.1089/ten.2006.0438 PMID:17961003

(2013). Science and society: Experts warn against bans on 3D printing. *Science*, *342*(6157), 439. PMID:24163835

Shafiee, A., & Atala, A. (2016). Printing technologies for medical applications. *Trends in Molecular Medicine*, *22*(3), 254–265. doi:10.1016/j.molmed.2016.01.003 PMID:26856235

Shi, S. (2009). RhBMP-2 microspheres-loaded chitosan/collagen scaffold enhanced osseointegration: An experiment in dog. *Journal of Biomaterials Applications*, *23*(4), 331–346. doi:10.1177/0885328208090013 PMID:18667455

Stolzing, A., Jones, E., McGonagle, D., & Scutt, A. (2008). Age-related changes in human bone marrow-derived mesenchymal stem cells: Consequences for cell therapies. *Mechanisms of Ageing and Development*, *129*(3), 163–173. doi:10.1016/j.mad.2007.12.002 PMID:18241911

Sun, C., Fang, N., Wu, D.M., & Zhang, X. (2005). Projection micro-stereolithographyusing digital micro-mirror dynamic mask. *Sensor Actuat a-Phys, 121*, 113–120.

Sun, W., Starly, B., Nam, J., & Darling, A. (2005). Bio-CAD modeling and its applications in computer-aided tissue engineering. *Comput Aided Design, 37*(11), 1097–1114.

Ting, Z. (2017). Biomimetic design and fabrication of multilayered osteochondral scaffolds by low-temperature deposition manufacturing and thermal-induced phase-separation techniques. *Biofabrication*, *9*(2), 25–21. PMID:28462906

Tsimbouri, P. M., Childs, P. G., Pemberton, G. D., Yang, J., Jayawarna, V., Orapiriyakul, W., ... Dalby, M. J. (2017). Stimulation of 3D osteogenesis by mesenchymal stem cells using a nanovibrational bioreactor. *Nat. Biomed. Eng.*, *1*(9), 758–770. doi:10.103841551-017-0127-4

Tsuruga, E., Takita, H., Itoh, H., Wakisaka, Y., & Kuboki, Y. (1997). Pore size of porous hydroxyapatite as the cell-substratum controls BMP-induced osteogenesis. *Journal of Biochemistry*, *121*(2), 317–324. doi:10.1093/oxfordjournals.jbchem.a021589 PMID:9089406

Vaccaro, A. R. (2002). The role of the osteoconductive scaffold in synthetic bone graft. *Orthopedics*, *25*(5Suppl), 571–578. PMID:12038844

Ventola, C. L. (2014). Medical applications for 3D printing: Current and project uses. *Pharm. Ther.*, *39*(10), 704–711. PMID:25336867

Walthers, C. M., Nazemi, A. K., Patel, S. L., Wu, B. M., & Dunn, J. C. Y. (2014). The effect of scaffold macroporosity on angiogenesis and cell survival in tissue-engineered smooth muscle. *Biomaterials*, *35*(19), 5129–5137. doi:10.1016/j.biomaterials.2014.03.025 PMID:24695092

Wernike, E. (2010). VEGF incorporated into calcium phosphate ceramics promote vascularisation and bone formation in vivo. *European Cells & Materials*, *19*, 30–40. doi:10.22203/eCM.v019a04 PMID:20178096

Whang, K., Thomas, C. H., Healy, K. E., & Nuber, G. (1995). A novel method to fabricate bioabsorbable scaffolds. *Polymer, 36*(4), 837–842. doi:10.1016/0032-3861(95)93115-3

Williams, J. M., Adewunmi, A., Schek, R. M., Flanagan, C. L., Krebsbach, P. H., Feinberg, S. E., ... Das, S. (2005). Bone tissue engineering using polycaprolactone scaffolds fabricated via selective laser sintering. *Biomaterials, 26*(23), 4817–4827. doi:10.1016/j.biomaterials.2004.11.057 PMID:15763261

Xia, Y. (2013). Selective laser sintering fabrication of nano-hydroxyapatite/poly-ε-caprolactone scaffolds for bone tissue engineering applications. *International Journal of Nanomedicine, 8*, 4197–4213. PMID:24204147

Yandell, K. (2013). Organs on demand. *Science, 27*, 38–45.

Young, M. F. (2003). Bone matrix proteins: Their function, regulation, and relationship to osteoporosis. *Osteoporosis International, 14*(Suppl 3), S35–S42. doi:10.100700198-002-1342-7 PMID:12730768

Yu, Y. (2016). *Three-dimensional bioprinting using self-assembling scalable scaffold-free "tissue strands" as a new bioink.* Academic Press.

Zein, I., Hutmacher, D. W., Tan, K. C., & Teoh, S. H. (2002). Fused deposition modeling of novel scaffold architectures for tissue engineering applications. *Biomaterials, 23*(4), 1169–1185. doi:10.1016/S0142-9612(01)00232-0 PMID:11791921

Zeltinger, J., Sherwood, J. K., Graham, D. A., Müeller, R., & Griffith, L. G. (2001). Effect of pore size and void fraction on cellular adhesion, proliferation, and matrix deposition. *Tissue Engineering, 7*(5), 557–572. doi:10.1089/107632701753213183 PMID:11694190

Zhang, C., Hu, Y.-Y., Cui, F.-Z., Zhang, S.-M., & Ruan, D.-K. (2006). A study on a tissue-engineered bone using rhBMP-2 induced periosteal cells with a porous nano-hydroxyapatite/collagen/poly(L-lactic acid) scaffold. *Biomedical Materials (Bristol, England), 1*(2), 56–62. doi:10.1088/1748-6041/1/2/002 PMID:18460757

Section 3
Prosthesis:
Design, Machining, and Optimization

Chapter 5
Design of a Prosthetic Ankle Complex:
A Study in Biomimetic System Design

Dheeman Bhuyan
https://orcid.org/0000-0001-9772-0028
Girijananda Chowdhury Institute of Management and Technology, India

Kaushik Kumar
Birla Institute of Technology, India

ABSTRACT

Nature has, over a large span of geological time, engineered near perfect solutions to most problems humans face today. Motion of the limbs is one such area, and the cutting edge in the development of effective prostheses is biomimetics. Limb prostheses have been used by mankind for the better part of known history, and most of the technology currently available in prosthetics is not exclusively new. However, modern prosthetics either are uncomfortable—and the lack of flexion affects the gait of the patient—or too expensive for a large segment of the populace. This chapter seeks to study the mimicry of physiological systems through the design for an ankle prosthesis that includes a passive damper and mimics the shape and behavior of the natural ankle joint.

DOI: 10.4018/978-1-5225-8235-9.ch005

INTRODUCTION

The human body is a near perfect machine evolved over millions of years. The limbs of the body are engineered to withstand the wear and tear inflicted upon it and repair most of the damage that may occur. However, there may be certain etiologies where the repair of the limb is not possible. Under such circumstances the removal of the limb is the preferred option. The amputation of a limb may be the caused by various etiologies with diabetes and trauma being exceedingly common. The absence of a limb may also be the result of congenital defects.

The loss or absence of a limb is one of the most traumatic experiences a person may have to go through. As such, the prosthetic has to not only to deliver renewed functionality which is aesthetically pleasing and features effective cosmesis, but it also should serve to improve the wearer's quality of life by fulfilling his sense of wholeness. In as much, it becomes not just a medical device but takes on the added role of being an emotional comfort.

Taking a look at the history of prostheses, it is seen that the history of prosthetics is tinged with the colours of human development, especially those who have been left with something missing, either by birth, accidents or otherwise. Prosthetics, over time became synonymous with hooks and wooden stumps, worn by reel pirates. While it may have been perfectly feasible for seafarers to have a hook or a wooden stump for a prosthetic owing to the relative lack of resources at sea, the image popularised by Hollywood representations may be an over-reach.

It has been seen that some of the most effective solutions to human problems come from the mimicry of nature. Over the course of millions of years of evolution, nature has engineered near perfect systems to perform various functions and the human body is no exception. Mimicking the physiological foot has long been the goal of medical and engineering professionals for many years. Today, the modern versions of primitive peg leg have emerged, integrating the cutting edge of technology and showing promising visions for the future.

BRIEF BACKGROUND

The Prosthetic Leg

In order to understand the pedigree of the modern prosthetic design, it is necessary to trace its path through history. Indian literature from around 1500BC has documented the use of artificial legs (Vanderwerker, 1976; Dellon & Matsuoka, 2007). The first documented prosthetic leg was found in Pompeii dating back to 300 BC (Seymour, 2002).

Lower limb prostheses have been romanticized by Hollywood flicks showing pirates wearing wooden stumps and iron hooks. While it may have been perfectly feasible for seafarers to have a hook or a wooden stump for a prosthetic owing to the relative lack of resources at sea, the image popularised by Hollywood representations may be an over-reach.

The dark ages followed by the middle ages of Europe saw little to no development and the next watershed events in this timeline came in the sixteenth century when Ambroise Pare contributed major advances in prosthetics such as mechanical, hinged hands, and locking knee joints. One of his designs is shown in Figure 1. The American Civil War saw numerous casualties and this drove the need to develop newer and more effective prosthesis. The next watershed events in the development of prosthetics came during the World Wars followed by the Korean and Vietnam conflicts.

Modern prosthetics are much more advanced than the wooden stumps and hooks that were the original prosthetic limbs. The most advanced designs feature electronic control with computer interfaces and bionics

Biomimetic Design

The term biomimetics, coined by Otto H Schmitt (Schmitt 1969), represents the studies and imitation of nature's methods, mechanisms and processes. Nature's capabilities are far superior in many areas to human capabilities, and adapting many of its features and characteristics can significantly improve our technology (Bar-Cohen, 2005; Vincent 2001). Biomimetic design i.e. nature inspired design solutions to engineering problems has been practiced on an *ad hoc* basis throughout history (Glier, McAdams & Linsey, 2011). The usage of formal tools and principles to generate these solutions is a fairly recent development. Biomimetic design uses biological phenomena

Figure 1. Artificial leg invented by Ambroise Pare (middle sixteenth century)
Source: Malgaigne (1841)

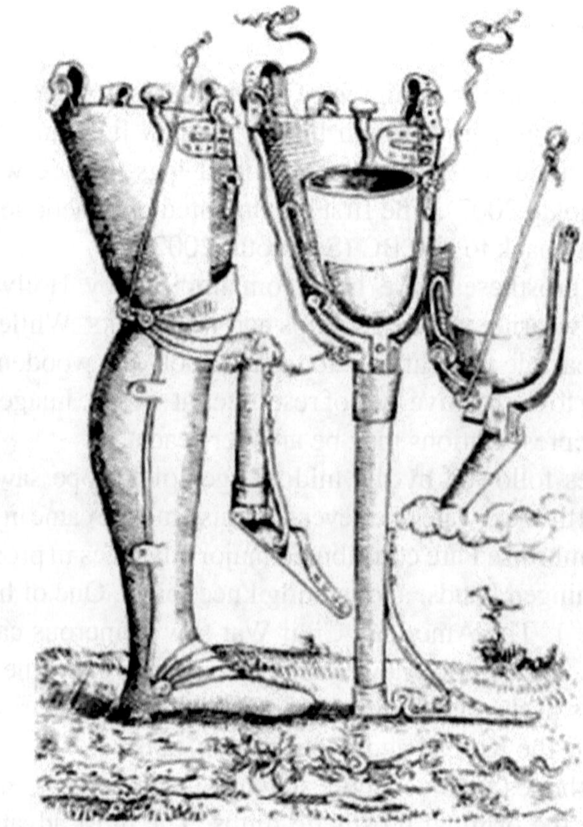

and their mimicry to inspire design solutions. Examples of these can be seen throughout history e.g. the myth of Icarus.

Evolution is the development of "experimental" solutions to nature's problems and the improvement and further adaptation of the successful ones and it has been an ongoing process. Proponents of biomimetics argue that over the course of 3.85 billion years of evolution, the designs of our natural environment and its inhabitants have been honed to near perfection by the need for survival (Benyus, 2009).

During the process of evolution, principles of physics, chemistry, mechanics, materials science, mobility, control, sensors, and many other fields that we recognize as science and engineering, came into play to develop viable solutions. Solutions developed at the nano and micro scales were also scaled up to macro and mega scales. The accumulated information is coded into the genetic structures of living organisms and passed from one generation to another. It must be noted here that even though an organism may not be wholly optimized for its particular environment, the goal in nature is to survive long enough to be able to reproduce.

As such the adaptation of ideas from biology can involve copying the complete appearance and function of specific creatures (Bar-Cohen, 2006) e.g. the inspiration for powered flight came from birds and was achieved by using human-developed capabilities, and the design and function of fins used by divers, was copied from the legs of water creatures like seals. Further, biologically made structures have numerous advantages and the honeycomb is one such example. Bees create the honeycomb for its efficient packing configuration and, for its low weight and high strength; the same structural shape of the honeycomb is used to produce many aircraft parts (Bar-Cohen, 2006). Table 1 shows an example of systems derived from the mimicry of nature, either in function or in form.

Table 1. Characteristic similarities of biology and engineering systems (Bar-Cohen, 2006)

Biology	Engineering	Bioengineering, biomimetics, bionics and biomechanics
Body	System	Systems with multifunctional materials and structures are developed emulating the capability of biological systems
Skeleton and bones	Structure and support struts	Support structures are part of every man-made system
Brain	Computer	Advances in computers are being made emulating the operation of the human brain
Intelligence	Artificial intelligence	There are numerous aspects of artificial intelligence that have been inspired by biology including augmented reality, autonomous systems, computational intelligence, expert systems, fuzzy logic, etc
Senses	Sensors	Computer vision, artificial vision, radar, and other proximity detectors all have direct biological analogies. However, at their best, the capability of the man-made sensors is nowhere near as good as biosensors
Muscles	Actuators	Electroactive polymers are actuators with functional similarity to natural muscles
Electrochemical power generation	Rechargeable batteries	The use of biological materials to produce power will offer mechanical systems enormous advantages

THE PHYSIOLOGICAL ANKLE JOINT

A total of thirty three joints between twenty six individual bones, including the long bones of the lower limbs, make up the foot – ankle complex. The ankle joint or "talocrural joint" is a synovial hinge joint that is made up of the articulation of 3 bones, namely the tibia, the fibula and the talus, or the ankle bone. The articulations are between the talus and the tibia and the talus and the fibula. The "mortise" is the concaved surface formed by the tibia and fibula. The mortise is adjustable and is controlled by the proximal and distal tibiofibular joints (Norkin & Levangie, 1992). Figure 2(a) shows the dorsiplantar projection of the human foot and 2(b) shows the lateral view of the ankle joint.

The nature of the ankle joint complex is such that it mainly allows for hinge-like movements of the foot i.e. dorsiflexion and plantarflexion. Strong ligaments firmly anchor the distal end of the fibula to the larger distal end of the tibia creating a deep bracket-shaped socket. Of the shape of the talus, it can be said that it is shaped like a half cylinder tipped onto its flat side, with the two ends facing laterally and medially respectively. Stabilization of the ankle joint is achieved by the medial and lateral ligaments

Figure 2. (a) Dorsiplantar foot (b) Lateral ankle joint
Source: Smith (2006)

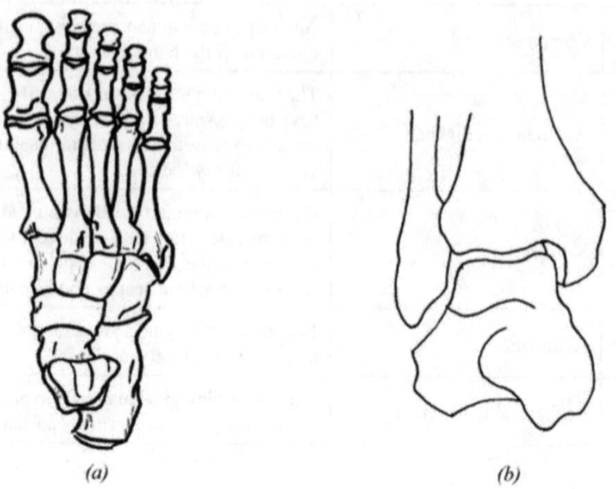

Functional Anatomy

The ankle complex comprises three articulations: the taloclural joint, the subtalar joint, and the distal tibiofibular syndesmosis. These three joints work in concert to allow coordinated movement of the rear foot. Rear foot motion is often defined as occurring in the cardinal planes as follows: sagittal-plane motion (Plantarflexion - Dorsiflexion), frontal-plane motion (inversion-eversion), and transverse-plane motion (internal rotation-external rotation) (Hertel, 2002).

Taloclural Joint Anatomy

The talocrural, or tibiotalar, joint is formed by the articulation of the dome of the talus, the medial malleolus, the tibial plafond, and the lateral malleolus. The shape of the talocrural joint allows torque to be transmitted from the lower leg (internal and external rotation) to the foot (pronation and supination) during weight bearing. This joint is sometimes called the ''mortise'' joint and, in isolation, may be thought of as a hinge joint that allows the motions of plantar flexion and dorsiflexion. The axis of rotation of the talocrural joint passes through the medial and lateral malleoli. It is slightly anterior to the frontal plane as it passes through the tibia but slightly posterior to the frontal plane as it passes through the fibula. Isolated movement of the talocrural joint is primarily in the sagittal plane, but small amounts of transverse and frontal plane motion also occur about the oblique axis of rotation (Lundberg et al., 1989).

In an in vivo study of loaded ankles in the closed kinetic chain, 30° of physiologic plantar flexion (actual motion) from the neutral position was composed of 28° sagittal-plane movement (plantar flexion), 1° transverse-plane movement (internal rotation), and 4° frontal-plane movement (inversion) (Lundberg et al., 1989). Comparatively, 30° of physiologic dorsiflexion (actual motion) in the closed kinetic chain was composed of 23° sagittal-plane movement (dorsiflexion), 9° transverse-plane movement (external rotation), and 2° frontal-plane movement (eversion) (Lundberg et al., 1989).

Under fully loaded condition of the ankle complex, primary stabilization against excessive talar rotation and translation is provided by the articular surfaces (Hertel, 2002).

Human Gait and Ambulation

The lower limb is of particularly critical importance when in consideration of human ambulation. Taking into account the extreme complexity of the foot – ankle assembly, it may be said that perhaps the most significant parts are the ankle and the subtalar joints. Studies have shown that the internal/external movements of foot ankle complex are equally contributed to by the ankle and subtalar joints (Seigler et al., 1988).

Potentially there are 6 degrees of freedom in all joints.

3 plane rotation:

1. Abduction-adduction.
2. Internal-external.
3. Flexion-extension.

3 plane translation:

1. Medial-lateral.
2. Compression-distraction.
3. Anterior-posterior

These are shown by Figure 3.

The foot ankle complex provides three different rotations in the sagittal plane about three different points (Leardini et al., 2014). Studies related to gait analysis have shown that a dorsiflexor momement is demonstrated at the striking of the heel. This can be explained as the eccentric contraction of the dorsiflexors in order to control rotary motion of the foot, thereby preventing the foot from slapping onto the ground (Das et al., 2018).

The second phase of movement is carried out by the eccentric contraction of the dorsiflexors which allows a forward progression of the shank over the foot, thereby resulting in a plantarflexor moment. In the third phase, the plantarflexion moment continues along with concentric contraction of plantarflexors towards toe-off (Das et al., 2018). It needs to be noted that the pattern of the ankle kinetics always remains same irrespective of the walking speed with the only change being an increase in magnitude.

1. It helps in descending the foot to the floor by rotation about the heel which remains in contact with the foot initially i.e. from terminal part of swing phase to foot lying parallel(flat)to the ground;

Figure 3. Motions of the foot
Source: Masum et al. (2014)

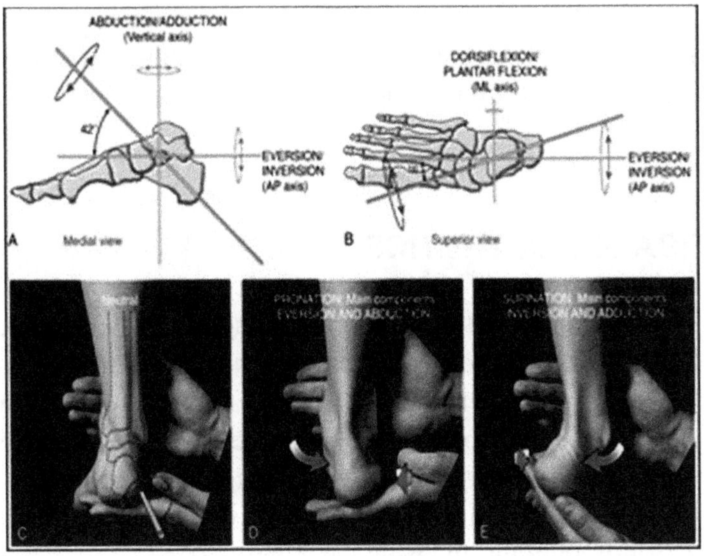

2. Forward motion is continued by rotation of ankle joint during the period in which foot remains flat to ground and the shank advances;
3. The power generation during push off phase happens through rotation about metatarsophalangeal joints.

Gait Cycle

There are two phases of the human gait as shown in Figure 4:

- Stance phase
- Swing phase

The stance phase begins with the striking of the heel and progresses till toe off. It constitutes about 60-62% of the gait cycle. The stance is subdivided into three phases.

1. Controlled dorsiflexion (constituting about 38% of gait cycle beginning with foot flat to maximum dorsiflexion)
2. Controlled plantar flexion (constituting about 12% of gait cycle starting from heel strike and ending with foot flat)

3. Powered plantar flexion (constituting about 10-12% of gait cycle starting from maximum dorsiflexion till toe-off).

Swing phase occurs when the foot is raised from the ground and it continues till the heel strike the ground of the same foot. It accounts for 40% of the gait cycle

TRANSTIBAL PROSTHETICS

Transtibial amputations, also known as "below knee" or "BK" amputations are among the most frequently performed major limb amputations. Statistically, about half of all major lower limb amputations are transtibial, and, in the past several decades, this amputation level has been emphasized in education and training for surgery, prosthetics and rehabilitation. Because of this, many individuals with transtibial amputations successfully achieve rehabilitation at or near their pre-amputation levels (Marshall, 2016).

Figure 4. Human gait cycle
Source: Leardini et al. (2014)

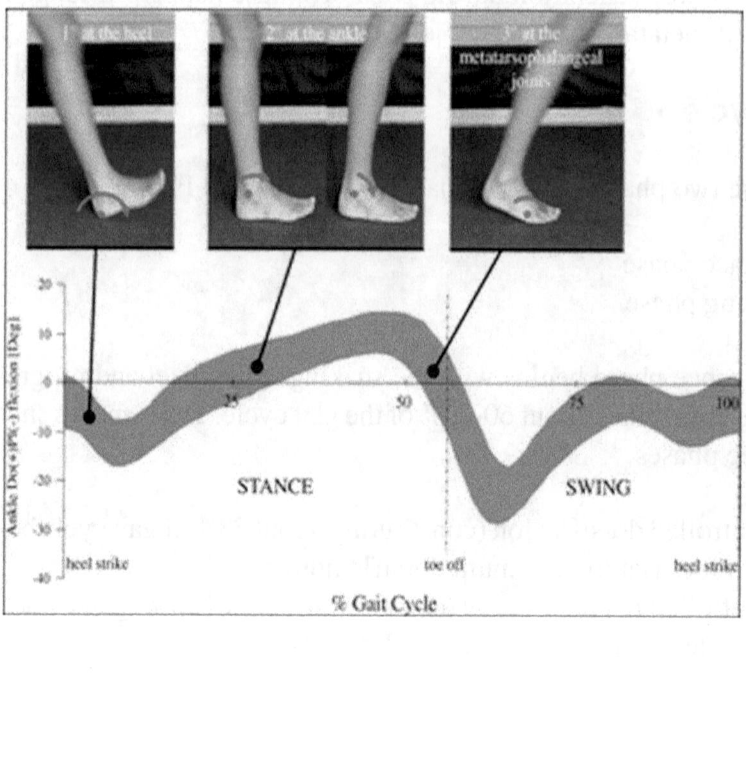

A person who has undergone a transtibial amputation retains the knee joint. This is a major advantage. Whenever possible, a surgeon wants to preserve a healthy knee joint because it provides a transtibial amputee with many functional advantages not available to those who have undergone a transfemoral amputation or a knee disarticulation (amputation through the knee joint). Not only does a healthy knee provide the power to lift and lower, it is also helpful in maintaining overall balance. The knee is very important in transfers, such as on and off the toilet, in and out of bed, and up and down stairs, and it also gives us greater ability to push forward, slow down, and walk on slopes and stairs.

For the transtibial amputee, the major challenge is replacing the foot and ankle. We typically think of our ankles as pushing down and pulling up, but their major roles are accommodation, shock absorption and motion. Our foot adjusts to uneven and different surfaces. We can move from concrete to gravel and still stand or walk steadily, and the foot lets us know when there's a change in the surface and responds rapidly to nerve signals to accommodate it. This ability of the foot to feel position and surface is called proprioception. It's the sensation that tells us the foot's relation to the ground, whether the ground slopes up or down, and whether it's hard or soft, slippery or dry, rough or smooth. Without a foot and ankle, we lose the feeling, the sense of positioning, and shock absorption. The partial foot amputation preserves a small bit of this ability, but all of it is lost with a transtibial amputation.

Prosthetic feet generally can be designed to be soft and accommodating or firm and spring like, but not both. A prosthetic foot that's soft and accommodating usually remains that way, while a prosthetic foot that's made to provide the firmer foundation needed for push off and the spring like propulsion of stored energy is often described as too "stiff" for less vigorous uses.

The construction of a prosthesis depends largely on is function. While cosmetic hands are concerned purely with appearance, prosthetic legs are substitutes for a major structural part of someone's body and have to bear their entire weight. Typically, a prosthetic arm or leg is made from a strong and durable but lightweight material such as carbon fiber, covered with foam padding (for comfort) or flesh-colored plastic. The weight of prosthetic limbs is a very important factor. Given that, the two legs amount to 30–40 percent of a person's total body weight, and the two arms about 10 percent, it is clearly seen why prosthetic limbs need to be much lighter: one would quickly get tired moving prosthetic limbs that weighed as much as natural ones.

The comfort and effectiveness of a prosthesis is largely governed by how well it fits onto the remaining part of the patient's own limb, which is called their residual limb (or sometimes, informally, the "stump"—a term some people understandably find offensive, though it is, nevertheless, widely used in the medical world). The connecting part of a prosthesis is called the socket and it's carefully molded around a plaster cast taken from the residual limb. The fit of a socket has to be precise or the new limb may damage the residual one, causing discomfort or tissue damage and perhaps even making it impossible to wear the prosthesis for a time. A patient's residual limb is likely to change shape and size over months and years so new sockets will be needed from time to time. More precisely fitting sockets can now be made by scanning a patient's residual limb with lasers and cutting-edge techniques such as 3D printing are also now being used.

A variety of artificial foot designs is available, each having its advantages and disadvantages. Feet currently available can be divided into two classes

- **Articulated:** Those with moving joints.
- Non-articulated.

Those with moving joints generally require more maintenance and are slightly heavier than most of the non-articulated kind. Articulated feet may have one or more joints.

Prosthetic Ankle Joints

Prosthetic components seek to emulate the shock absorption functions of the physiologic foot and ankle, but do not have mechanisms to do so effectively. The prime reason is that they lack sufficient triplanar rotary motion or variable loading stability. In general, prosthetic foot/ankle mechanisms either attempt to emulate the shock absorbing lower limb motion during the first rocker, or attempt a completely different shock absorption approach (Anonymous, ?).

However, despite the fact that prosthetic limbs have been around for millennia, there does not exist enough evidence to establish precise criteria for the prescription of prosthetic ankle-foot mechanisms in individuals with a lower limb amputation (Hofstad et al., 2004).

It has been recommended that practitioners take into account availability, patient functional needs, the type of knee mechanism to be prescribed and the inter-relationship with ankle-foot mechanisms, and cost (Hofstad et al., 2004).

The Single Axis Foot

The single-axis foot (Figure 5) features only one joint and provides for ankle action that is controlled by two changeable rubber bumpers, either of which can be changed to permit more or less motion as needed. This design is typically described as a low activity foot.

The articulated single-axis foot enhances knee stability through an ankle joint that allows the foot to move up and down. The faster the full sole of the foot is in contact with the ground, the more stable the prosthesis becomes. This is especially useful for users with higher levels of amputation i.e. from the knee to the hip, who need active control the prosthesis to prevent the knee from buckling, and the single-axis ankle-foot mechanism reduces the effort required. However, the single-axis ankle joint increases the weight of the prosthesis. It requires periodic servicing and is more expensive than most SACH foot models.

The Multi Axis Foot

A multi-axis foot is mostly prescribed for people who have to walk on uneven surfaces. A multi axis foot allows some motion about all three axes of the ankle. It is, slightly heavier than the other types of feet and requires more maintenance as well. However, daily activities involving normal walking along with the ability to demonstrate varied cadence is possible with multi axis feet. Figure 6 shows an example of the Multi Axis Foot.

Figure 5. Single axis foot
Source: MedicalExpo (n.d.)

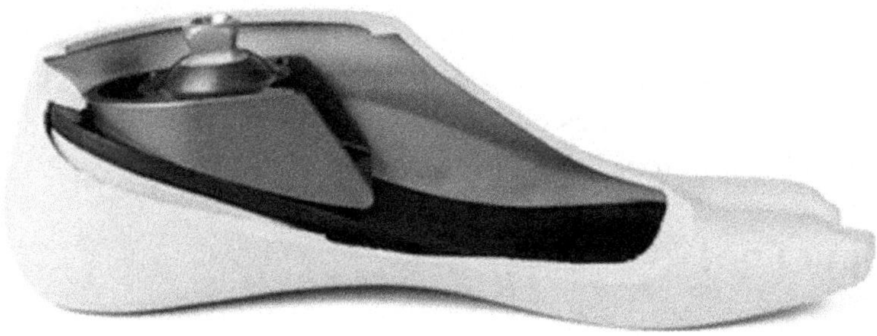

Figure 6. Multi axis foot
Source: Custom Prosthetics (n.d.)

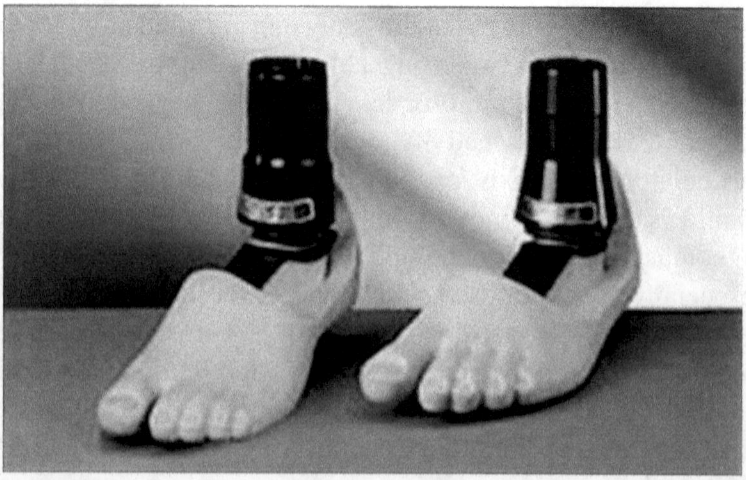

The SACH Foot

The simplest design of non-articulated prosthetic feet is the SACH (solid ankle-cushion heel) Foot (Figure 7). The design has a rigid keel while ankle action is provided by the soft rubber heel. The heel compresses during the early part of the stance phase of walking, under load. The rubber heel wedges are available in three densities: soft, medium, and hard.

The SAFE Foot

The SAFE (stationary attachment flexible endoskeletal) Foot has the same action as the SACH foot along with the ability for the sole to conform to slightly irregular surfaces and thus makes it easier for the amputee to walk over uneven terrain. Feet of this type make walking easier because of the flexibility, and are sometimes called "flexible keel" feet. Figure 8 shows a cross sectional diagram of the SAFE foot.

The Jaipur Foot

Developed in 1968, the Jaipur Foot is a handmade prosthetic foot designed to meet the demands of the lifestyle in developing countries. Design was initially based on the SACH foot design. However it digressed from the SACH

Figure 7. Pediatric SACH foot
Source: Willow Wood (n.d.)

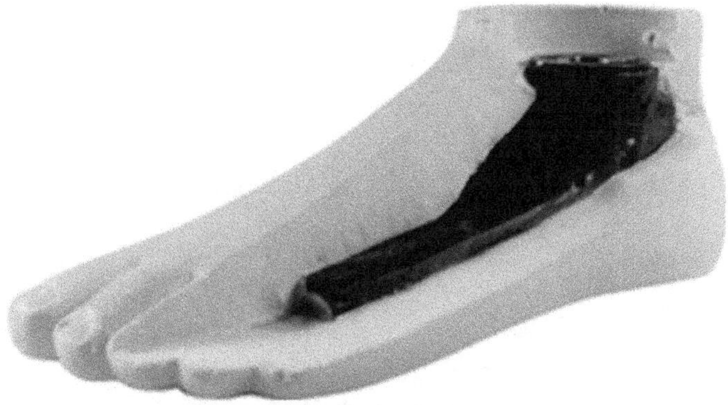

Figure 8. Cross-section of the S.A.F.E. foot throughout its length in a parasagital plan
Source: Campbell and Childs (1980)

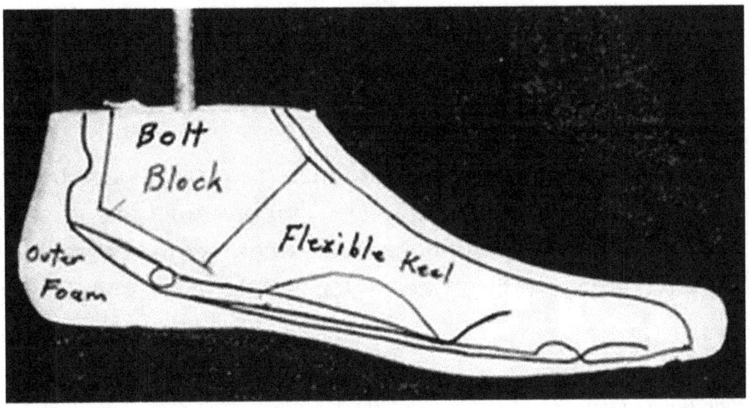

design owing to multiple factors such as weight and non - sustainability in local conditions. In the conditions of the Indian Subcontinent, the Jaipur foot has seen unprecedented success as it is affordable and light weight. Figure 9 shows a Jaipur foot.

Dynamic Response Feet

In recent years, there has been a major change in the new designs for artificial feet. Most of these new models are capable of absorbing energy in a "flexible" keel during the "roll-over" part of the stance phase. This enables them to spring back immediately to provide push-off, or assistance in getting the toe off of

Figure 9. The Jaipur Foot
Source: Jaipur Foot.org (n.d)

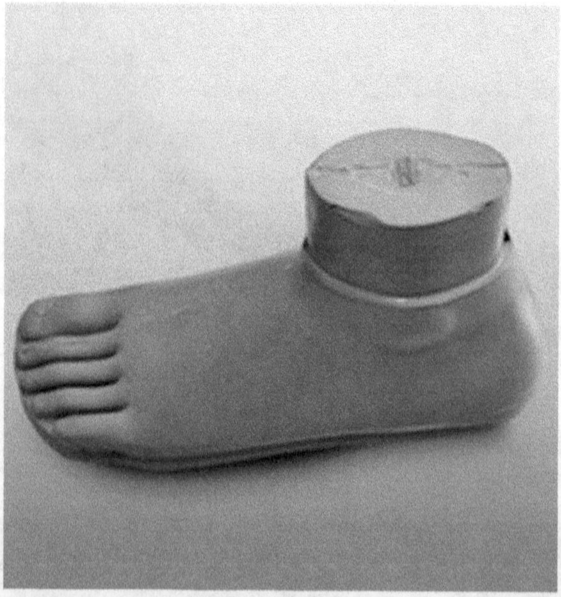

the ground, to start the swing phase. Although the original idea behind these designs was to provide an active athlete with more function, amputees who are a lot less active have also found these designs useful. These designs are often called "dynamic response" feet and one of these is shown in Figure 10.

Figure 10. Dynamic Elastic Response foot
Source: Human Biomechanics and Control Lab (2007)

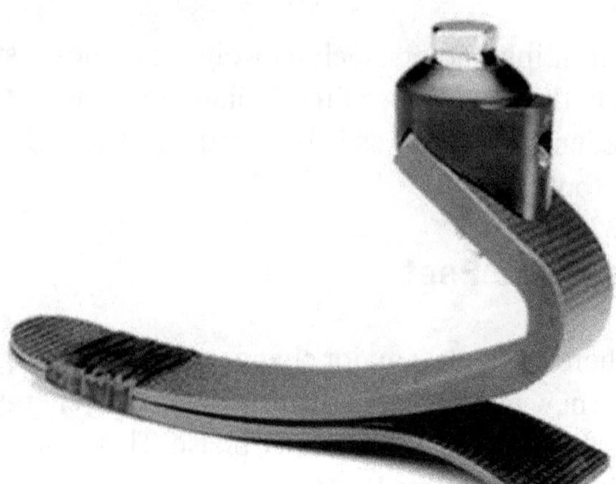

Comparison During Level Walking and Incline/Decline Walking

In individuals with a transtibial amputation, there was found to be a slight trend towards a greater stride length when walking with the Flex-foot in comparison to the SACH foot. During level treadmill walking there were no differences in energy cost in either the individuals with a traumatic or vascular transtibial amputations. However, when walking speed was increased or when subjects walked on a decline or incline treadmill, the energy cost was lower when walking with an energy-storing foot than with the SACH foot. Studies indicate that the individual with a transtibial amputation who is active and is able to walk on inclines and declines could benefit from an energy-storing prosthetic foot (Hofstad et al., 2004).

Comparisons Between Various Designs

Multiple studies have been conducted comparing the performance of various designs and have shown marked differences between natural gait and the gait of an amputee with a transtibial prosthesis. Also the gait changes with respect to the design of the foot being used.

In a study involving amputees with Single Axis and SACH foot prostheses, interchanging the prosthetic foot on a prosthesis did not appear to have a significant effect on the gait patterns of unilateral below-knee amputees. The ankle of the prosthetic foot during the foot flat phase of gait showed a significant statistical and clinical difference (Macke et al., 2006).

It has been seen that in high activity individuals with a transfemoral amputation, there is limited evidence for the superiority of the Flex foot during level walking compared with the solid-ankle cushioned heel (SACH) foot in respect of energy cost and, gait efficiency. This benefit has only been confirmed in individuals with a transtibial amputation during decline and inclines walking and increased walking speeds.

In individuals with a transtibial amputation, there was found to be a slight trend towards a greater stride length when walking with the Flex-foot in comparison to the SACH foot. During level treadmill walking there were no differences in energy cost in either the individuals with a traumatic or vascular transtibial amputations. However, when walking speed was increased or when subjects walked on a decline or incline treadmill, the energy cost was lower when walking with an energy-storing foot than with the SACH foot. Studies indicate that the individual with a transtibial amputation who is active and is able to walk on inclines and declines could benefit from an energy-storing prosthetic foot (Macke et al., 2006).

There is insufficient evidence from high quality comparative studies for the overall superiority of any individual type of prosthetic ankle-foot mechanism, al-though there is a small trend towards the Flex-foot in comparison with the SACH foot for greater stride length and lower energy cost in individuals with a transtibial amputation, and improved gait efficiency and lower energy cost in high activity individuals with transfemoral amputation. In prescribing prosthetic-ankle foot mechanisms for individuals with a lower limb amputation, practitioners should take into account availability, patient functional needs, patient mobility level, type of knee mechanism to be prescribed and the inter-relationship with ankle-foot mechanisms, and cost (Macke et al., 2006). Table 2 shows a comparison between various designs of prosthetic feet with regards to the stride characteristics.

THE NEW DESIGN

Some of the driving factors behind the design were the need for simplicity and ease of manufacture on the part of the industry and proper flexion and gait as close to the natural gait along with reduced weight and ease of maintenance on the part of the wearer.

The various parts of the joint were designed such that most of the joint can be cast in the same mould and then polished for surface finish, or may be machined out of a single stock, with the exception of the damper.

Table 2. Stride characteristics, free-paced walk (Torburn et al.,1990)

	Mean (standard deviation)		
	Velocity (m/min)	**Stride length (meters)**	**Cadence (steps/min)**
SACH	66.9 (15 .5)	1 .35 (0 .14)	98 .1 (12 .6)
Flex-Foot	69.3 (17 .6)	1 .40 (0 .16)	98 .0 (13 .8)
STEN	70.4 (12 .3)	1.41 (0 .09)	99 .8 (11 .6)
SEATTLE	72 .0 (12 .6)	1 .42 (0 .11)	100.7 (10 .8)
CC II*	73 .2 (13 .0)	1 .42 (0 .09)	102 .3 (11 .4)
Normal	81 .6 (9 .41)	1 .51 (0 .14)	108.2 (9 .1)

*(CC II = Carbon Copy II)

Ankle Joint Assembly

The prosthetic ankle joint (Bhuyan & Kumar, 2017), along with a representative foot, as depicted in Figures 11 and 12, has limited dorsiflexion – plantarflexion, by allowing a foot or a foot keel to pivot about a horizontal medial – lateral axis to accommodate the incline.

The ROM prosthetic foot and the prosthetic ankle joint, have limited dorsiflexion – plantarflexion (up – down) pivoting to accommodate different terrain, by allowing a foot or a foot keel to pivot about a horizontal medial – lateral (side to side) axis to accommodate the incline. For example, the foot keel can pivot in dorsiflexion if an upward incline is encountered and in plantarflexion if a downward incline is encountered.

The prosthetic foot or foot keel can accommodate an elongated forefoot keel. The forefoot keel can extent from the toe location of a natural foot to the heel location of the natural foot. The ankle joint is coupled pivotally between the shank and the prosthetic foot. The shank has a standard attachment affixed to the end to allow coupling to the socket which will receive the residual limb of the amputee.

Figure 11. Perspective view of entire assembly

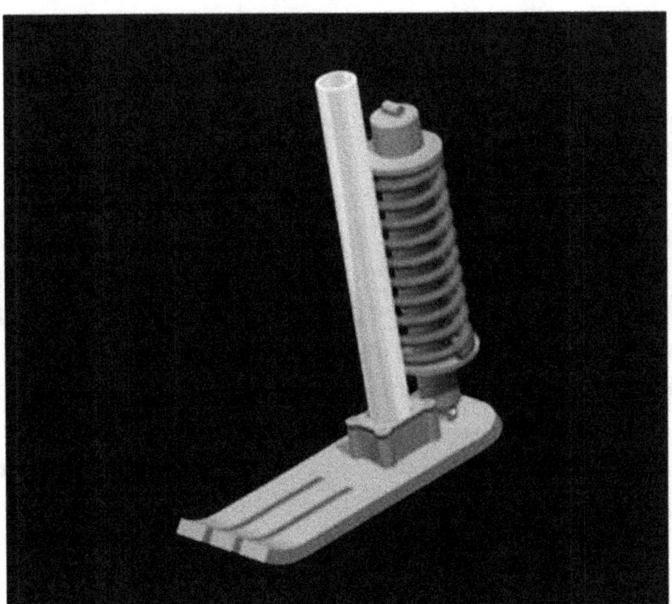

Figure 12 (a) Side view of entire assembly (b) Front view of entire assembly (c) Top view of entire assembly

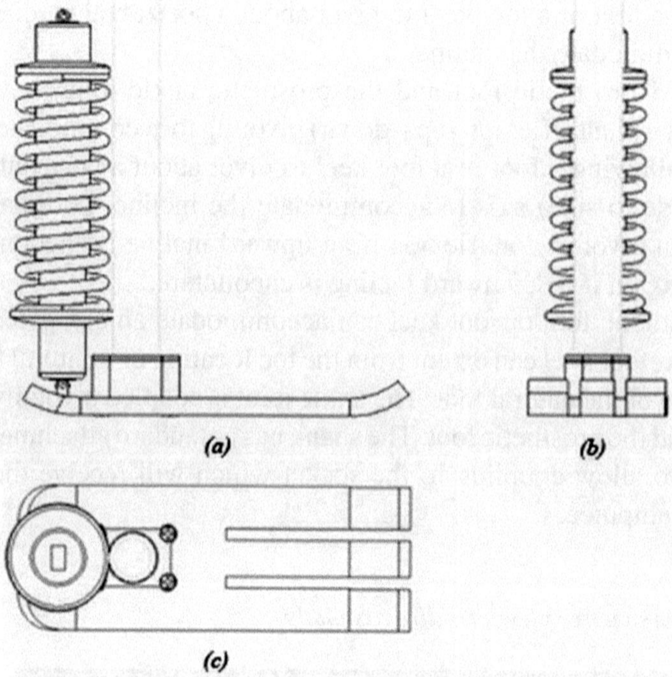

The prosthetic ankle joint has a lower housing or hub attached to the prosthetic foot. The lower housing or hub is coupled pivotally to the shank at the pivot axis. The pivotal coupling of the shank and the prosthetic ankle joint is achieved by the shaping of the lower housing or hub and the shank end. The coupling may include associated suitable bushings and pins.

The inside surfaces of the lower housing or hub are coated with suitable chemical compounds to reduce friction and give a more natural gait and/or feel to the ankle joint. The guide rail on the end of the shank fits into the slot in the lower housing or hub. The entire assembly is closed off by the upper cover plate. A bushing is affixed between the housing and the cover plate. The entire prosthetic ankle joint is affixed to the foot by suitable means, an example of which is nuts and bolts.

The damper – spring arrangement, is coupled to the prosthetic foot or foot keel. The coil spring is customized and has its stiffness suited to the needs of the amputee. The coil spring is coaxially coupled with the damper by the flanges. The damper – spring arrangement is coupled to the prosthetic foot or foot keel pivotally along a horizontal medial – lateral (side to side) axis, located parallel to the pivotal axis of the prosthetic ankle joint and rearwardly. The coupling may include suitable associated bushings and pins.

The damper selected for this design was reverse engineered from existing automotive dampers (Bhuyan, 2018). It is a twin tube design which provides greater range of motion for the entire assembly without compromising on the damping.

Motion of the Joint During Gait

On heel strike, the forefoot keel moves in plantar flexion (toe moving downwards), against the spring and pushing the rebound chamber of the damper up. Thus causing the hydraulic fluid contained in the working chamber of the damper to move though the piston valve and the pressure within the working chamber will close the foot valve of the damper.

At midstance, the forefoot keel moves in dorsiflexion (toe moving upwards) along the spring and causing the rebound chamber to lower and drawing hydraulic fluid through the piston valve. The foot valve opens and allows fluid from the rebound chamber to enter the working chamber of the damper to allow for the pressure difference and to prevent aeration of the hydraulic fluid.

At toe-off, the forefoot keel is pulled in plantar flexion (toe moving downwards), against the spring and pushing the rebound chamber of the damper up. Thus causing the hydraulic fluid contained in the working chamber of the damper to move though the piston valve and the pressure within the working chamber will close the foot valve of the damper.

During swing phase, the spring forces the rebound chamber of the damper down, pulling the forefoot keel into dorsiflexion (toe moving upwards).

SOLUTIONS AND RECOMMENDATIONS

The advantages offered by this design over the existing designs are numerous. Most significant being ease of manufacture and personalization, thereby reducing costs. Also, the inverted mortise of the joint allows the same range of motion as the physiological ankle. Greater flexion is achieved by mimicking the physiologic ankle joint, leading to ease o use and reduced energy expenditure.

CONCLUSION

The complications caused by the loss of control and power added to the psychological trauma of lost limbs plays havoc with the rehabilitation of the patient. A prosthesis is meant not only to deliver renewed functionality and is an aesthetically pleasing and effective cosmesis, but it also serves to improve the wearer's quality of life by fulfilling his sense of wholeness. A prosthesis hence serves as much as a medical device as it does as an emotional comfort. Many ideas and inventions, such as the fixed-position foot, have been worked on, explored and further developed, while others have become obsolete, such as the use of iron in prostheses. Modern prosthetics are much more advanced than the wooden stumps and hooks that were the original prosthetic limbs.

As the art progresses and science comes ever closer to recreating nature, the ultimate goal of prostheses design should be to return as much function as possible to the amputee. As such the mimicry of physiological systems provides the most elegant solutions to the many problems posed.

REFERENCES

Bar-Cohen, Y. (2005). *Biomimetics—Biologically Inspired Technologies*. Boca Raton, FL: CRC Press. doi:10.1201/9780849331633

Bar-Cohen, Y. (2006). Biomimetics—using nature to inspire human innovation. *Bioinspiration & Biomimetics*, *1*(1), 1–12. doi:10.1088/1748-3182/1/1/P01 PMID:17671297

Benyus, J. M. (2009). *Biomimcry. Innovation Inspired by Nature*. Harper Collins Publishers.

Bhuyan, D. (2018). Designing of a Twin Tube Shock Absorber: A Study in Reverse Engineering. In Design and Optimization of Mechanical Engineering Products (pp. 83 – 104). Hershey, PA: IGI Global. doi:10.4018/978-1-5225-3401-3.ch005

Bhuyan, D., & Kumar, K. (2017). *Indian Patent application no. 1319/ KOL/2015*. Kolkata: India Indian Patent.

Campbell, J. W., & Childs, C. W. (1980). The S.A.F.E. Foot. *Orthotics and Prosthetics*, *34*(3), 3–16.

Das, A., Baruah, J., & Bhuyan, D. (2018). The Anatomy of the Foot-Ankle Complex and The Mechanics of Walking: A Brief Review. *Asian Journal of Convergence in Technology, 4*(1).

Dellon, B., & Matsuoka, Y. (2007, March). Prosthetics, Exoskeletons, and Rehabilitation: Now and for the Future. *IEEE Robotics & Automation Magazine*, 30–34. doi:10.1109/MRA.2007.339622

Dixon, J. C. (2007). *The Shock Absorber Handbook* (2nd ed.). John Wiley and Sons Ltd. doi:10.1002/9780470516430

Glier, M. W., McAdams, D. A., & Linsey, J. S. (2011). Concepts in Biomimetic Design: Methods and Tools to Incorporate Into a Biomimetic Design Course. *Proceedings of the ASME 2011 Design Engineering Technical Conferences & Computers and Information in Engineering Conference, 7.*

Hertel, J. (2002). Functional Anatomy, Pathomechanics, and Pathophysiology of Lateral Ankle Instability. *Journal of Athletic Training*, *37*(4), 364–375. PMID:12937557

Hofstad, C. J., van der Linde, H., van Limbeek, J., & Postema, K. (2004). Prescription of Prosthetic Ankle-Foot Mechanisms after Lower Limb Amputation. *Cochrane Database of Systematic Reviews*, (1): CD003978. doi:10.1002/14651858.CD003978.pub2 PMID:14974050

Houdaille, M. (1908). *Improvements in or Relating To Shock-Absorbing or Dash-Pot Apparatus for Motor Vehicles and the Like.* France Patent number FR394081-A.

Houdaille, M. (1909). *Shock-absorbing apparatus.* United States Patent Number US933076 A.

Human Biomechanics and Control Lab. (2007). *Dynamic Elastic Response Foot* [Electronic image]. Retrieved January 2016. From http://www-personal.umich.edu/~artkuo/Lab/2008/06/elastic-preload-energy-storage-in.html

Leardini, A., O'Connor, J. J., & Giannini, S. (2014). Biomechanics of the natural, arthritic and replaced human replaced human ankle joint. *Journal of Foot and Ankle Research*, *7*(1), 8. doi:10.1186/1757-1146-7-8 PMID:24499639

Lundberg, A., Goldie, I., Kalin, B., & Selvik, G. (1989). Kinematics of the Ankle/Foot Complex: Plantarflexion and Dorsiflexion. *Foot & Ankle*, *9*(4), 194–200. doi:10.1177/107110078900900409 PMID:2731829

Macke, S., Misra, R., Sharma, A., & Prahalad, C.K. (2003). *Jaipur Foot: Challenging Convention.* University of Michigan Business School Case Study Series.

Malgaigne, J. F. (1841). *The Complete Works Of Ambroise Paré: Reviews and Collations on All Previous Editions*. Paris: J. B. Baillière.

Marshall, J. (2015). *The History of Prosthetics*. Retrieved 16 April 2016 from http://unyq.com/the-history-of-prosthetics/

Masum, H., Bhaumik, S., & Ray, R. (2014). Conceptual Design of a Powered Ankle-Foot Prosthesis for Walking. *Procedia Technology*, *14*, 228–235. doi:10.1016/j.protcy.2014.08.030

MedicalExpo. (n.d.). *K2 Prosthetic Foot* [Electronic image]. Retrieved January 2016. From http://www.medicalexpo.com/prod/college-park/product-74912-660646.html

Norkin, C. C., & Levangie, P. K. (1992). *Joint Structure & Function: A Comprehensive Analysis* (2nd ed.). Philadelphia: F.A. Davis Co.

Paul E Leimkuehler Online Learning Center, American Academy of Orthotists and Prosthetists. (n.d.). Retrieved January 2016 from http://www.oandp.org/

Prosthetics, C. (n.d.). *Multi Axis Foot* [Electronic Image]. Retrieved January 2016 from http://www.customprosthetics.com/lowerextremity.html

Schmitt, O. H. (1969). Some interesting and useful biomimetic transforms. *Proc. 3rd Int. Biophysics Congress*, 297.

Seymour, R. (2002). *Prosthetics and Orthotics: Lower Limb and Spinal.* Lippincott Williams & Wilkins.

Siegler, S., Chen, J., & Schnek, C. D. (1988). The Three Dimensional Kinematics and Flexibility Characteristics of the Human Ankle and Subtalar Joints-Part I: Kinematics. *Journal of Biomechanical Engineering*, *110*(4), 364–373. doi:10.1115/1.3108455 PMID:3205022

Smith, S. (2006). *SCS Continuing Education, Basic Structure and Function of the Ankle and Foot*. Retrieved January 2016 From www.ceuarmy.com/BSFAFpdf.pdf

Torburn, L., Perry, J., & Ayyappa, E. (1990). Below-knee amputee gait with dynamic elastic response prosthetic feet: A pilot study. *Journal of Rehabilitation Research and Development*, *27*(4), 369–384. doi:10.1682/JRRD.1990.10.0369 PMID:2089148

Vanderwerker, E. E. Jr. (1976). A Brief Review of the History of Amputations and Prostheses. *Inter-Clinic Information Bulletin*, *15*(5), 15–16.

Vincent, J. F. V. (2001). Stealing ideas from nature. In S. Pellegrino (Ed.), *Deployable Structures* (pp. 51–58). Vienna: Springer. doi:10.1007/978-3-7091-2584-7_3

Wood, W. (n.d.). *Pediatric SACH Foot* [Electronic image]. Retrieved January 2016 from http://www.willowwoodco.com/products-and-services/pediatric/feet/sach

Chapter 6
Experimental Investigation on ECMM With Nimonic 75 Alloy for Prosthetic Component

Pankaj Charan Jena
https://orcid.org/0000-0002-3837-7626
Veer Surendra Sai University of Technology, India

Barsarani Pradhan
Veer Surendra Sai University of Technology, India

Sudhansu Ranjan Das
Veer Surendra Sai University of Technology, India

D. Dhupal
Veer Surendra Sai University of Technology, India

ABSTRACT

Electrochemical micromachining is an advanced technology of recent trends of machining of hard and electrically conductive materials in micrometer and sub-micrometer scale. This manufacturing technique finds application in many technologically demanding industries: locomotive, biomedical, electronics, etc. However, due to very small inter-electrode gap, there is some limitation in using this machining process. This chapter aims at developing an optimized model for flow analysis of electrolyte in inter-electrode gap to obtain optimal process parameter for machining. Experimentation has been done to associate the findings of optimized output in ECMM such as material removal rate (MRR), overcut, and depth. Influence of voltage, feed rate, concentration, pulse on/pulse off ratio, and IEG investigated and finally optimized using response surface method. The effect of the process parameters are also analyzed using ANOVA.

DOI: 10.4018/978-1-5225-8235-9.ch006

INTRODUCTION

Historical Background of Electrochemical Machining

Currently Biomedical instruments are more micro in size and high accuracy. Manufacturing and selecting suitable machining process of such instruments are a challenge for present researchers. Electrochemical process is one of the advanced machining processes and can be possible to manufacture micro sized medical instruments like micro passages for surgical equipment, nozzles and tubes for dentist equipment, etc.

It is a machining process of metal removal generally used in mass production based on electrochemical process. Usually the ECM process machines hard materials, otherwise challenging to machine by conventional method. This method of machining is known as the reverse of anodizing or electroplating as a basic principle. In ECM process, the work piece is machined by controlling anodic dissolution at its atomic level. In which the desired shape of tool as high current at low potential variance through an electrolyte is imprinted on the work piece. The electrolyte is generally water based neutral salt solution. Because of its ability to machine hard materials at greater accuracy, ECM is considered as one of the advanced machining technology and is used in the fields of aerospace, defense, aeronautics, medical equipment. Recently ECM is also finding its application in the field of automobile & turbomachinery because of its inherent advantages low tool wear, lower thermal mechanical stress on work piece and more precision machining in difficult to cut materials by other non-traditional machining processes.

Why Electrochemical Micromachining (ECMM)

As the world is moving towards miniaturized, competent and superiority products, micromachining technique will play a very vital role in realizing the potential the miniaturization era where all products are getting smaller with better efficiency. Micromachining plays a crucial role in technologically demanding industries like medical, electronics, computer, and aerospace industry where complex shapes, holes, slots of micro dimension need to be made on a work piece with high accuracy. Material removal of the dimension ranging between 1.0 micrometers to 999.0 micrometers comes under micromachining. Using conventional micromachining for producing these shapes has its own share of limitations, which include high tool wear rate, thermal stress, and imperfect surface finish. To overcome these limitations, researchers are exploring new non-conventional micromachining technique. One such technique is Electrochemical micromachining (ECMM) having advantages like tool having no wear, stress-free surfaces, machining electrically conductive material regardless of physical as well as chemical property, bright surface finish. ECMM is worked on anodic suspension at atomic level in electrolyte. In spite of having so many advantages, ECMM is not widely used process as it faces some challenges like generating hydrogen bubble which adverse effects on MRR, the impact of variation in tool geometry, the impact of flow of electrolyte on surface finish and rate of machining etc. Researchers are working on how to tackle all these problems in order to get ECMM workable in more area of machining in most optimum way. When the work piece is of simple shape it is easy to define machining variable within IEG but it becomes problematic to define the same when the work piece is of complex shape. This problem can be solved by studying the flow pattern of electrolyte. This information in turn will help to avoid the passivation, which is one of the major problems in ECMM related to complex shape machining. Another problem, which is associated with ECMM, is generation of hydrogen gas at cathode. As electrolyte passes through cathode, it absorbs hydrogen gas generated at cathode. Due to this absorption, electrical conductivity of electrolyte decreases. As MRR and surface finish in ECMM is directly dependent on the electrical conductivity of the electrolyte, a decrease in it will hamper the machining rate and surface finish of work piece. In order to avoid all these, we need to know the source, effects, & pattern of hydrogen bubble generation. How it affect various critical parameters and overall machining performance. As discussed above, there is a lot which needs to be investigated in order to make ECMM more widely used machining technique.

Comparative Studies of ECM and ECMM

Although there is no major difference between the working principle of ECM and ECMM it can be differentiated with respect to these major machining characteristics (Table 1).

Table 1. Comparison of ECM and ECMM

Major Machining Characteristics	(ECM)	(ECMM)
Voltage	10-30 V	< 10
Current	150-10000 A	< 1 A
Current Density	20-200 A/ cm^2	75-100 A/ cm^2
Power supply -DC	Continuous/Pulsed	Pulsed
Frequency	Hz-kHz range	KHz-MHz range
Electrolyte flow	10-60 m/s	< 3 m/s
Electrolyte temperature	24- 65^0C	37- 50^0C
Electrolyte type	Salt Solution	Natural salt or dilute acid/alkaline solution
Electrolyte concentration	> 20g/l	< 20 g/l
Size of the tool	Large to medium	Micro
Inter-electrode gap	100-600µm	5-50µm
Operation	Maskless	Mask/maskless
Machining rate	0.2-10mm/min	5µm/min
Side gap	> 20µm	< 10µm

WORKING PRINCIPLE

ECMM uses the principle of Faraday laws of electrolysis; it states that "Weight of substance produced during electrolysis is proportional to current passing, length of time the process used and the equivalent weight of material which is deposited".

For satisfactory material removal rate, the tool gap is needed to be maintained very minimum. The electrolyte flow has been done at very high pressure for the recirculation. The electrolyte should have the respective properties- high electrical conductivity, non-toxicity, non-corrosive, high specific heat, and chemically stable, low viscosity.

Major Factors Affecting in ECMM

Tool and Work-Piece

The tool is connected with the negative terminal of the power supply and is termed as the cathode whereas work piece is connected with the positive terminal of the power supply and is termed as the anode. In the presence of pressurized electrolyte between anode and cathode with a pre-set temperature and pressure, the anodic dissolution occurs which removes materials from work-piece. Generally, the anodic dissolution is more than the cathodic dissolution, which is being cleared from electrochemistry leads to increase in lifespan of the tool.

Electrolyte

In case of electrochemical micromachining process, electrolyte plays the most essential role. The most important function performed by the electrolyte is as follows:

1. Bring to an end the electrical circuit for operation and permitting large current to pass.
2. The required electrochemical reaction is being sustained.
3. The metal sludge is being carried away, which is the reason for generation of heat at the zone of machining.

Temperature Control

The conductivity of the electrolyte varies with the variation in temperature, as the conductivity of the electrolyte is directly proportional to the temperature of the electrolyte. Therefore, electrolyte temperature must be constant throughout the machining operation. The electrolyte temperature range must be in between 37^0 and 50^0 to avoid vaporization by the increase in temperature and decrease in material removal rate by lower temperature.

Micro Tool Feed Rate

For maximum material removal rate and minimum overcut, micro tool feed rate plays an important role. Optimum feed rate helps in controlling the micro-spark generation in between electrodes. It is important to maintain 0.005 to 0.05 mm inter-electrode gap throughout the micromachining process for better accuracy and precision.

Micro-Tool Design

The recent study for micro tool design procedures was mainly directed to the numerical study to the inverse boundary problem which is mostly applied to the numeric technics such as finite element method (FEM) where "Correction Factor" concept has been adoptedto modify the tool design and shape. Electrochemical etching and Wire-EDG are used for developing the micro tool. Materials used for ECMM should be chemically inert material, electrically conductive, high corrosion resistance. An insulation coating of SiC /Si_3N_4 for the tool material by means of chemical vapor deposition (CVD) is preferred for reducing the stray current effect, which leads to better accuracy and reduced tool wear as well as overcut.

Nature of Power Supply

There, are two types of power supply that is, full wave rectified DC supply and pulsed DC power supply. In case of the full wave rectified power supply current efficiency decreases due to increase in contamination in between inter-electrode gap. Therefore, that pulsed DC power supply is mainly preferred in case of electrochemical micromachining for the increase in current density, which directly leads to increase in material removal rate.

Micro Sparks Phenomena

An occurrence of micro-spark in the gap between electrodes may not be completely neglected. Generally, these micro-sparks occurs due to heat generation across IEG and the when the anode and cathode come in, contact with each other. But this phenomenon can be neglected up to a certain extent by:

- Movement of micro-tool
- Circulation of electrolyte
- Monitoring and controlling inter-electrode gap

Material Removal Rate (MRR)

The MRR can be quantified using Faraday's law given as;

$$m = \frac{ItA}{\rho z F} \tag{1}$$

In case of alloy the equation (1) can be modified as;

$$Q = \frac{100}{\rho F}\left(\frac{1}{\sum_i \left(\frac{x_i z_i}{A_i}\right)}\right) \tag{2}$$

Advantages of ECMM

1. Tool wear in the case of ECMM is minimum.
2. The complicated geometrical shape can be machined easily and more accurately.
3. No heat-affected zone is obtained.
4. Work-piece can be machined easily.
5. ECMM deburring can deburr difficult to access areas of parts.
6. Brittle materials can be machined easily.
7. The excellent surface finish of 0.05-0.4 μm can be achieved during ECMM.

Limitation of ECMM

1. Large amount of energy is consumed during the machining process.
2. During the removal of hydrogen, gases that are generated in machining process safety issue found.
3. This process is not appropriate for non-conductive material and difficulty in management and holding brine solution (electrolyte).

Application of ECMM

1. Medical, micro tools, mini robots, biomedical implants, utensils etc.
2. Inkjet printer nozzle plate.
3. High accuracy holes in turbine blades.

4. 3D micromachining.
5. Machining of micro holes, slots with the complex configuration.
6. Metal masking

Safety in ECMM

The ECMM of metals is related to numerous hazard factors. The impact of the harmful gases and pressurized canned products created over the span of ECMM.

1. The danger of an electric stun.
2. Impact due to electromagnetic field
3. Risk of burning if short circuit occurs.
4. Danger of attack of electrolyte during machining
5. The threat of a blast of flame.
6. Mechanical elements.

LITERATURE REVIEW

A comprehensive literature study on electrochemical micro machining is carried out. The history of ECM goes way back to 1969 when it was first experimented. The advancement of technology demanded microstructure, so the electrochemical micro machining comes into account. This section includes few reach work related to electrochemical micro machining (ECMM). This chapter contains review on parametric studies of ECMM, experimental investigation on ECMM, Flow analysis study of ECM. Based on the review objective and scope of the present study has been established.

Study on Parameters of ECMM

Ghoshal et al. (2015) have fabricated micro-feature containing high aspect ratio on anticorrosive and high strength material with the help of coated electrode. In addition, experimental investigation has done for finding the effect of vibration occurs on the micro tool. Bhattacharyya et al. (2017) has investigated the MRR and overcut by considering the input parameter pulse on time as 10-15 ms, electrolyte concentration as 15-20 g/l and voltage range as 6-10 V. In this paper, effect of micro-sparks on the material removal rate has investigated. Pillai et al. (2017) have investigated the process parameters of electrochemical micro machining process of nimonic -75 alloy as work piece material, tungsten carbide as the tool material and a combination of hydrofluoric acid, sodium bromide and ethylene as electrolyte. In this paper duty cycle, given voltage, feed rate of micro tool has considered as input parameter to observe the output as material removal rate, overcut and conicity. TOPSIS method has considered as optimization method. In this paper a brief idea about electro chemical micro machining is given. It contains the area of application of titanium, challenges in machining, difficulties in anodic dissolution, process parameters ECMM for mask less machining of titanium.

Study on ECMM Experimentation

Munda et al. (2008) have examined the effect of material removal and radial overcut through response surface methodology by considering input parameter as pulse on/off time 1.0, machining voltage 3 V electrolyte concentration 15g/voltage frequency of 42.118 Hz and tool vibration frequency of 300Hz. Here it has found that the ground of irregularities is due to the nature of pulse voltage. Cole et al. (2017) have optimized the machining parameters of electrochemical micro machining for Zr-based bulk metallic glass. Here Taguchi method was used for showing the effect of surface roughness, effect of duty cycle, effect of electrolyte concentration, effect of voltage. In this method 0.4l/min, 1:10, 2.235-3V taken as electrolyte flow rate, duty cycle, voltage respectively. Ghoshal et al. (2017) in the report more emphasis has given to the scan feed rate calculation at different machining parameters. Scan feed rate plays an important role in microchannel formation for reduction of overcut. Liu et al. (2017) have done their investigation on internal features of micro holes machined in electro chemical machine. In the present report, effect of feed rate on the machining efficiency has shown. Bhattacharyya et al. (2017) Has done the experimental work on electrochemical micromachining by taking the machining parameter as 55Hz frequency, 20 g/l electrolyte concentration and 55Hz frequency. Stray current and on-line pulse pattern has found as the grounds for micro-sparks generated. Anasane et al. (2017) have publicized the excellent properties of titanium chemical as well as physical when used as electrode in mask-less electrochemical micromachining for micro milling of microgrooves. Machining parameter such as pulse frequency, machining voltage and micro-tool feed rate has been taken for the analysis of width overcut, length overcut and taper angle. Munda et al. (2003) have done their experiment on electrochemical micro machining for weakening stray-current and micro-spark effect for the enhancement of material removal rate with controlled parameter. Here surface response methodology is used for the design of experiment. Bhattacharyya et al. (2017) have scrutinized electrochemical micro machining process for significant material removal rate and not as much of overcut at various machining parameters.

Objective and Scope of the Study

It is observed that past researchers have discussed various approaches to understand MRR as well as current density distribution in ECMM. They have used different tool geometry for these analyses. In case, complicated micro tool geometry and work pieces, it is very difficult to know the machining variables within the IEG as it is in micro level. However, there is a need to understand about those parameters, the impact of their variation in the IEG as well as in different materials by proper experimental investigation. In this work copper tool has considered on Nimonic-75 work piece material.

EXPERIMENTAL WORK

The present chapter contains experiment that has been steered in the electrochemical machine set up available in the production-engineering laboratory of VSSUT Burla.

ECMM SET UP

Tool post of electrochemical machine set up used for the experiment has shown Figure1.The detail specification for machining of micro hole is gives below in the Table 2.

The electrochemical machining set up consists of three sub classifications. Those are as follow:

1. Machining cell
2. Control panel
3. Electrolyte circulation system

Machining Cell

The machining cell of electrochemical micro machining system is associated with stepper motorized x-axis, y-axis and z-axis movement of tool, an electrolyte dispensing arrangement with attached flow meter, job-fixing arrangement, machining chamber with transparent window. All components material used in machining operations chosen in such a way that, they possess corrosion resistant property.

Tool post image of the ECMM set up is shown in the Figure 1. It is used to hold the tool post connected with the 3- axis fixture arrangement for allowing x, y and z axis movement to the tool.

Table 2. Specifications for machining of micro hole

Tool area	:	300 square mm
Cross head stroke	:	40 mm
Tool feed motor	:	Stepper motor

Figure 1. Tool Post of ECMM set up

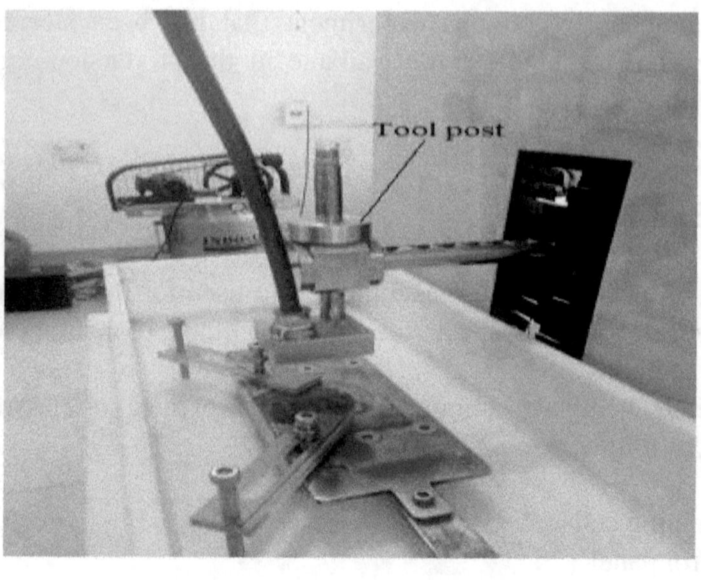

Preparation of Tool, Workpiece and Electrolyte

For performing the operation in the electrochemical machine for machining micro holes, 260 micron thick cylindrical copper with flat end has taken as electrode as shown in Figure 2. For experiment, nimonic 75 alloy has taken as work-piece material. Work piece material is of size (2.5×2.5×1) cm shown in the Figure 2. Preparation of electrolyte solution plays an important role in the process of electrochemical micro machining. Electrolyte solution is prepared by mixing water and sodium nitrate salt. Therefore, for the experiment 10 liter water has taken. For preparation of three levels of electrolyte solution, that is 10gm/l, 20gm/l and 30gm/l, 100 grams of salt, 200 grams of salt, and 300 grams of salt have mixed with water respectively in room temperature.

Taguchi Experimental Design and Analysis

The result of experiment depends upon clear and accurate output from the experimental data for accomplishing this design of experiment is used. It is based on drawing getting conclusion from observations when observations are not exact but may vary. Secondly, design of experiment provides appropriate method for collection of experimental data. In conventional design of experiment single variable is look after while other variable remain constant. This type of experiment provide only experimental result based on the response of chosen variable under certain settings. Limitation: it doesn't provide the effect of change in value of other variable simultaneously. In order to take into account all the possible combination of influencing factors

Figure 2. Material (a) Tool and (b) Work piece material

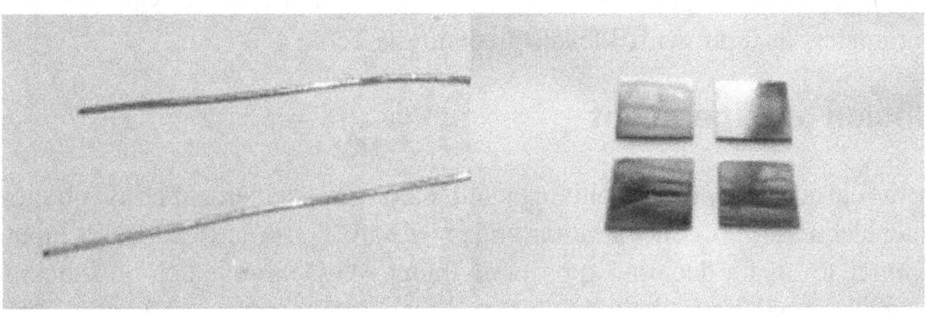

(a) (b)

Table 3. Components classification for experimental investigation

Component	Material	Shape
Tool	Copper	Cylindrical flat end
Work piece	Nimonic75 alloy	Square shaped
Electrolyte	$NaNO_3$	-

in the experiment a very large number of trials need to be done. In order to get out of this problem one can use a part of combined factors that will produce most of the information related to experiment. In view of absence of generally lead procedure, analysis of result in this method is difficult to get. One method to get out of this problem is Taguchi method.

Taguchi method is based on engineering fundamentals rather than statistical approach. Orthogonal array are used in Taguchi design for conductance of experiment. For designing of experiment first appropriate OA's are selected, parameters and outputs are assigned to the assigned columns. For making the task of assignment of parameters simple, linear graphs and triangular Tables are used. By analyzing the main effect of each of the parameter optimum condition is identified. The information of impact of individual parameter is most important in identifying the control parameters, which need to be put in production process. In order to determine how much each parameter contributes, the analysis of variance (ANOVA) is applied to the finding of the experiment, which is a statistical treatment. By studying ANOVA Table one can determine the parameters, which needs to be controlled for a given analysis. ANOVA is a method of data analysis used in Taguchi method. In order to identify significant parameters, standard ANOVA is conducted on S/N ratio. In case of optimum value of quality with least variation, value of S/N ratio is high.

The experiment designed for the machining process by considering five parameters as input with 3 levels given in the Table 4.

Design of Experiment

In the current study five machining parameters are considered such as voltage, inter electrode gap, concentration, and pulse on/off ratio and feed rate as input in three levels for deciding appropriate range of machining factors. Taguchi L_{27} orthogonal array method is selected for achieving the experiments. The

Table 4. Parameters and its levels for Experiment

Sl.no	Machining parameters	Symbol	Units	Levels		
				Level-1	Level-2	Level-3
1	voltage	v	Volt	3	6	9
2	Concentration	c	gm/lt	10	20	30
3	Inter electrode gap	i	micron	10	15	20
4	Pulse on time/ pulse off time	d	nil	15/10=1.5	10/5=2.0	5/2=2.5
5	Feed rate	f	*12 micron / min	1	2	3

machining attribute decided for the present study are overcut, depth of hole and material removal rate.

Procedure for Experimentation

The initial weight of the work piece is first measured using a precision electronic balance and again final weight is being measured after machining of a single hole to calculate the MRR. The copper tool was fitted to the tool holder and work piece material is fixed to the worktable for machining. Then all input parameters (voltage, current, feed rate, pump flow rate, pulse on time, and pulse off time) for the machining is set. For machining of micro holes current, flow rate and machining time has kept fixed as 1 amp, 2.5 m/s, 240 secs respectively. After each machining, the data saved at USB and transferred to computer, which is in; excel format and the weight of the work piece being noted. The depth travelled by the tool is found from the machine itself, as the stepper motor is connected with the encoder and the tool travel before machining is set as zero so we can say that the depth calculated by the machine is correct. The image in the Figure 3 contains the workpiece during micro machining process. Figure 4 is showing the result and input parameters settings during machining process.

Optical Microscope Images

Optical microscope is also known as light microscope. It used to magnify images of small objects. Here optical microscope is used to visualize the outer diameter of the micro hole to find the overcut. By the use of optical

Figure 3. Workpiece during machining

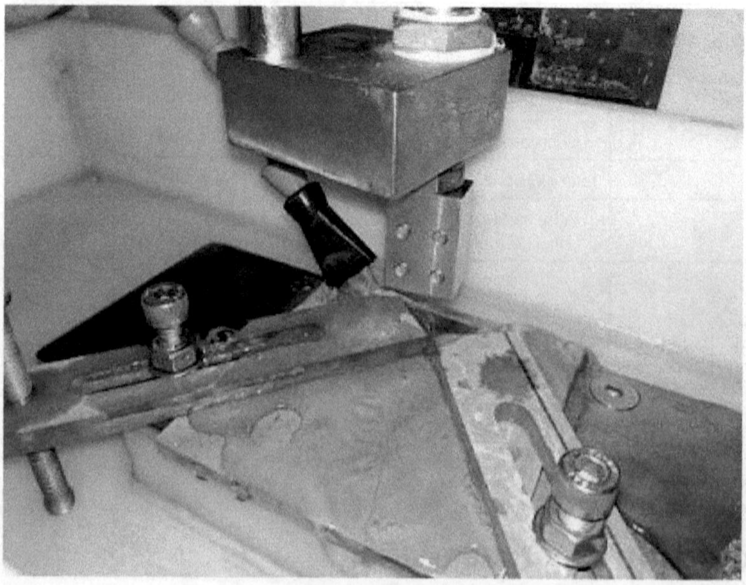

Figure 4. Control panel during machining

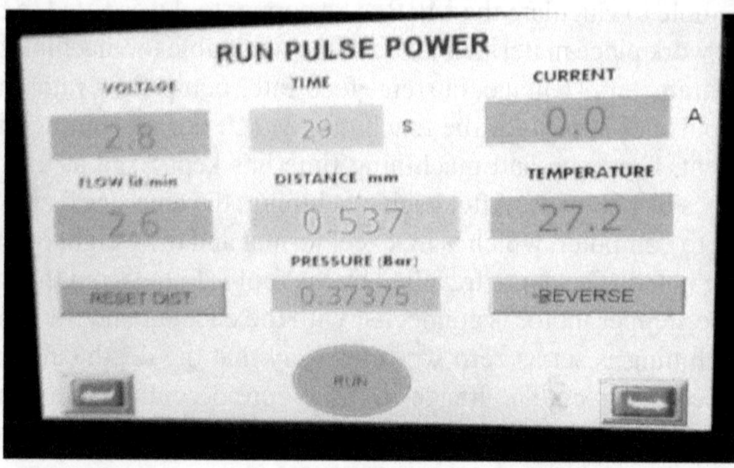

microscope, microstructure has also been captured. An image of heat-affected zone near the machined surface was captured as well as grain expert analysis was also done to know the effect of micro grains after machining of micro holes.

Table 5. Observation table by L27 Orthogonal Array

Sl.no	Voltage (volts)	IEG (micron)	Concentration (gm/lt)	Pulse on / pulse off	Feed rate (*12 micron/ mm)	DEPTH (mm)	OVERCUT (micron)	MRR (gm/min)
1	3	10	10	1.5	1	0.0017	580	0.001464
2	3	10	10	1.5	2	0.019	610	0.001529
3	3	10	10	1.5	3	0.023	683	0.001644
4	3	15	20	2.0	1	0.022	590	0.001588
5	3	15	20	2.0	2	0.034	613	0.001618
6	3	15	20	2.0	3	0.042	665	0.001762
7	3	20	30	2.5	1	0.027	672	0.0016
8	3	20	30	2.5	2	0.057	729	0.00175
9	3	20	30	2.5	3	0.059	760	0.00185
10	6	10	20	2.5	1	0.019	614.2	0.0019
11	6	10	20	2.5	2	0.031	688	0.00205
12	6	10	20	2.5	3	0.0554	780.5	0.00215
13	6	15	30	1.5	1	0.027	750	0.0026
14	6	15	30	1.5	2	0.059	816	0.0027
15	6	15	30	1.5	3	0.07515	899	0.0028
16	6	20	10	2.0	1	0.029	638.6	0.0029
17	6	20	10	2.0	2	0.041	736	0.003
18	6	20	10	2.0	3	0.052	791	0.0031
19	9	10	30	2.0	1	0.026	970	0.00315
20	9	10	30	2.0	2	0.055	1007	0.0032
21	9	10	30	2.0	3	0.066	1072	0.00325
22	9	15	10	2.5	1	0.026	603	0.0034
23	9	15	10	2.5	2	0.058	641	0.00345
24	9	15	10	2.5	3	0.076	732	0.0035
25	9	20	20	1.5	1	0.026	725.7	0.00365
26	9	20	20	1.5	2	0.056	831	0.0037
27	9	20	20	1.5	3	0.077	897	0.00375

Over cut is calculated after observations under Optical microscope.

Figure 5. Work piece after machining

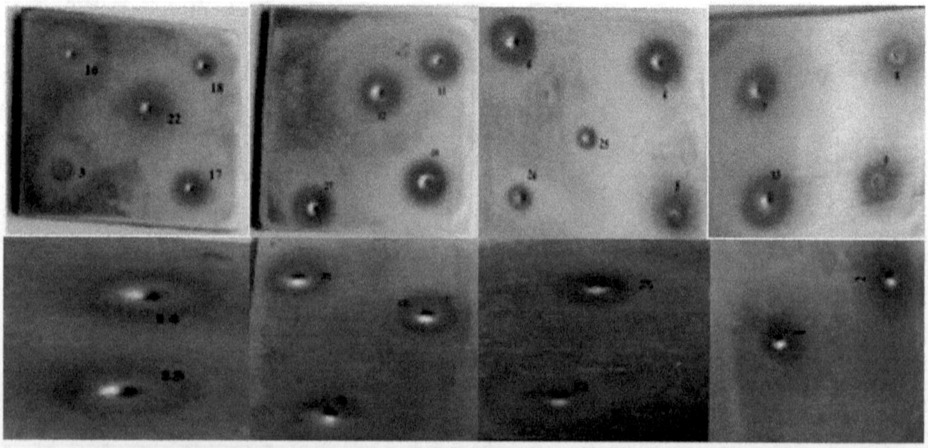

Figure 6. Optical microscope images after machining

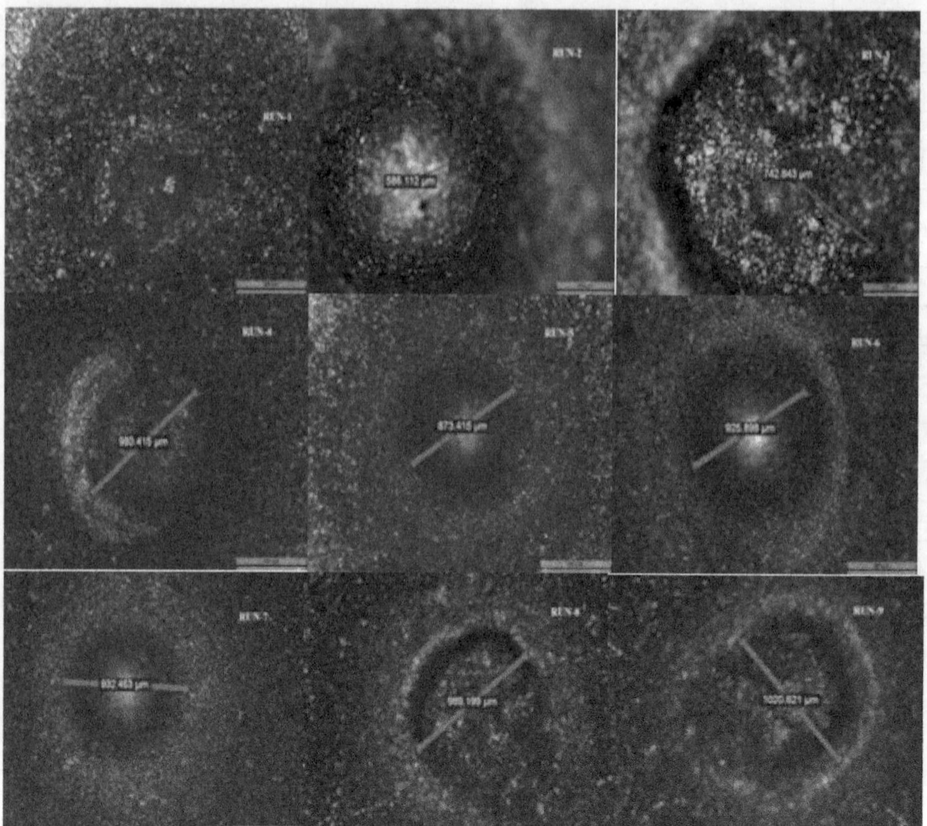

Sample Calculation

$$\text{MRR}=\frac{W_{t=0}-W_{t=2\,\min}}{t}\text{ in gm/min)} \quad (1)$$

where t= machining operation time =2 min is observed.

EXPERIMENTAL RESULT

Effect on Depth

The Figure 7 Shows the effect of voltage (v), inter electrode gap (i), concentration of electrolyte (c), pulse on /off ratio (d), feed rate (f) on the output depth obtained from the software MINITAB-17. Figure 8 shows the S/N ratio plot for the effect of depth analysis.

From the Figure 7 and Figure 8, it has been agreed that with the increase in voltage from 3V to 9V depth is increasing, with the increase in inter electrode gap depth is increasing but the variation in depth from 15 micrometer to 20 micrometer is very small. With increase in molar concentration of electrolyte

Figure 7. Main plot for depth

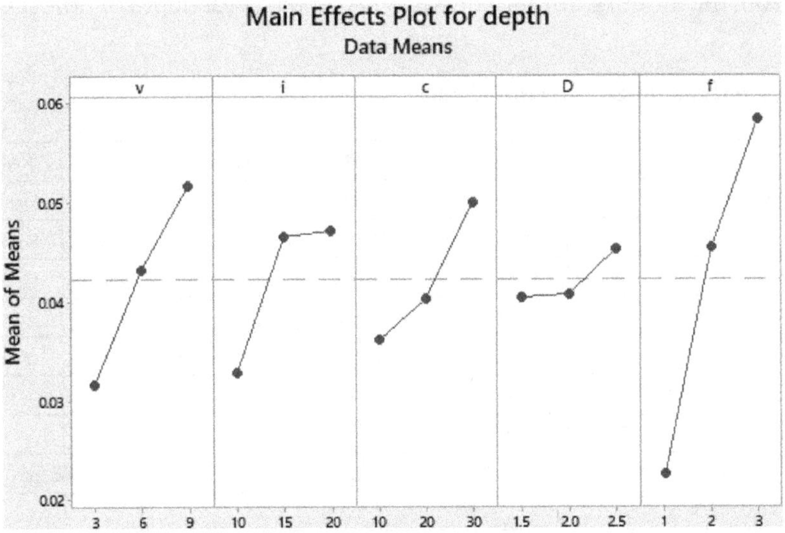

Figure 8. Main plot for S/N ratio for depth

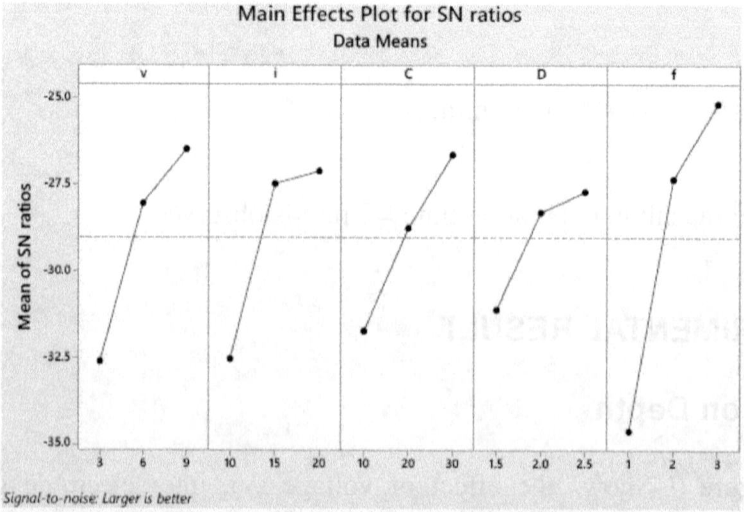

the depth of the hole in increasing. The feed rate pulse on/ off ratio for the machining has less effect on the depth of the micro hole, although with increase in pulse on /off ratio depth is also increasing. Feed rate for the machining has major effect on the depth of the hole. From the Figure 8, it is concluded that change in feed rate can greatly affect the tool travel.

From the Table 6, from the values of P it can be clearly said that voltage, inter electrode gap, concentration of electrolyte, feed rate has more significant result for finding of depth. As the P-values is less than the significant level 0.05. From the model summary of ANOVA analysis for depth of hole it is clear

Table 6. Analysis of variance for depth

Source	DF	Adj-SS	Adj-MS	F-Value	P-Value	Remarks
v	2	0.001839	0.00920	18.42	0.000	Significant
i	2	0.001168	0.000584	11.69	0.001	Significant
c	2	0.000924	0.000462	9.62	0.002	significant
d	2	0.000137	0.000069	1.38	0.281	-
f	2	0.000799	0.002954	59.16	0.000	significant
Error	16	0.000799	0.000050			
Total	26	0.010775				

S	R-sq	R-sq (adj)	R-sq (pred)
0.0070658	92.59%	87.95%	78.89%

that the model fits the data up to r-sq. value of 92.59%, standard deviation for the model between fitted value and data point is approximately 0.0070658 units. The predicted response for the model, which is given by r-sq. (pred), is 78.89%. It defines that the predicting ability of the model is around 78.89%.

The regression equation drawn from the MINITAB-17 for depth analysis is as follows:

Regression Equation

Depth = 0.04219 - 0.01056 v_3 + 0.00098 v_6 + 0.00958 v_9 - 0.00929 i_10 + 0.00438 i_15+ 0.00492 i_20 - 0.00601 c_10 - 0.00193 c_20 + 0.00793 c_30 - 0.00177 d_1.5- 0.00142 d_2.0 + 0.00318 d_2.5 - 0.01956 f_1 + 0.00336 f_2 + 0.01620 f_3

From the response Table 7, the rank of the process parameters for maximizing depth of hole is feed rate, voltage, inter electrode gap, electrolyte concentration as per larger is better concept. Therefore, feed rate plays important role in maximizing the depth of micro hole. Increase in feed rate leads to faster machining. Whereas variation of pulse on/ off ratio less important role in comparison to voltage, feed rate, pulse on/off ration and concentration of electrolyte.

Effect on MRR

From the main effect plot for MRR plotted in Figure 9 and Figure 10, it is observed that voltage is affecting more for increased MRR. More the supply of voltage more the material removal rate is observed. Material removal rate is increased steadily with increase in voltage from 3V to 9V.

Table 7. Response table for depth analysis

Level	V	i	c	d	f
1	0.03163	0.03290	0.03619	0.04043	0.02263
2	0.04317	0.04657	0.04027	0.04078	0.04556
3	0.05178	0.04711	0.05013	0.04538	0.05839
Delta	0.02014	0.01421	0.01394	0.00435	0.03576
Rank	2	3	4	5	1

Figure 9. Main effect plot for MRR

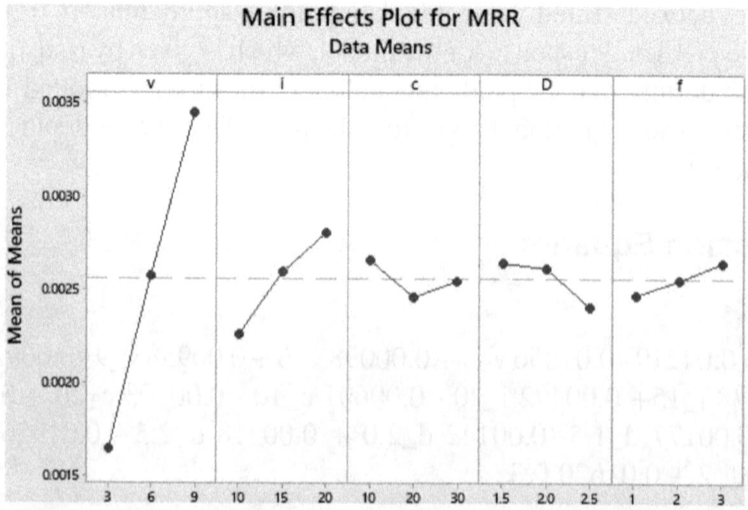

Figure 10. Main effect plot for S/N ratio for MRR

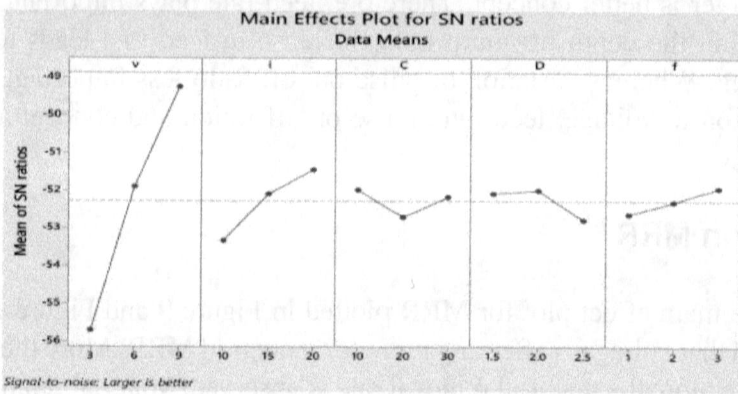

From the analysis of variance Table 8 it is been observed that all the factors selected for machining plays vital role for better machining. All the P-values from the analysis is been found as 0.000 which is less than 0.05. It means all factors are significant for the model. The standard deviation value is 0.0000336 unit is very less means all values considered for the experiment meets the model assumption. From the above value of model summary, it is clear that the model taken for analysis is 99.69% correct.

The Regression Equation for MRR is as follows:

Table 8. Analysis of variance for MRR

Source	DF	Adj-SS	Adj-MS	F-Value	P-Value	Remarks
v	2	0.000015	0.000007	6512.65	0.000	Significant
i	2	0.000001	0.000001	619.45	0.000	Significant
c	2	0.000000	0.000000	82.66	0.000	Significant
d	2	0.000000	0.000000	140.35	0.000	Significant
f	2	0.000000	0.000000	59.61	0.000	significant
Error	16	0.000000	0.000000			
Total	26	0.000017				
S	R-sq.	R-sq.(adj)	R-sq. (pred)			
0.0000336	99.89%	99.82%	99.69%			

MRR = 0.002558 - 0.000913 v_3 + 0.000020 v_6 + 0.000892 v_9 - 0.000298 i_10 + 0.000044 i_15 + 0.000254 i_20 + 0.000108 c_10 - 0.000094 c_20 - 0.000013 c_30 + 0.000091 d_1.5 + 0.000061 d_2.0 - 0.000152 d_2.5 - 0.000085 f_1 - 0.000002 f_2 + 0.000088 f_3

The Table 9 describes the rank of the parameter from 1- 5 in terms of factor affecting the material removal rate.

Effect on Overcut

The Figure 11 contains the main plot for overcut by plotted by MINITAB-17. Figure 12 contains the S/N ratio plot MINITAB-17. From the S/N plot of the overcut, the quality characteristics can be identified that which factor is effecting for getting more overcut due to machining.

The Figure 11 contains the main plot for overcut by plotted by MINITAB-17. From the analysis, it has found that with the increase in pulse electrolyte

Table 9. Response Table for MRR

Level	V	i	c	d	f
1	0.001645	0.002260	0.002665	0.002649	0.002472
2	0.002578	0.002602	0.002463	0.002619	0.002555
3	0.003450	0.002811	0.002544	0.002406	0.002645
Delta	0.001805	0.000551	0.000202	0.000243	0.000173
Rank	1	2	4	3	5

Figure 11. Main effect plot for overcut

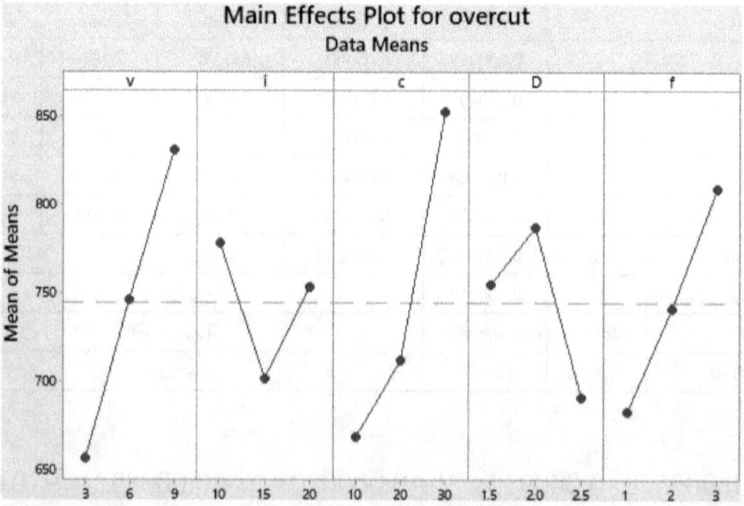

Figure 12. Main effect plot for S/N ratio of overcut

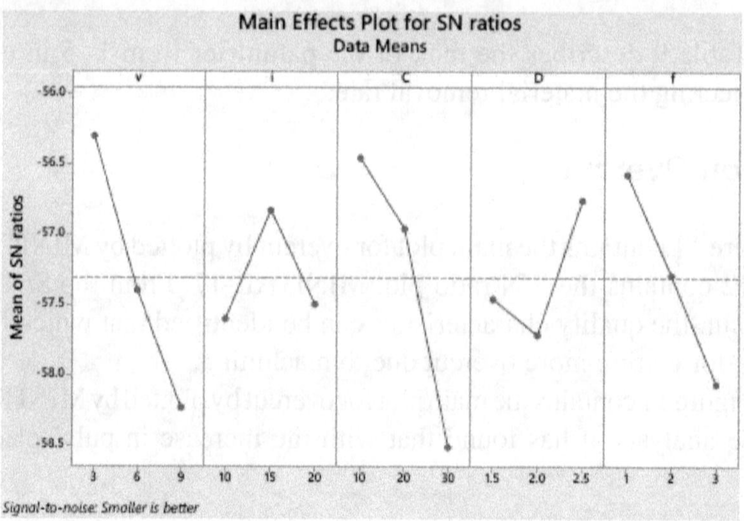

concentration, feed rate and voltage the overcut increases. However, with the increase in inter electrode gap and pulse on/off ratio value of overcut diminishing.

Table 10 contains the analysis of variance values for overcut. From the taguchi analysis it has been found that all the parameters for machining micro holes are significant and the prediction for the analysis is 95.79% correct.

Table 10. Analysis of variance for overcut

Source	DF	Adj-SS	Adj-MS	F-Value	P-Value	Remarks
v	2	138149	69074.6	164.17	0.000	Significant
i	2	28018	14008	33.29	0.000	Significant
c	2	167530	83764.8	199.08	0.000	Significant
d	2	42830	21414.9	50.90	0.000	Significant
f	2	71816	35907.9	85.34	0.000	significant
Error	16	6732	420.8			
Total	26	455074				

S	R-sq	R-sq(adj)	R-sq (pred)
20.5125	98.52%	97.60%	95.79%

The regression equation for the overcut is as follows:

Regression Equation

Overcut = 744.22 - 88.44 v_3 + 1.70 v_6 + 86.74 v_9 + 34.08 i_10 - 43.22 i_15 + 9.14 i_20 - 75.93 C_10 - 32.62 C_20 + 108.56 C_30 + 10.41 D_1.5 + 42.73 D_2.0 - 53.14 D_2.5- 61.61 f_1 - 3.00 f_2 + 64.61 f_3

Multiobjective Optimisation

Multi objective optimisation is done by using surface response analysis in MINITAB-17. The result for the surface response is as follows:

The analysis for multi-objective optimization for L27 orthogonal array by Taguchi method is done by response surface methodology (RSM). The

Table 11. Response analysis for overcut

Level	V	i	C	d	f
1	655.8	778.3	668.3	754.6	682.6
2	745.9	701.0	711.6	787.0	741.2
3	831.0	753.4	852.8	691.1	808.8
Delta	175.2	77.3	184.5	95.9	126.2
Rank	2	5	1	4	3

Figure 13. Multi-objective optimization result

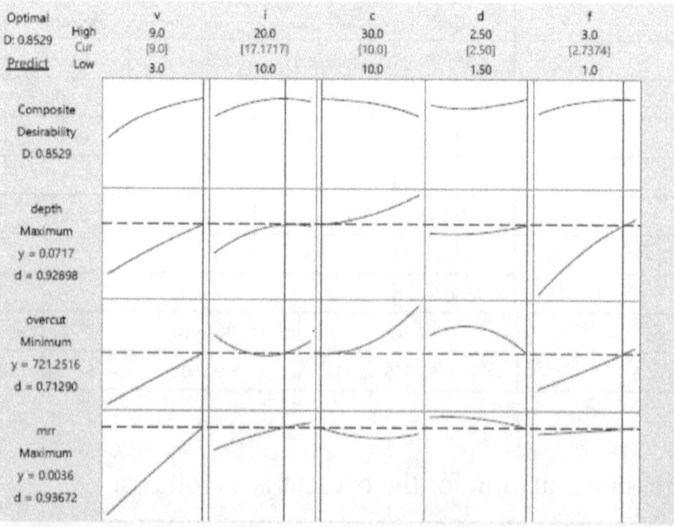

result for optimization is got by maximizing MRR, minimizing overcut and maximizing depth of hole value. The predicted value for input parameters for getting optimum value is shown in the above Figure 13. The prediction for desirability is 0.8529. The confirmatory test is done after the optimization which is shown in the Table 12. The error percentage is given in Table 13.

GRAPHS AND CONTOUR PLOTS

Line Plots Surface Plots and Contour Plots

In the Figure14 counter plot, surface plot and line plot is obtained from MINITAB-17 in between MRR vs. IEG vs. Voltage. From the Figure14 it is cleared the with increase in voltage material removal rate increases with change in IEG gap

In the Figure15 counter plot, surface plot and line plot is obtained from MINITAB-17 in between Overcut vs. IEG vs. Voltage. From the Figure15 it is cleared that with increase in voltage overcut increases with change in IEG gap.

In the Figure16 counter plot, surface plot and line plot is obtained from MINITAB-17 in between Depth vs. IEG vs. Voltage. From the Figure16 it is cleared that with increase in voltage depth increases with change in IEG gap.

Table 12. Confirmatory test result

v	i	C	d	F	Mrr	overcut	depth
9	18	10	2.5	3	0.00322	649	0.065

$$\text{Error}\left(\text{in percentage}\right) = \frac{\text{theoritical value} - \text{experimental value}}{\text{theoritical value}} \times 100$$

Table 13. Error percentage result

Output parameters	MRR	Overcut	Depth
Error percentage	10.5	9	8

Figure 14. MRR vs. IEG vs. voltage

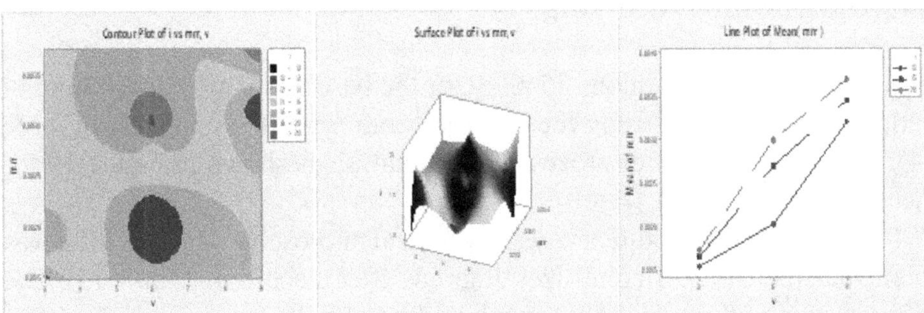

Figure 15. Overcut vs. Voltage vs. IEG

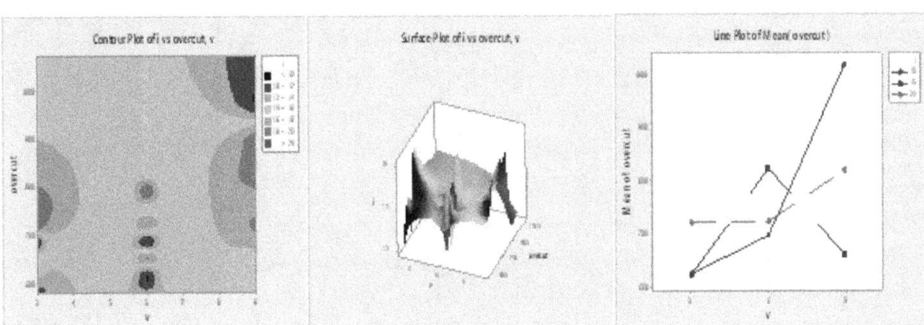

Figure 16. Depth vs. Voltage vs. IEG

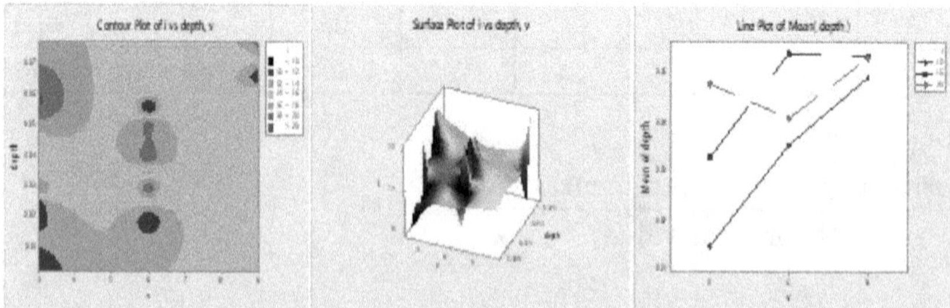

Probability Plots for MRR, Depth and Overcut

Figure 17 obtained from the MINITAB-17 is the probability plot for the output of the machining material removal rate, overcut and depth of the machined hole.

Micro Structure Analysis

The grain analysis of nimoni-75 alloy for the base metal after machining in optical microscope by using the software grain expert is conducted (Table 14). From the image after processing the analysis is shown in Figure 19 for the experiment no.22.

From the microstructure analysis by optical microscope (Figure 20) it was found that, there are different sizes of grains after machining (Table 15). The different size of the grains is shown by different color.

Figure 17. Probability plots for MRR, overcut and depth

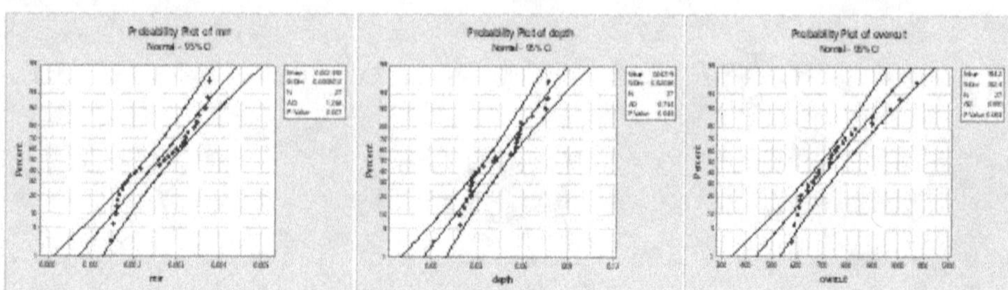

Figure 18. Base metal after machining for heat-affected zone

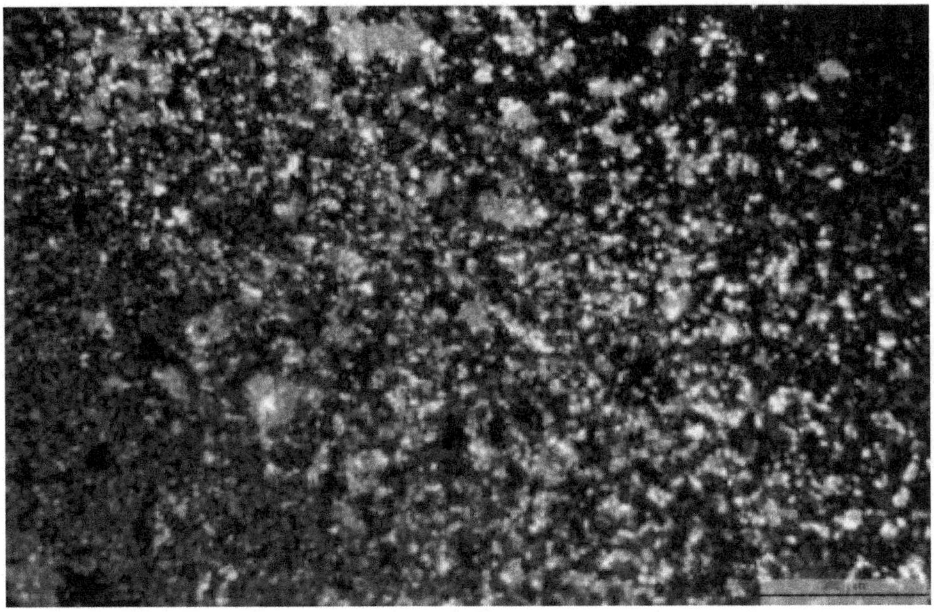

Table 14. Grain analysis by optical micro scope

Grain Number	6.495	Result	-
Experiment	Grain size analysis	Observation	-
Preparation	-	Technologist	adkp
Specimen	Nimonic-75	Calibration:	1 pixel = 1.06 Microns
Keywords	-	Scanned Area:	889708.0411
Analysis Date:	19-04-2018		

CONCLUSION

This work is based on machining of micro holes by electro-chemical micro machine with a cylindrical flat end tool, is giving idea of effect on distribution of velocity, pressure pattern, variation of profile of temperature, current density distribution. In this analysis, work-piece material is NIMONIC-75 nickel super alloy, Cupper is taken as the tool material and Sodium Nitrate is taken as the electrolyte.

Figure 19. Original and processing image by optical microscope of base metal of run 22

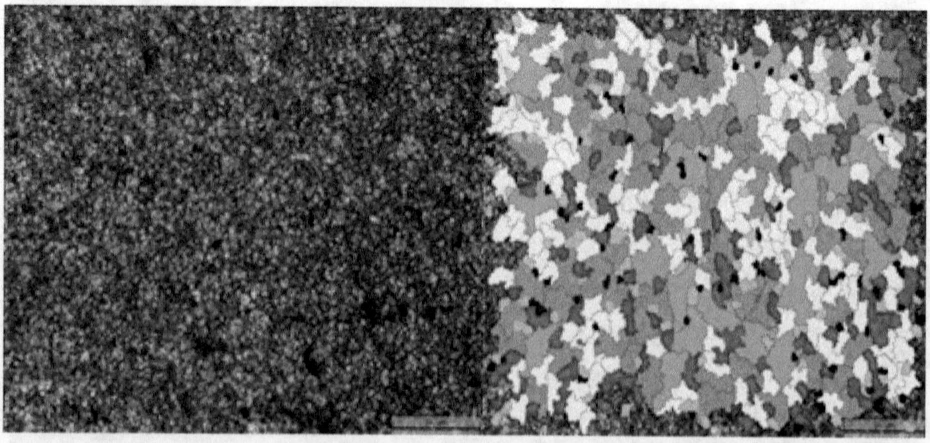

Figure 20. Grain structure analysis of base metal of RUN 22

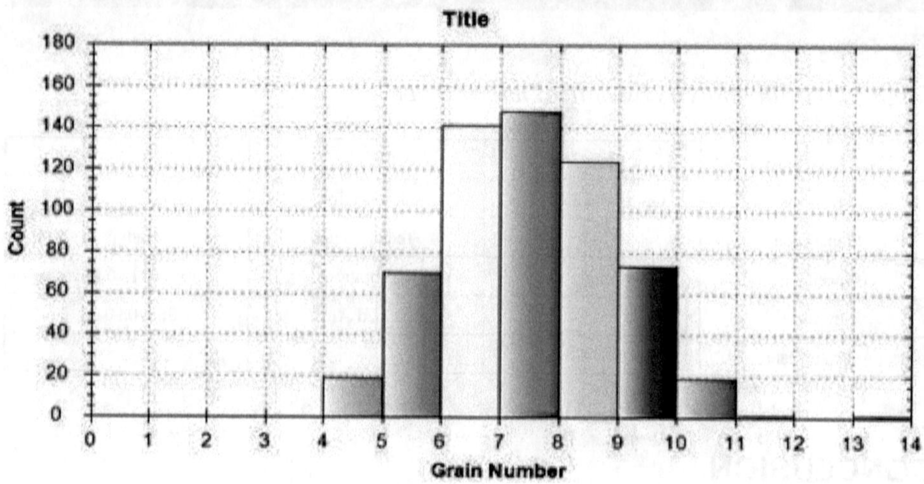

Table 15. Grain counts of microstructure

Total Count	596
Mean	7.481169482
Total	4458.777011
Oversize Count	0

The experiment has been conducted by taking the five input parameters such as voltage, electrolyte concentration, pulse on/off ratio, feed rate, inter electrode gap. The input parameters for the experiment were chosen on the basis references. The output parameters for the experiments are material removal rate (MRR), Depth of the hole, Overcut. The output parameters were analyzed by using Taguchi-ANOVA strategy in MINITAB-17.0 software.

1. It can be concluded from above discussion that, a more concentrated electrolyte gives better MRR as well as surface finish as it offers a low resistance to flow of machining current through it for the specific operating voltage.
2. Depth of the machined hole increases with increase in voltage, feed rate, concentration, whereas pulse on/off ratio and inter electrode gap has less effect on the machining deep hole.
3. Material removal rate increases with the increase in voltage and feed rate but decreases with increase concentration, inter electrode gap, and pulse on/off ratio.
4. Overcut of the hole increases with increase in voltage, molar concentration of electrolyte and feed rate whereas decreases with increasing pulse on /off ratio and inter electrode gap.
5. The multi objective optimization using response surface analysis showed the optimum conditions with voltage 9V, 10gm/l and 17.1717 micrometer inter electrode gap, 2.5 pulse on /off ratio (pulse on time 5 millisecond and pulse off time-2 millisecond) and 2.7374 *12 micron/ min for best output, which will give maximum depth, minimum overcut and maximum material removal rate.

REFERENCES

Anasane, S. S., & Bhattacharyya, B. (2017). Electrochemical Micromachining of Titanium and Its Alloys. In Non-traditional Micromachining Processes (pp. 337–365). Cham: Springer. doi:10.1007/978-3-319-52009-4_9

Anasane, S. S., & Bhattacharyya, B. (2017). Experimental investigation into micromilling of microgrooves on titanium by electrochemical micromachining. *Journal of Manufacturing Processes*, *28*, 285–294. doi:10.1016/j.jmapro.2017.06.016

Bhattacharyya, B., Malapati, M., & Munda, J. (2005). Experimental study on electrochemical micromachining. *Journal of Materials Processing Technology*, *169*(3), 485–492. doi:10.1016/j.jmatprotec.2005.04.074

Bhattacharyya, B., & Munda, J. (2003). Experimental investigation into electrochemical micromachining (ECMM) process. *Journal of Materials Processing Technology*, *140*(1-3), 287–291. doi:10.1016/S0924-0136(03)00722-2

Bhattacharyya, B., & Munda, J. (2003). Experimental investigation on the influence of electrochemical machining parameters of machining rate and accuracy in micromachining domain. *International Journal of Machine Tools & Manufacture*, *43*(13), 1301–1310. doi:10.1016/S0890-6955(03)00161-5

Cole, K. M., Kirk, D. W., Singh, C. V., & Thorpe, S. J. (2017). Optimizing electrochemical micromachining parameters for Zr-based bulk metallic glass. *Journal of Manufacturing Processes*, *25*, 227–234. doi:10.1016/j.jmapro.2016.11.015

Ghoshal, B., & Bhattacharyya, B. (2015). Vibration assisted electrochemical micromachining of high aspect ratio micro features. *Precision Engineering*, *42*, 231–241. doi:10.1016/j.precisioneng.2015.05.005

Ghoshal, B., & Bhattacharyya, B. (2016). Electrochemical micromachining of microchannel using optimum scan feed rate. *Journal of Manufacturing Processes*, *23*, 258–268. doi:10.1016/j.jmapro.2016.05.003

Liu, G., Li, Y., Kong, Q., & Tong, H. (2017). Research on ECM process of micro holes with internal features. *Precision Engineering*, *47*, 508–515. doi:10.1016/j.precisioneng.2016.10.006

Munda, J., & Bhattacharyya, B. (2008). Investigation into electrochemical micromachining (ECMM) through response surface methodology based approach. *International Journal of Advanced Manufacturing Technology*, *35*(7-8), 821–832. doi:10.100700170-006-0759-0

Munda, J., Malapati, M., & Bhattacharyya, B. (2007). Control of micro-spark and stray-current effect during ECMM process. *Journal of Materials Processing Technology*, *194*(1-3), 151–158. doi:10.1016/j.jmatprotec.2007.04.112

Pillai, H. P., Sampath, S. C., Elumalai, R., Hariharan, S., & Natarajan, Y. (2017). Influence of Process Parameters on Electrochemical Micromachining of Nimonic 75 Alloy. In *ASME 2017 International Mechanical Engineering Congress and Exposition* (pp. V002T02A007-V002T02A007). American Society of Mechanical Engineers.

Chapter 7
Correction of Artifacts and Optimization of Atomic Force Microscopy Imaging:
A Case of Thin Aluminum Films for Prosthetic Applications

Fredrick M. Mwema
University of Johannesburg, South Africa

Esther T. Akinlabi
University of Johannesburg, South Africa

Oluseyi P. Oladijo
https://orcid.org/0000-0003-1650-6244
Botswana International University of Science and Technology, Botswana

ABSTRACT

Acquisition of experimental data from atomic force microscopy (AFM) sometimes has artefacts that distort the information contained in the image. Such artefacts can be very delirious especially for sensitive applications such as in biomedical and microelectronics. This chapter illustrates the correction of the artefacts resulting from tapping mode imaging. It also shows the application of Taguchi optimization technique for reducing artefacts during AFM imaging. Using AFM images of Al films, Fourier filtering is illustrated as a useful technique for correcting the artefacts. Taguchi optimization is shown to determine the optimal scan rate, scan size, integral and proportional gains in minimizing the size and number of artefacts at the imaging stage. The correction technique is shown to improve the morphological information of the AFM images while the Taguchi method is effective for determining the best imaging conditions for AFM analysis.

DOI: 10.4018/978-1-5225-8235-9.ch007

Box 1. Graphical abstract

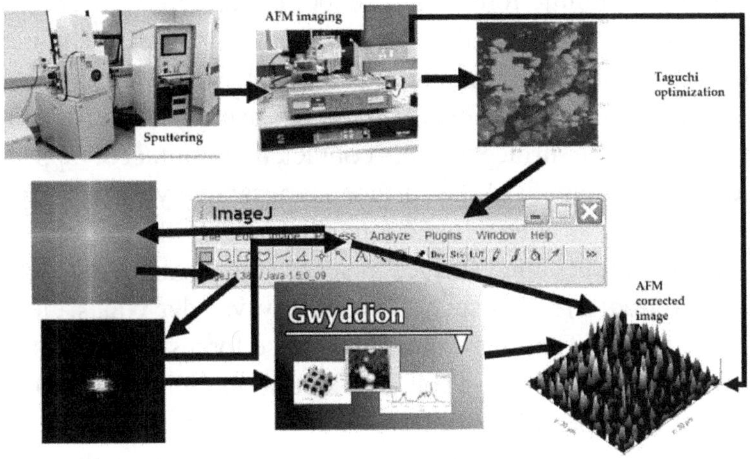

INTRODUCTION

Atomic force microscopy (AFM) is one of the scanning probe microscope (SPM) techniques that provides lateral information and heterogeneity of surface topography at the nanoscale level, and its resolution can reach atomic measurements for perfectly flat surfaces (Anandhan 2003). The major advantage of AFM microscopy over the other microscopy techniques (such as optical, SEM, TEM, etc.) is that it does not require the tedious surface preparation, and therefore, it finds applications in a wide spectrum of nanomaterials including metals, polymers, composites and biological materials (Bandyopadhyay 2008). The versatility of AFM technology is further enhanced by its capability to image in different media, including vacuum, fluid and gas environment and as such its application cuts across all disciplines from life to physical sciences and engineering. It is possible to capture the atomic arrangement or molecules of various surfaces; for instance, at images of 5 nm scale, the crystallographic structure of materials in both life and physical sciences can be studied (Eaton and West 2010). The other advantage of AFM is that it can image nearly all types of materials' surfaces; be it very hard (metals, ceramics or polymers) or soft (animal cells, very thin lone standing films or genetic molecules).

The above advantages are attributable to the unique design and operating mechanism of the atomic force microscope. Unlike, SEM, TEM or optical microscopes, which uses light to capture images, AFM scans ('touches') the surface of the sample under imaging (Eaton and West 2010; Jacobs, Junge, and Pastewka 2017). In operation, the AFM tip (usually having a radius range of 2-100 nm) scans the surface through contact, non-contact or tapping mode. The detection and imaging of the surface topography by the AFM probe are based on the concept of inter-atomic force distance as illustrated in Figure 1. As the tip nears the specimen surface, it senses the distance-dependent (also known as inter-atomic) forces such as a capillary, van der Waals, electrostatic and magnetic forces. The measurement of these forces in AFM is based on Hooke's principle (force as a product of deflection and spring constant of the AFM cantilever beam). As the tip scans over the surface, the resultant tip-sample forces make the cantilever to deflect according to the topography of the surface under analysis. The AFM assembly is fitted with position photosensors, which use a laser to detect any deflections and raster motions of the cantilever. Also, AFM facilities consist of piezo-vibrator that is meant to oscillate the tip at a range of frequencies or near the natural frequency for tapping mode operation.

To achieve accurate feedback from the raster scans of the AFM probe and cantilever deflections, the proportion-integral-derivative (PID) gains should be optimised during AFM imaging. Integral and proportional gains are the most significant PID controls for feedback optimisation in AFM imaging. Too low gain results in inaccurate control of the set point and poor surface tracking whereas too high gains lead to interference and hence electrical noise in the image. The feedback is also affected by scan rate of the probe as it determines the time of PID loop to adjust the feedback variables to the set point. Too fast scan rate means that the controller does not have enough time to adjust the variables to the set point and therefore the output topography values deviate from the actual measurements. Besides the PID controls, the quality of AFM imaging is affected by external factors such as non-linearity of the piezo-scanner, tip distortion to the sample and vibrations of the AFM facility (Bowen and Doneva 2000).

When the above factors are not controlled during AFM imaging, artefacts may arise and degrade the quality of information of the micrographs. Some of these artefacts can be noticed during imaging and avoided while others may never be noticed, and the user may end up analysing them as part of the surface features resulting in 'false' characterizations. AFM artefacts can be classified into five categories, namely scanner, probe, vibration, external noise

Figure 1. Illustrating force-distance curve for AFM (Bandyopadhyay, 2008)

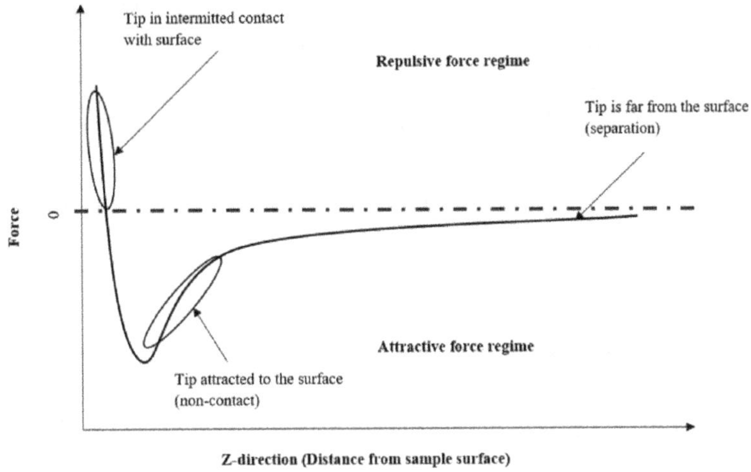

and image analysis artefacts (Eaton and West, 2010). The probe artefacts may be caused by the use of worn out tip and usually results in strange shapes of the topography (Eaton and West, 2010; Gołek, Mazur, Ryszka, & Zuber, 2014). Sometimes the image structures may appear falsely too large, small or too circular or irregular. Vibration from external sources such as buildings and acoustics cause disturbance onto the tip and scanner which may lead to that noise being registered as surface features. The vibrations can also be caused by the improper combination of PID controls resulting in poor tracking and hence producing artefacts on the AFM images.

These artefacts are more pronounced in thin films prepared through physical vapour deposition techniques than chemical methods because of relatively higher roughness (Jacobs, Jungle, & Pastewka, 2017). For example, the roughness of pure aluminium thin films deposited by radio frequency (rf) magnetron sputtering was shown to be more than 20 nm and containing structures having an average height of more than 350 nm (Mwema, Oladijo, Sathiaraj, & Akinlabi, 2018). Surfaces with high root mean square values are difficult to scan in AFM and therefore prone to artefacts. The paper uses a two-fold approach to deal with artefacts in AFM imaging of thin films and coatings: (1) Firstly, it illustrates the use of flattening, bandpass and fast Fourier transform filtering techniques to correct the artefacts and improve the morphological information of the AFM images. Such FFT filtering technique was earlier used by Bowen and Doneva (Bowen and Doneva, 2000) for pore correction in cyclopore membranes, but their procedure did not include flattening prior the filtering process as it is in the present case. (2) Secondly, the application Taguchi optimization method during AFM imaging of thin aluminium film is illustrated to show the best combination of parameters of AFM measurement to reduce these artefacts. The choice of Al films in this work is because of their application as interlayer for Ti-based alloys for medical applications (Garbacz, Wieciński, Adamczyk-Cieślak, Mizera, & Kurzydłowski 2010) and high roughness when deposited on metallic substrates (Mwema et al., 2018).

MATERIALS AND METHODS

The thin aluminium films used in this study were deposited by rf magnetron sputtering system which is part of the HHV TF-500 thin film deposition facility whose pictorial view is shown in Figure 2. The facility also houses thermal spray and electron beam deposition techniques. This sputtering system can form thin films on three substrates per run. The target material was 99.99% purity aluminium (circular plate with a diameter of 75 mm and 3 mm thickness). The sputtering was carried out for 2 hours for all the samples and allowed to cool inside the sputtering chamber for at least 12 hours. The details of this experiment were described in our earlier work (Mwema et al., 2018). The reason for the choice of the aluminium films in this case is because they are widely used as both functional films (biomedical interlayers, optics and microelectronics), and surface protectors against corrosion (Mwema, Oladijo, Akinlabi, & Akinlabi, 2018) and that aluminium films deposited by sputtering are prone to artefacts during AFM microscopy due to high roughness. Furthermore, the surface topography of these films was reported elsewhere in our work (Mwema et al., 2018), and therefore the results of that previous study can be used to validate the filtering procedure used here for correcting the artefacts in AFM micrographs.

Taguchi Method

The thin aluminium films' imaging was undertaken using Veeco Dimension 3100 AFM facility at scan sizes 30x30 μm, 5x5 μm and 1x1 μm at resolutions of 256x256 pixels. Further details of the AFM microscopy of this work is contained in reference (Mwema et al., 2018). For Taguchi optimization of the measurement process, the imaging was taken under varying scan rate, proportional and integral gain as indicated in Table 1. The Taguchi steps applied in this work to determine the optimal AFM measurement parameters are summarized in the chart in Appendix Figure 12. Taguchi method is a very powerful tool widely used in various fields of engineering and science to optimize systems and design of experiments. Through this technique, the number of experiments can be reduced significantly and the parameters for desired output can be determined. The reason for its choice in this work is because it minimises the number of the experiments or measurement undertaken in an optimization process and still provide reliable solutions to engineering problems. It uses loss function to compute the difference between the collected data and the expected output. From this function, the signal-to-noise (S/N) ratio of the data is determined for each combination of parameters (Kivak, 2014). Usually, there are three modes of Taguchi evaluations for any system performance, viz. lower-the-better; nominal-the-best and higher-the-better as detailed in the literature (Kivak, 2014). In this study, we used four factors (scan rate, scan size, proportional and integral gains) and three levels, resulting in a mixed level Taguchi L_{18} orthogonal array ($2^1 \times 3^3$) shown in Table 2. The choice of these parameters was motived by their significant influence on the AFM imaging and formation of artefacts. The objective of the analysis, in this case, was to minimize the artefacts in AFM images for aluminium films. The artefacts were evaluated by section analysis of the obtained images from which the average maximum height deviations (H) was computed for the artefacts. The maximum height of the artefacts was used as measure of size of the artefacts. As such, we used the *low-the-better* mode of quality analysis as represented by the equation (1) below.

$$\eta = \frac{S}{N} = -10\log\left[\frac{1}{n}\sum_{i=1}^{n} y_i^{\,2}\right] \tag{1}$$

where y_i is the H values computed from the AFM images in the ith experiment in the Orthogonal Array (OA) and n represents the number of measurements in that experiment. In this case, five H values were obtained for each experiment and the average determined for statistical accuracy.

Correction of Artefacts

The images with a higher density of artefacts were deliberately selected for this work to demonstrate data correction of the AFM images using flattening,

Figure 2. Pictorial view of HHV TF-500 film deposition apparatus

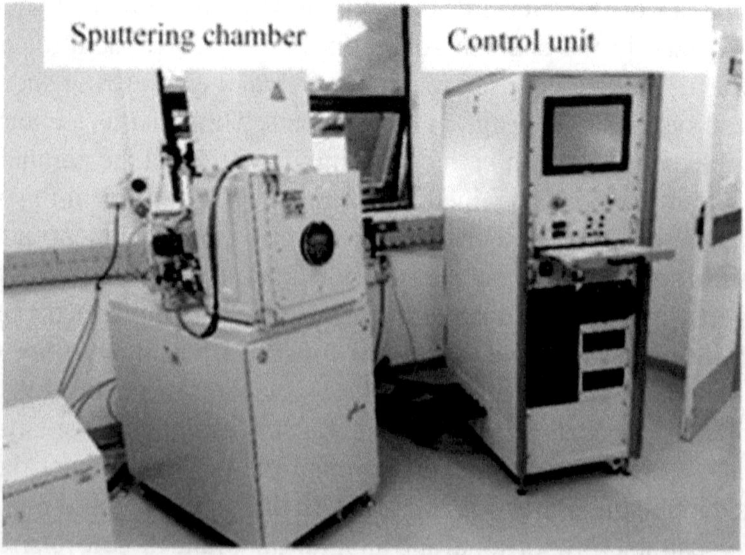

bandpass and fast Fourier (FFT) filtering techniques. The methodology of implementing the correction is illustrated by the flow chart in Figure 2. Further details of the specific image analysis functions used during this process are illustrated in the diagram in Appendix Figure 13. In principle, FFT decomposes images into waves (spatial frequencies) corresponding to various features of the real image. The FFT process produces a power spectrum of the image with the central white patch indicating low frequencies that corresponds to the large features of the image and dark background showing high-frequency region corresponding to finer details of the image (Buchko, Kozloff, & Martin, 2001). Sometimes bright features observed isolated (asymmetrical) on the power spectrum of the FFT image. These features are associated with peaks in the real image, and they could represent the actual periodicity of surface morphologies of the structures or noise of the image related to artefacts in AFM images (Bowen & Doneva, 2000). In the current work, bandpass and FFT filtering techniques have been implemented in image analysis to remove the asymmetrical features and noise from the power spectrum, thereby correcting the artefacts in AFM micrographs of thin aluminium films.

Table 1. Atomic force microscope measurement variables and their levels in tapping mode

Parameters	Symbol	Level 1	Level 2	Level 3
Scan rate (Hz)	SR	1	2	
Scan size (μm)	SS	1×1	5×5	30×30
Integral gain	IG	0.4	0.6	1.0
Proportional gain	PG	0.6	0.8	1.2

Figure 3. Image analysis methodology used for correcting AFM artefacts in this work

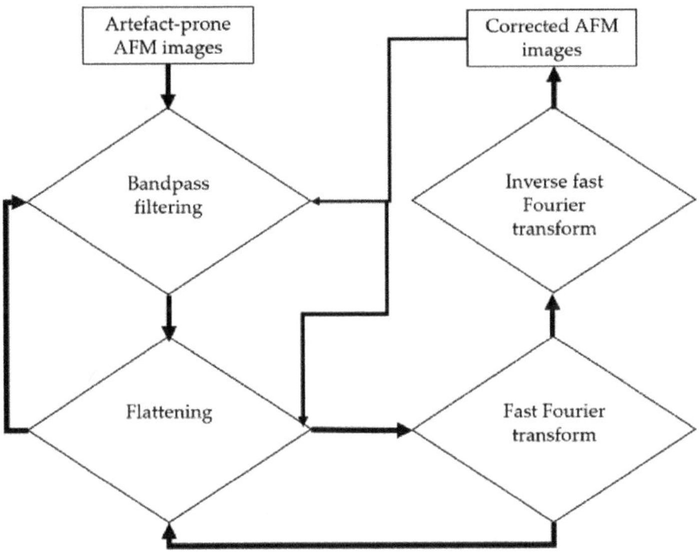

RESULTS

The results of this study are presented under two subsections, one for the correction of artefacts and the other for optimization of measurement, through Taguchi method, during AFM imaging.

Correction of Artefact-Prone Images

Figure 4 shows AFM images (30x30 μ m.) of thin aluminium films deposited on stainless steel substrates by rf magnetron sputtering at 150 W for 2 hours. These images were taken during the optimization stage of the AFM imaging.

Table 2. Factorial design of Taguchi L_{18} (2^1x3^3) orthogonal array

Experiment No.	Factor SR	Factor SS	Factor IG	Factor PG
1	1	1	1	1
2	1	1	2	2
3	1	1	3	3
4	1	2	1	1
5	1	2	2	2
6	1	2	3	3
7	1	3	1	2
8	1	3	2	3
9	1	3	3	1
10	2	1	1	3
11	2	1	2	1
12	2	1	3	2
13	2	2	1	2
14	2	2	2	3
15	2	2	3	1
16	2	3	1	3
17	2	3	2	1
18	2	3	3	2

The black arrows shown in the images indicate some artefacts. These artefacts are attributed to blunt tip apex and the improper parameters such as scan rate, tip amplitude/force, integral/proportional gain, etc., which causes poor tracking of the AFM probe in tapping mode operation. As reported in our earlier AFM analysis (Mwema et al., 2018) and in the literature (Mwema et al., 2018), aluminium films prepared through sputtering have considerably high roughness and very large scan size can lead to poor tracking hence causing such artefacts. Poor tracking resulted in vibrations of the cantilever leading to very high noise (shown by arrows) to be detected by the AFM scanner. These images were recorded at optimized PID controls more specifically the set point, integral and proportional gains as illustrated by the scope trace of height micrographs in Figure 4 (as inset). These images cannot be used for accurate measurement or qualitative analysis of the thin films due to the very high density of artefacts. To eliminate these artefacts and show the better morphology of the surface structures of aluminium films, flattening technique was used to process the images and then passed through a low-pass filter prior to fast

Fourier transform filtering. The corrected images are shown in Figure 5. Figure 5(a) illustrates the 3D image after flattening and bandpass filtering; in which the excess noise was removed. The corresponding FFT power spectrum of the image is shown in Figure 5(c) and it is observed that the spectrum is symmetrical but with very bright features (indicated by arrows) off the central region. The bright features represent the noise in Figure 5(a).

The FFT filtering, in this case, involved removing these bright features in the high-frequency regions of the image as shown in Figure 5(d). As shown, the occasional bright areas were iteratively filtered from the dark (high frequency) regions and then inverse fast Fourier transform (IFFT) was applied to produce a corrected image of the surfaces. The value of roughness on the corrected image (Figure 5(b)) was computed to be 29.96 nm, which is within the range (30.718±4.02 nm) reported earlier for the same sample from more accurate AFM images (Mwema et al., 2018). The morphological features are also similar to those observed in our earlier work on AFM analysis of the same samples (Mwema et al., 2018).

The similar procedure was applied to AFM image taken at scan size of 5x5 μm. of aluminium films deposited on mild steel substrates (Figure 6). The original AFM images had edge artefacts that mostly results in 'dragging' and elongation of the surface features. These artefacts mostly result in asymmetrical FFT power spectrum and filtering, in this case, involved removing the asymmetry with careful attention to the long wavelengths of the spectrum. The filtering removed the dragging effect of the surface features and clearer morphologies comparable to those reported from accurate AFM images of the films (Mwema et al., 2018). The roughness value of this image

Figure 4. (a) 3D and (b) 2D Tapping AFM images (30x30 μ.) of thin aluminium films prepared by rf magnetron sputtering. (Insert) shows the scope trace for the image

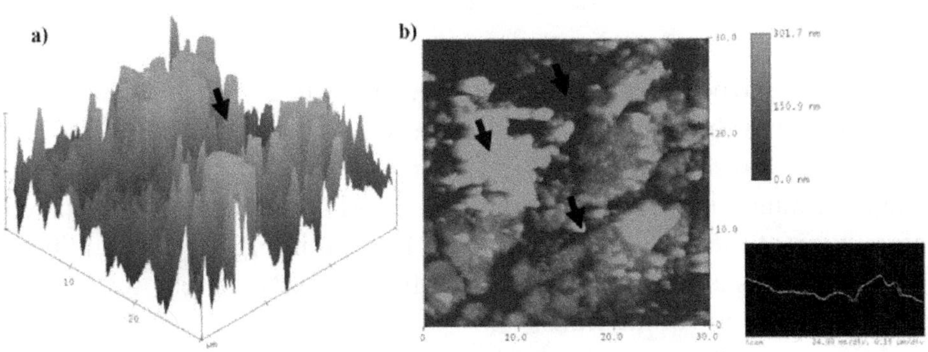

Figure 5. Illustrating fast Fourier transform filtering of AFM image shown in Figure 4

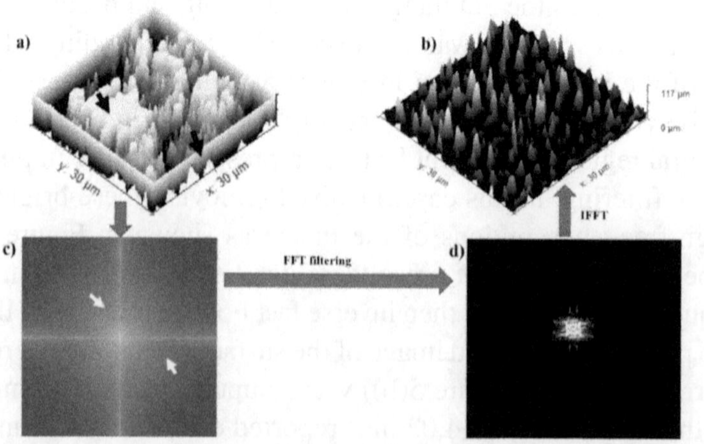

Figure 6. Fast Fourier transform filtering of 5x5 µm AFM micrographs of thin aluminium films on mild steel substrates deposited at 150 W rf power

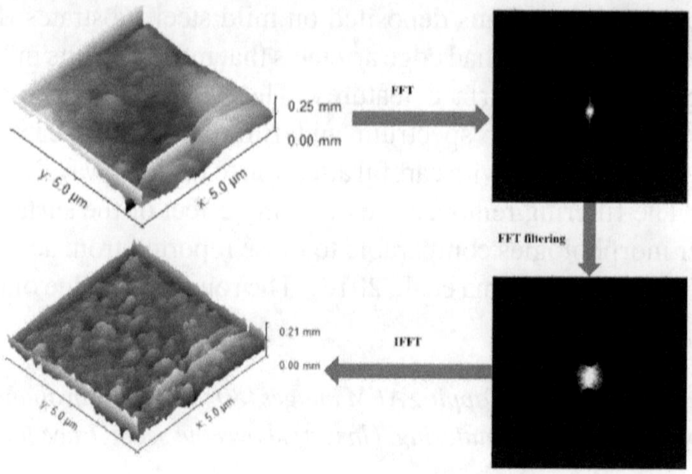

was computed to be 33.59 nm which is comparable to 27.59±6.84 nm, which was reported in the accurate AFM microscopy (Mwema et al. 2018). The technique was further applied in correcting the artefacts in 1x1 µm AFM images of aluminium films deposited on Ti6Al4V substrates and detailed information of the surface structures can be seen in Figure 7. In addition, the filtering was able to remove the scan line artefacts, thereby revealing a clearer morphology of the films.

Figure 7. Fast Fourier transform filtering of 1x1 μ. AFM micrographs of thin aluminium films on Ti6Al4V substrates deposited at 150 W rf power

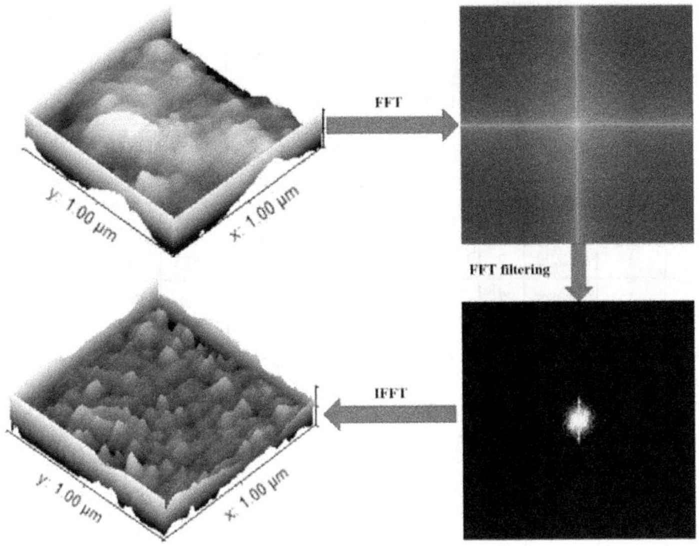

Results of Taguchi Optimization for Reduction of Artefacts in AFM Imaging

The maximum height deviation values (H) were determined from each combination of parameters according to Table 2 and the experimental values obtained, and their corresponding signal-to-noise ratios are shown in Table 3. The artefacts, in this case, were quantified by measuring the maximum height of the undesirable features for five different measurements for each experiment and the signal-to-noise ratios were determined from the means of the five measurements using equation 1 as tabulated in Table 3.

The influence of each AFM parameter (scan rate (SR), scan size (SS), integral gain (IG) and proportional gain (PG)) on the maximum heights of the surface artefacts was investigated using S/N response table shown in Table 4. The S/N response table shows the optimum levels of the measurement which gives the smallest values of the artefact quantity (H). These optimal levels are further illustrated by the graphs in Figure 8.

Table 3. Experimental results and S/N ratio values of the mean height deviations, H

Experiment No	Control Factors (AFM Parameters)				Height Deviations, H (nm) Measurements					Means of H Values (nm)	S/N ratio (dB) for Mean H
	SR (Hz)	SS (μm)	IG	PG	1	2	3	4	5		
1	1	1	1	1	120.0	106.0	102.0	98.4	94.5	104.18	-40.3864
2	1	1	2	2	84.3	88.4	82.4	79.4	80.1	82.92	-38.3798
3	1	1	3	3	150.0	150.3	140.4	120.9	112.5	134.82	-42.6517
4	1	2	1	1	83.0	88.4	89.2	92.7	85.3	87.72	-38.8682
5	1	2	2	2	89.0	90.3	98.1	100.3	101.1	95.76	-39.6360
6	1	2	3	3	84.8	79.1	85.3	89.1	88.1	85.28	-38.6242
7	1	3	1	2	120.6	119.3	123.5	126.1	115.6	121.02	-41.6610
8	1	3	2	3	125.3	120.9	128.5	122.4	125.1	124.44	-41.9011
9	1	3	3	1	129.5	130.8	125.9	128.2	130.2	128.92	-42.2072
10	2	1	1	3	87.4	93.2	94.1	92.5	88.1	91.06	-39.1905
11	2	1	2	1	86.5	90.1	85.0	86.1	88.6	87.26	-38.8182
12	2	1	3	2	89.5	80.3	88.9	90.0	89.2	87.58	-38.8557
13	2	2	1	2	104.1	103.8	104.0	103.6	104.5	104.00	-40.3407
14	2	2	2	3	114.5	113.4	115.6	117.1	114.0	114.92	-41.2085
15	2	2	3	1	118.9	115.6	116.9	118.0	119.4	117.76	-41.4205
16	2	3	1	3	127.1	128.9	130.1	126.9	126.4	127.88	-42.1366
17	2	3	2	1	130.5	128.5	124.6	135.4	130.1	129.82	-42.2700
18	2	3	3	2	159.4	160.5	158.9	159.3	158.9	159.40	-44.0498

DISCUSSION

Artefact Corrections

Through FFT filtering, different AFM artefacts such as those arising from external and internal noise, edge overshoot, light interference and tip inaccuracies can be corrected to achieve useful information from the image (Gołek et al., 2014). As illustrated in Figure 6, for example, the artefact arose from various sources and of which the most significant of all the other aspects where the light interference. In such cases, the FFT power spectra are characterized by asymmetrical peaks along either X or Y direction. To correct such image, the filtering process involves, therefore, removing those picks to make the power spectrum symmetrical and expose the actual features of the topography. A similar procedure was reported earlier for correction of artefacts o AFM images to reveal actual sizes of pores in membranes (Bowen & Doneva, 2000). The artefact correction procedures are iterative and should be done carefully to ensure the results are as close as possible to the expectations of the measurement. As reported in the literature (Eaton & West, 2010), image analyses processes can introduce artefacts to AFM images and therefore the correction process should be carefully observed to avoid creating rather than correcting the artefacts. The process of artefact correction maybe useful to samples of very high roughness such as aluminium films prepared through magnetron sputtering, silicon carbide prepared by evaporation and so forth. However, when many detailed analyses such as those reported by Ţălu, Bramowicz, Kulesza and Solaymani (2018) are to be undertaken on the AFM micrographs, it is advisable to obtain accurate images by optimizing the AFM measurement through Taguchi method as illustrated in this paper.

Taguchi Optimization of AFM Imaging

The Taguchi optimization on the effect of scan rate (SR), scan size (SS), integral gain (IG) and proportional gain (PG) on the maximum height of features considered as artefacts in the AFM images revealed the optimal combination of measuring parameters for reduction of artefacts (Figure 8 and Table 4). Figure 8 shows the plots of the means of signal-to-noise ratios for different parameters and levels. These plots provide a quick identification of the optimal levels for each parameter. The images with fewer artefacts were obtained at scan rate, scan size, integral and proportional gains of 1 Hz, 1x1 μm, 0.6 and 0.8 respectively at which the maximum height of the artefacts was the minimum (~ 82.92 nm). A confirmation experiment under these parameters was undertaken and the results summarized in Table 5. As Table 5 indicates, the five sets of measurements undertaken confirm the Taguchi methodology of reducing artefacts in AFM imaging. The use of maximum height (H) to indicate the size of surface features has been reported in the literature and it is undertaken through section analysis of the AFM micrographs (Mwema et al., 2018). The changes in the maximum height of artefacts with the AFM parameters are represented by contour plots in Figure 9, 10 and 11. As observed in Figure 9, increase in scan rate and size results in large sizes of the artefacts. The observation agrees with the results reported in the literature on AFM artefacts (Gołek et al. 2014; Shen, Dan, Fei, & Gan, 2018, 2017). The effects of integral and proportional gains are insignificant on the size of artefacts as compared to scan size and rate as seen in the contour plots.

However, proper choice of PID controls (integral and proportional gains) is crucial for optimum tracking of the probe onto the surface of the sample, that means that there is a specific combination of these gains at which artefact-free images can be observed (Bandyopadhyay, 2008; Hussain, Khurshid, Jianmin, & Hui, 2017). This is the reason for the oval-shaped central region seen on the contour plot for integral gain and proportional gain versus the maximum height of the artefacts. The oval shape indicates the region of the lowest height of the artefacts and it can occur anywhere depending on the nature of the surface under analysis.

Table 4. S/N ratios for each parameter

Levels	Scan Rate (Hz)	Scan Size (μm)	Integral Gain	Proportional Gain
1	**-40.48***	**-39.71***	-40.43	-40.66
2	-40.92	-40.02	**-40.37***	**-40.49***
3		-42.37	-41.30	-40.95
Delta	0.44	2.66	0.93	0.46
Rank	4	1	2	3

*The optimal levels of the AFM measurement parameters

Figure 8. Effect of scan rate (SR), scan size (SS), integral gain (IG) and proportional gain (PG) on the average S/N ratio for maximum height values (H) of artefacts

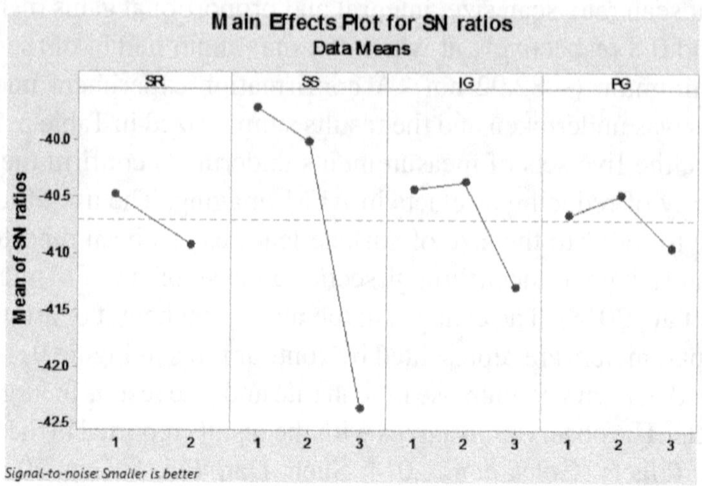

Table 5. Confirmatory experiment at the optimal parameters from the Taguchi modelling

Experiment No.	The Maximum Height of Features
1	90.1
2	79.4
3	81.9
4	80.8
5	81.6
Mean	82.76

Figure 9. Effect of scan rate, scan size and integral gain on the maximum height of artefacts features

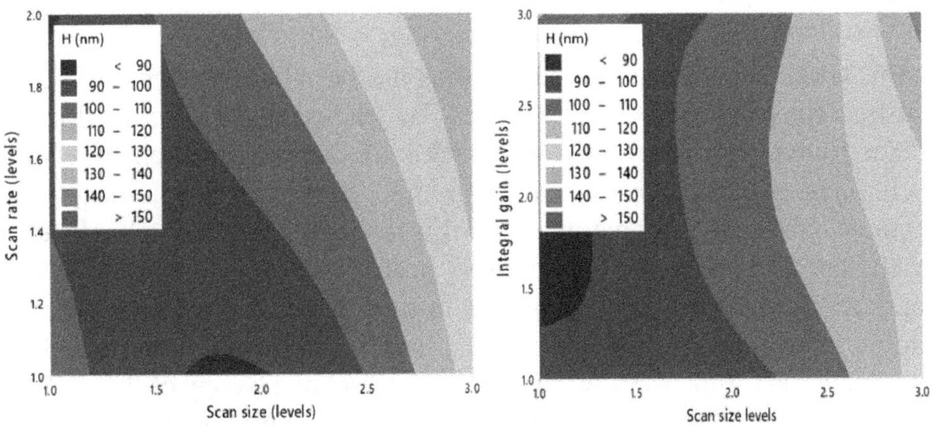

Figure 10. Effect of scan rate, proportional and integral gains on the maximum height of artefacts features

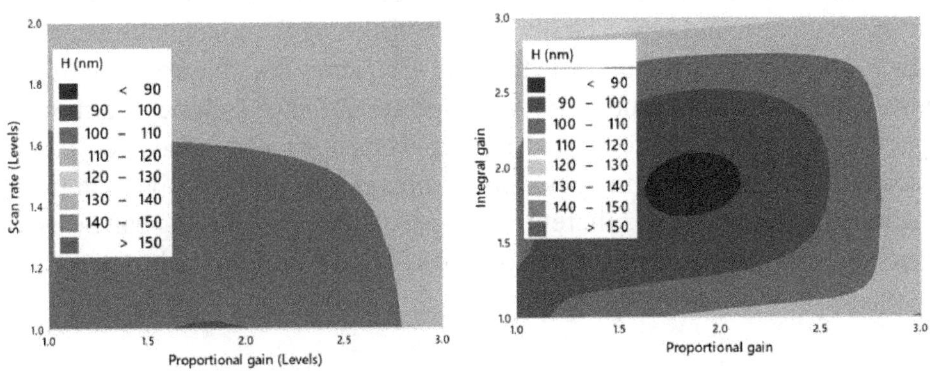

Figure 11. Effect of scan rate, scan size, proportional and integral gains on the maximum height of artefacts features

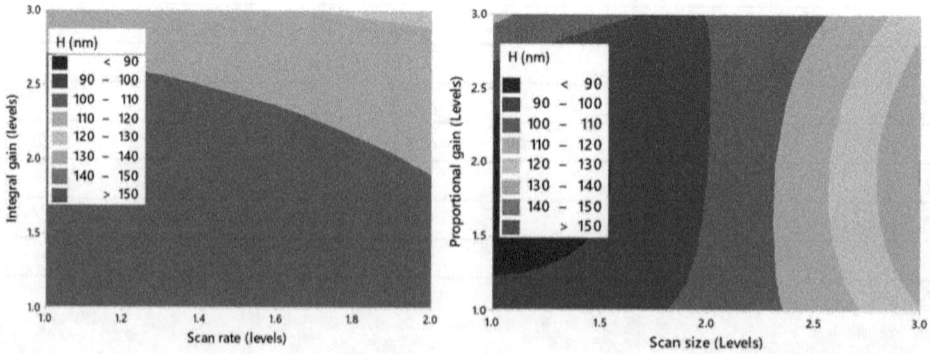

CONCLUSION

In this article, the thin aluminium coating has been used as a case study to illustrate the correction of artefacts in AFM microscopy. The reason for the choice of aluminium prepared by sputtering is that high roughness characterizes such films (when deposited on metallic substrates) and usually getting accurate nanoscale information in AFM is difficult. The work is motivated by the application of Al as interlayers in Ti-based alloys for biomedical applications and thin film conductors in sensors and microelectronics for various industrial uses. Choosing correct scan size of such films during AFM imaging is very important. As such, atomic force microscopy of these films is prone to artefacts leading to elongated features and noisy images. Such artefacts lead to asymmetry in power spectrum after fast Fourier transform of those images. The paper has shown that AFM artefacts can be corrected through flattening, bandpass filtering followed by fast Fourier filtering. It is illustrated that FFT filtering can correct the elongation of structures (artefacts) and scan lines. The objective of filtering is to isolate the central white low-frequency region from the high-frequency dark background of the power spectrum. An accurate AFM image should have symmetrical power spectrum about the white central region. The roughness values computed from the corrected AFM images were comparable with those obtained from accurate micrographs. It is therefore suggested that FFT filtering can be used to correct artefacts from AFM micrographs of thin aluminium films prepared by magnetron sputtering.

Optimization of AFM measurements by Taguchi method revealed that different combinations of parameters influence the sizes of the artefacts during AFM analysis of aluminium thin films. In this paper, the input parameters to the Taguchi method were scan rate and size, integral and proportional gains whereas the response was a maximum height of the artefacts observed from the obtained AFM images. The optimal scan rate, scan size, integral and proportional gains were obtained as 1 Hz, 1x1 μm, 0.6 and 0.8 respectively. At these conditions, the AFM images contained minimum artefacts (phase image shown in Appendix Figure 14). Further analysis of the individual influence of the parameters on the artefacts of the films revealed that scan size and scan rate were most significant parameters compared to integral and proportional gains during AFM imaging. From this study, we can recommend that Taguchi, analysis of variance (ANOVA) and full factorial designs of AFM measurements for different thin films should be studied to comprehend the influence of different AFM parameters on the quality of the obtained micrographs. Furthermore, more AFM parameters and different tips under different measurement mediums should be investigated for optimization of the AFM imaging process.

ACKNOWLEDGMENT

We acknowledge the University Research Committee (URC) of the University of Johannesburg for sponsoring the PhD student working on this research. The assistance of Mr. Maphane Phalaneng of Department of Physics and Astronomy at Botswana International University of Science and Technology (BIUST) is also acknowledged. Finally, we thank Microscopy and Microanalysis Unit (MMU) staff at the University of Witwatersrand, Johannesburg, for allowing us to access and use their AFM facility.

CONFLICTS OF INTEREST

The authors declare no conflict of interest. The work is part of the ongoing research by the PhD researcher and it is submitted according to the postgraduate and publication regulations of the University of Johannesburg.

REFERENCES

Anandhan, S., De, P. P., De, S. K., Bandyopadhyay, S., & Bhowmick, A. K. (2003). Mapping of Thermoplastic Elastomeric Nitrile Rubber / Poly (Styrene-Co-Acrylonitrile) Blends Using Tapping Mode Atomic Force Microscopy. *Journal of Materials Science*, *8*(13), 2793–2801. doi:10.1023/A:1024416031172

Bandyopadhyay, S. (2008). Applications of Atomic Force Microscope (AFM) in the Field of Nanomaterials and Nanocomposites. In S. Seal (Ed.), *Functional Nanostructures Processing, Characterization, and Applications* (pp. 504–568). New York, NY: Springer-Verlag. doi:10.1007/978-0-387-48805-9_9

Bowen, W. R., & Doneva, T. A. (2000). Artefacts in AFM Studies of Membranes: Correcting Pore Images Using Fast Fourier Transform Filtering. *Journal of Membrane Science*, *171*(1), 141–147. doi:10.1016/S0376-7388(00)00297-0

Buchko, C. J., Kozloff, K. M., & Martin, D. C. (2001). Surface Characterization of Porous, Biocompatible Protein Polymer Thin Films. *Biomaterials Biomaterials*, *22*(11), 1289–1300. doi:10.1016/S0142-9612(00)00281-7 PMID:11336301

Eaton, P., & West, P. (2010). *Atomic Force Microscopy*. New York, NY: Oxford University Press Inc. doi:10.1093/acprof:oso/9780199570454.001.0001

Garbacz, H., Wieciński, P., Adamczyk-Cieślak, B., Mizera, J., & Kurzydłowski, J. K. (2010). Studies of Aluminium Coatings Deposited by Vacuum Evaporation and Magnetron Sputtering. *Journal of Microscopy*, *237*(3), 475–480. doi:10.1111/j.1365-2818.2009.03297.x PMID:20500421

Gołek, F., Mazur, P., Ryszka, Z., & Zuber, S. (2014). AFM Image Artifacts. *Applied Surface Science*, *304*, 11–19. doi:10.1016/j.apsusc.2014.01.149

Hussain, D., Khurshid, A., Jianmin, S., & Hui, X. (2017). Advances in the Atomic Force Microscopy for Critical Dimension Metrology. *Measurement Science & Technology*, *28*(1), 012001. doi:10.1088/0957-0233/28/1/012001

Jacobs, T. D. B., Junge, T., & Lars, P. (2017). Quantitative Characterization of Surface Topography Using Spectral Analysis. *Surface Topography: Metrology and Properties*, *5*(1), 13001.

Kivak, T. (2014). Optimization of Surface Roughness and Flank Wear Using the Taguchi Method in Milling of Hadfield Steel with PVD and CVD Coated Inserts. *Measurement: Journal of the International Measurement Confederation*, *50*(1), 19–28. doi:10.1016/j.measurement.2013.12.017

Mwema, F. M., Oladijo, O. P., & Akinlabi, E. T. (2018). Effect of Substrate Temperature on Aluminium Thin Films Prepared byRF-Magnetron Sputtering. *Materials Today: Proceedings*, *5*(9), 20464–20473. doi:10.1016/j.matpr.2018.06.423

Mwema, F. M., Oladijo, O. P., Akinlabi, S. A., & Akinlabi, E. T. (2018). Properties of Physically Deposited Thin Aluminium Film Coatings: A Review. *Journal of Alloys and Compounds*, *747*, 306–323. doi:10.1016/j.jallcom.2018.03.006

Mwema, F. M., Oladijo, O. P., Sathiaraj, T. S., & Akinlabi, E. T. (2018). Atomic Force Microscopy Analysis of Surface Topography of Pure Thin Aluminium Films. *Material Research Express*, *5*(4), 1–15. doi:10.1088/2053-1591/aabe1b

Shen, J., Dan, Z., Fei, H. Z., & Gan, Y. (2017). AFM Tip-Sample Convolution Effects for Cylinder Protrusions. *Applied Surface Science*, *422*, 482–491. doi:10.1016/j.apsusc.2017.06.053

Shen, J., Dan, Z., Fei, H. Z., & Gan, Y. (2018). AFM Characterization of Patterned Sapphire Substrate with Dense Cone Arrays: Image Artifacts and Tip-Cone Convolution Effect. *Applied Surface Science*, *433*, 358–366. doi:10.1016/j.apsusc.2017.10.077

Ţălu, Ş., Bramowicz, M., Kulesza, S., & Solaymani, S. (2018). Topographic Characterization of Thin Film Field-Effect Transistors of 2,6-Diphenyl Anthracene (DPA) by Fractal and AFM Analysis. *Materials Science in Semiconductor Processing*, *79*, 144–152. doi:10.1016/j.mssp.2018.02.008

APPENDIX

The Taguchi steps applied in this study are summarized in the flowchart in Figure 12.
The iterative image analysis in ImageJ software for correction of the AFM images was undertaken based on the flowchart in Figure 13.
The phase AFM image of the optimized measurements from Taguchi method is shown in Figure 14.

Figure 12 Taguchi method steps used in optimization of AFM measurement

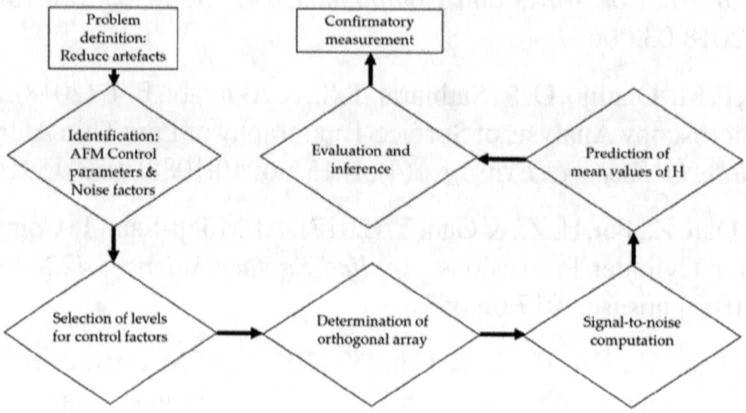

Figure 13 Image analysis procedure in ImageJ software used in this work

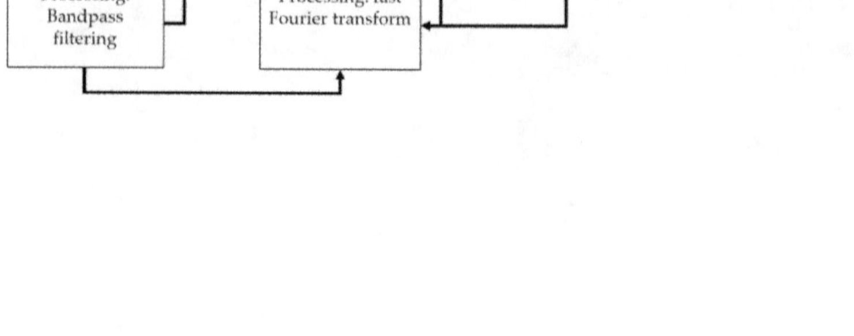

Figure 14 The phase image obtained at the optimal AFM conditions according to Taguchi optimization method in this work

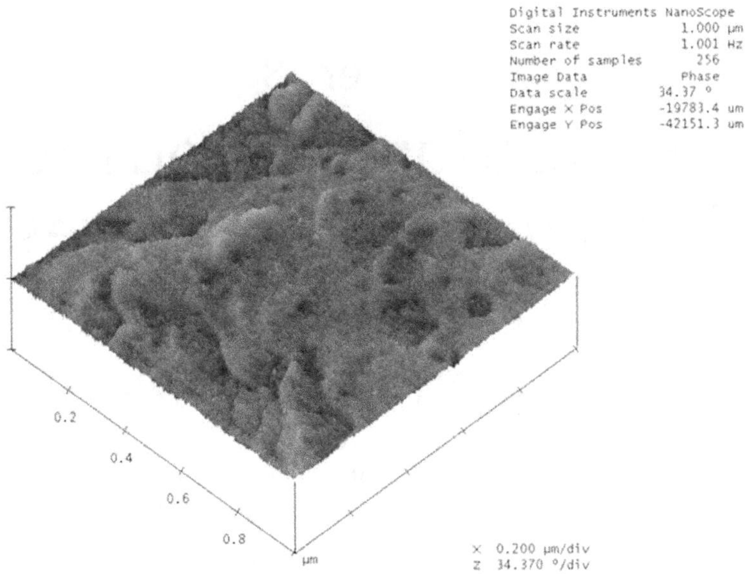

Chapter 8
Optimization Methods for Minimizing Induced Stress During Tensile Testing of Prosthetic Composite Materials

Kwame Anane-Fenin
University of Johannesburg, South Africa

Esther Titilayo Akinlabi
University of Johannesburg, South Africa

Nicolas Perry
Bordeaux University, France

ABSTRACT

The application of composite materials for prosthetic applications is the norm in recent times. Accurately characterizing the principal stresses during tensile testing is therefore essential. The low transverse compressive strength of most composite materials limits high clamping forces during tensile testing. Tabs are consequently critical for cushioning against grip pressure and surface damage. However, tabs tend to introduce induced stress concentrations. In this chapter, the induced stress concentrations are minimized via the optimization of tab design configurations. Stress concentration obtained via finite element analysis were used to develop a full factorial design for statistical analysis and compared with a Taguchi, Taguchi-multi response and Taguchi-genetic algorithm optimizations. It was established that to minimize the stress concentrations, low values of tab stiffness, thickness, and taper angle were required while the adhesive thickness was increased. The Taguchi and hybrid approaches were efficient and reduced the number of simulations from 32 to 8 (75% reduction).

DOI: 10.4018/978-1-5225-8235-9.ch008

INTRODUCTION

In the past decade, fibre reinforced composites have become the most notable materials for applications in orthotics and prosthetics. These composites are preferred due to their Lightweight, flexibility, corrosion resistance, fatigue resistance, energy storage, release properties ease of manufacture and aesthetics (Berry, 1987; Kadhim Oleiwi & Namah Hadi, 2016). Glass fibre over the years has consistently become the material of choice for prosthetic applications. Some of these applications include the manufacture of flexible composite keels, prosthetic limbs, prosthetic sockets and dental prosthesis. Recently Freedom Innovations introduced the Maverick™ Comfort AT, an all-terrain, fibreglass foot with an innovative Keel design which combines durability with flexibility (News Medical Life Science, 2017). Ali et al. (2016) also engineered a prosthetic limb for lower-limb amputees from glass fibre reinforced polymer composite and observed relatively good tensile and compressive properties.

Prosthetic sockets are designed to transfer a patient's weight to the ground by providing a structural interface between the human body and prosthetic part (Gerschutz, Haynes, Nixon, & Colvin, 2012). In industry, the standard procedure for fabrication of laminated prosthetic socket involves the application of acrylic polymer matrix to layers of a combination of conventional materials such glass fibre, carbon fibre, cotton or nylon around a mould (Campbell et al., 2012; Ganzert, 2012; Gerschutz et al., 2012; Phillips & Craelius, 2005; Slocumb, 2014). In accordance with industry standards, glass fibre is consistently regarded as suitable in relations to tensile strength (Campbell et al., 2012; Me, Ibrahim, & Tahir, 2012; Phillips & Craelius, 2005).

In dentistry, the most favourable reinforcement for resin composites are long continuous fibres placed on the tensile side of prosthetic components with the loading applied perpendicular to the fibre strands (Dyer, Lassila, Jokinen, & Vallittu, 2004; van Heumen, Kreulen, Bronkhorst, Lesaffre, & Creugers, 2008). Carbon fibre provides superior mechanical properties, however, the black appearance poses an esthetical disadvantage and therefore not favoured in the dental sector (Maruo, Nishigawa, Irie, Yoshihara, & Minagi, 2015). Glass fibre, on the other hand, provides not only enhanced mechanical properties but excellent biocompatibility, aesthetics and design flexibility for dental clinic or laboratory applications (Anusavis, 2013; Kanie, Fujii, Arikawa, & Inoue, 2000; Meriç, Dahl, & Ruyter, 2005; Vallittu, 2007). For the above reasons, Fibreglass is the most extensively utilized reinforcement in dental prosthesis.

The ability to correctly characterise the Principal forces and stresses within composite material used for the manufacture of orthotics and prosthetic products significantly assists in choice of the most appropriate material to meet the intended purpose (Berry, 1987). Tension and compression are the principal forces mostly considered. Conventional testing of the materials is carried out before and after manufacture. One of the primary tests for mechanical characterisation of composite materials is tensile testing. It is used to determine in-plane properties such as the modulus of elasticity, tensile strength and poison ratio of the considered material. The setup procedure requires the clamping of both ends of the sample with mostly serrated or coarse grips to limit slippage during testing. The application of axial loading, shear force and grip friction occur during the clamping (Adams, 2011;Adams & Adams, 2002; Alfano et al., 2011; Coguill & Adams, 1999). For most metals and their alloys, testing is carried out without the need for an intermediate medium between grips and test specimen. However, for fibre reinforced polymer composites such as non-crimp fabric composites, which characteristically possess low transverse compressive strength, tabs are a necessity (Alfano et al., 2011). The use of bonded tabs offers several advantages namely; high grip forces can be accommodated, and coarse grips which are required for friction can be used without the negative effects of surface damage and out-of-plane stress-induced damage. It must be noted that although tabs are standard practice, its presents some adverse effects such as the induction of high-stress concentrations at tab termination regions of test specimen during testing (Adams & Adams, 2002). Hart-Smith (1978) observed that the use and choice of tabs must be carefully considered or avoided if possible because it may not be necessarily better. The localised stress concentrations introduced during the use of bonded tabs can cause premature failures attributed to the reduced tensile properties of the specimen (Adams & Adams, 2002; Belingardi, Paolino, & Koricho, 2011; Hodgkinson, 2000; Joyce, Violette, & Moon, 2002).

Several tab geometric configurations have been proposed; these include the ASTM 3039/D3039M-14 (ASTM International, 2014) standards which advocates for the use of tapered tabs while the ASTM D5083 - 17 and ISO 527-1:2012 recommends the use of prismatic tabs. Belingardi et al. (Belingardi et al., 2011) proposed the use of a 30° bevel shaped tab design as it induced lower stress concentrations when compared with other designs. De Baere et al.(2009), observed that although tapered or chamfered tabs induced lower stress concentrations, the weak bonding between tab and specimen resulted in premature failures. Straight ended tabs were therefore recommended. Minimising induced stresses within the tab termination region through the optimisation of design and configuration parameters is critical to obtaining accurate characterisation results. For this reason, adoption of some statistical models developed for the analysis and optimisation of design and process parameters such as analysis of variance (ANOVA), regression techniques, multiple response optimisation, genetic algorithm optimisation and the Taguchi method can be exploited. The three optimisation techniques presented in this study provides validation to optimal solutions and alternatives for selection depending on the nature of the engineering problem. The complexity of the design problem determines which technique might be more suitable. For example, if the optimisation problem is no longer linear then a genetic algorithm approach might be most suitable for analysis. Furthermore, the study provides a comparative assessment of the complexities, advantages and limitation of each technique to serve as a guide.

MULTIPLE RESPONSE OPTIMISATION USING THE DESIRABILITY APPROACH

Multiple response optimisation techniques are superior as they are designed to overcome the limitations of the single response optimisations (Bhushan, 2013; Kuo, Li, & Wang, 2017). The desirability function is an integral component of the optimisation process, as it quantifies the optimal values. A gradient algorithm is employed to evaluate between a range of 0 and 1 the optimal desirability values (Balaji, Venkata Rao, Mohan Rao, & Murthy, 2018). Equations (1) – (3) are for evaluating individual desirabilities.

$$d_i = 0 \hat{y}_i < L_i \tag{1}$$

$$d_i = \left(\frac{\left(U_i - \hat{y}_i \right)}{\left(U_i - T_i \right)} \right)^{r_i} T_i \le \hat{y}_i \le U_i \tag{2}$$

$$d_i = 1 \hat{y}_i < T_i \tag{3}$$

The composite desirability which is the weighted geometric mean of all the individual desirabilities is calculated using equation (4):

$$D = \left(\prod\left(d_i^{w_i}\right)\right)^{\frac{1}{W}} \tag{4}$$

For cases where all responses have the same importance, the desirability is calculated using equation (5) as:

$$D = \left(d_1 \times d_2 \times \ldots \times d_i\right)^{\frac{1}{n}} \tag{5}$$

Where:

d_i = individual desirability for the ith response

D = Composite desirability

L_i = lowest acceptable value for i^{th} response

n = number of responses

r_i = weight of desirability function of ith response

T_i = target value of ith response

U_i = highest acceptable value for

w_i = Importance of ith response

W = sum of w_i or $\sum w_i$

$\hat{y}_t$ = value of ith response

Composite desirability (D) is used in assessing the optimal settings for a set of responses. The fundaments basis of this optimisation process was introduced by Derringer and Suich (1980). The desirability value lies between zero (0) and one (1) for which a value close to 1 is an indication of approaching acceptable responses from settings.

Multiple Objective Optimisation Using Genetic Algorithms

Genetic algorithms (GA) are classed in the evolutionary family of algorithms first developed by John Holland (1975) in accordance with Darwin's evolution theory. It is used to determine the optimal global solution for optimisation problems. To solve an optimisation problem, GA utilises the chromosomes of a population and not the decision variables. As such the decision variables are embedded within each chromosome for evaluating the objective functions. To ensure continuous production of new generations, selection of parent chromosomes for breeding based on fitness value is conducted with suitable candidates placed in a mating pool (Abarghooei, Arabi, Seyedein, & Mirzakhani, 2017). Production of new chromosomes is facilitated by the crossover operator which ensures that new offspring breeding is based on two by two (binary crossover) selection of parents (Affenzeller, Winkler, Wagner, & Beham, 2009; Sivanandam & Deepa, 2008; Sumathi & Surekha, 2016). Gene mutation of offspring is critical to obtaining an optimal solution as it introduces versatility within the new generation of the next population (Haupt & Haupt, 2004).

GA has superior advantages over many analytical methods available, mainly because it is not gradient based, and it inherently performs robust sampling of the model space (Yeng, Mahfouf, & Linkens, 2003). Furthermore, in comparison with other optimisation methods such as Monte-Carlo simulation, it explores sampling data using combinations, recombinations and crossover to provide better data fitting solutions.

Additionally, GA uses "the string" fitness approach to direct the search for a solution without requiring previous knowledge of the search space. GA is capable of handling diverse search spaces with noise, gaps and jumps. Noise dependency is minimised due to simultaneous searches from numerous points and directions within the search space by each string within the population (Goldberg, 1989; Gulsen & Smith, 1998; Tabassum & Mathew, 2014; Yeng et al., 2003).

Taguchi and Taguchi-Hybrid Methods

An optimisation based on the Taguchi method provides a powerful and unique process that is different from more traditional techniques (Wysk, Niebel, Cohen, & Simpson, 2000). In industry, it has contributed to the elimination of trial and error methodologies, reduction in manufacturing cost and a significant decrease in time loss. This has made the approach the focus of academic research and industrial applications geared at resolving quality and efficiency issues. The Taguchi design has widely been used as a powerful design tool for analysis in engineering. It significantly reduces the number of experiments using an orthogonal array design which minimises the influence of factors that are difficult to control. The Taguchi approach is a systematic and efficient method optimising manufacturing system parameters (Asiltürk & Akkuş, 2011; Kivak, Samtaş, & Çiçek, 2012; Palanikumar, 2011). The deviation between desired and experimental data is calculated using a loss function within the Taguchi method. Further conversion of the loss function to signal-noise (SN) ratio is then conducted (Asiltürk & Akkuş, 2011; Kivak et al., 2012). The lower-the -better, the higher-the-better and the nominal- the -best quality characteristics, are three conditions mainly used for the analysis of the SN ratio. It is determined from the S/N analysis for all levels of the process (Gupta, Singh, & Aggarwal, 2011; Kivak et al., 2012). The S/N ratio formulated as shown in equation (6).

$$\eta = \frac{S}{N_S} = -10\log\left[\frac{1}{n}\sum_{n}^{i=1} y_i^2\right] \tag{6}$$

Where n is the number of experimental or simulated observations and y_i is the *ith* experimental data observed (Mandal, Doloi, Mondal, & Das, 2011).

In a study by Abarghooei et al., (2017), the optimal parameter of a steady state stress semi-empirical model was determined by minimising the difference between model results and the experimental data using GA. Taguchi design of experiments (DOE) was used to generate the optimal GA parameters and combinations of parameters to improve the efficiency.

Kuo et al. (2017), performed multi-objective optimisation to determine the optimal parameter combination of cutting speed, feed rate and vibration frequency for drilling CFRP/Al stacks. They formulated a multi-objective model based on regression equations obtained from Taguchi analysis which identified the significant factors. Equal weights were assigned to each object implying equal importance.

Adams and Adams (2002) conducted a comprehensive study on the factors that affect the selection of tabbing materials, adhesives and tab design. The study also proposed a finite element methodology for analysing the stress concentration within the tab region. However, a robust approach to optimise the design configuration of tabs as a means for minimising the stress concentration was not adequately addressed. The most effective way of obtaining stress concentration is by finite element analysis (D. O. Adams & Adams, 2002; Belingardi et al., 2011; Hodgkinson, 2000). Therefore, this study utilises the FE approach proposed by Adams and Adams [2002] but further applies Taguchi DOE in combination with Multi-response and GA optimisations to develop a robust methodology suitable for the specific problem of tabbing but also adaptable for solving other parameter optimisation problems.

MATERIALS AND METHODS

Non-crimp fabric (NCF) composite plate manufactured by Chomarat was cut into sets of 0° and 10° fibre orientation test specimen for tensile testing in accordance with ASTM D3039. Rectangular tabs were fabricated from G-10 glass-epoxy with Hysol 907 two-part paste adhesive using the fixture shown in Figure 1. An MST Alliance RF/100 tensile testing equipment with a crosshead speed of 2mm/min and 100kN capacity was used.

Finite Element Analysis

Direct measurement stress concentration during testing is not possible. Therefore the only effective means is through the use of finite element analysis (Adams & Adams, 2002; Baere et al., 2009). The methodology proposed by Adams and Adams (2002) was used in this study. The finite element process is illustrated in Figure 2-4. G-10 glass fabric/epoxy with an elastic modulus of E=32.6 Gpa was selected as the low stiffness material, while the modulus of the tested non-crimp fabric composite E=132 Gpa was selected as the high stiffness material. A summary of the input parameters for the finite element analysis are presented in Table 1.

Figure 1. Tab bonding fixture

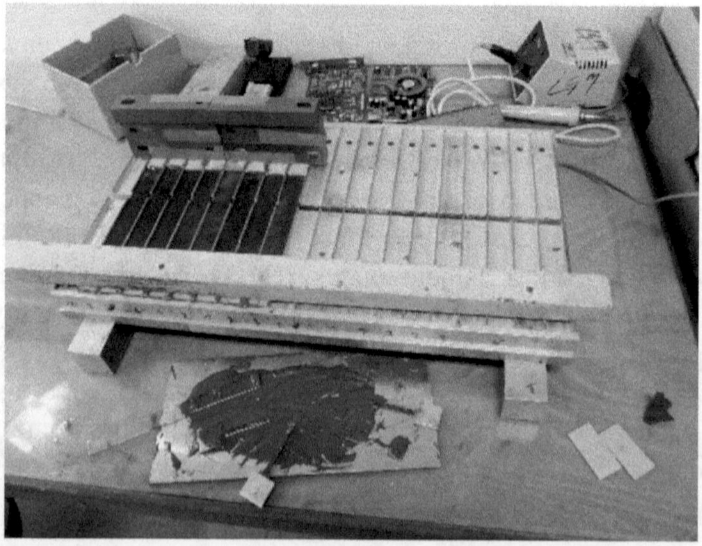

Figure 2. Finite element model configuration

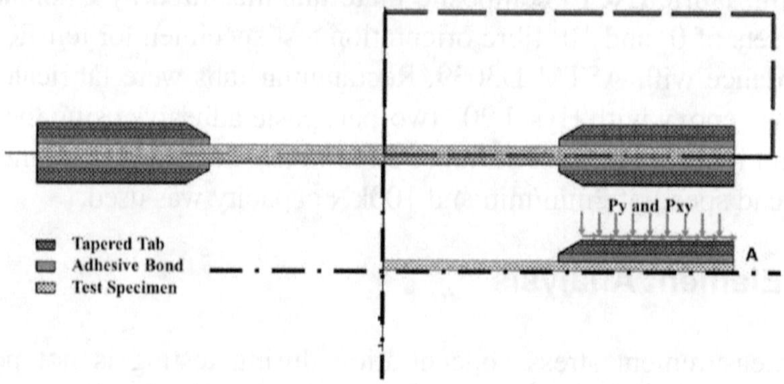

RESULTS AND DISCUSSION

Experimental Results

Mechanical characterisation after tensile testing of non-crimp fabric composite test specimen was achieved from the results of the tensile test as shown in Table

Figure 3. Bonded tab meshing

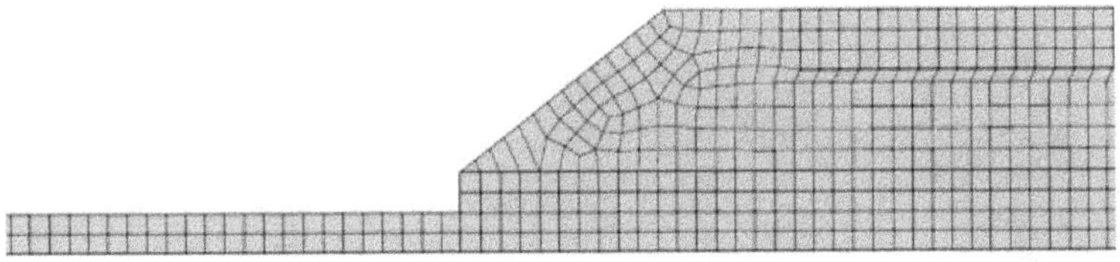

Figure 4. Finite element result showing the location of maximum stress concentration

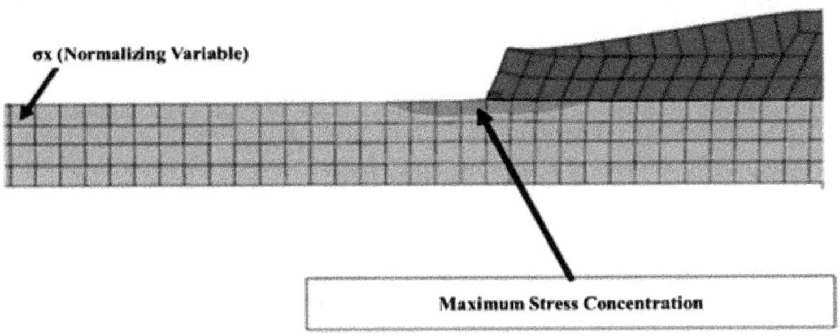

Table 1. Material input for finite element analysis

Material Properties	UD glass NCF-epoxy*	Tab Material (G-10 glass fabric-epoxy) **	Two-part Adhesive**
Ex (GPa)	132	32.6	3.17
Ey (GPa)	10	6.9	
Ez (GPa)	10	6.9	
Vxy	0.307	0.06	0.31
Vyz	0.307	0.06	
Vxz	0.307	0.06	
Gxy (GPa)	6.5	3.45	
Gyz (GPa)	66	10	
Gxz (GPa)	6.5	3.45	

*Experimental results from tensile testing
**Source [1]

2. The results were used as input for the finite element analysis. The stress-strain and shear (stress-strain) plots for 0° and 10° specimen are presented in (Figure 5 and Figure 6) and Figure 7 respectively. Figure 8 shows the shear failure of the 10° G-10 glass-epoxy specimen.

Figure 5. Stress-strain curve for 0° test specimen

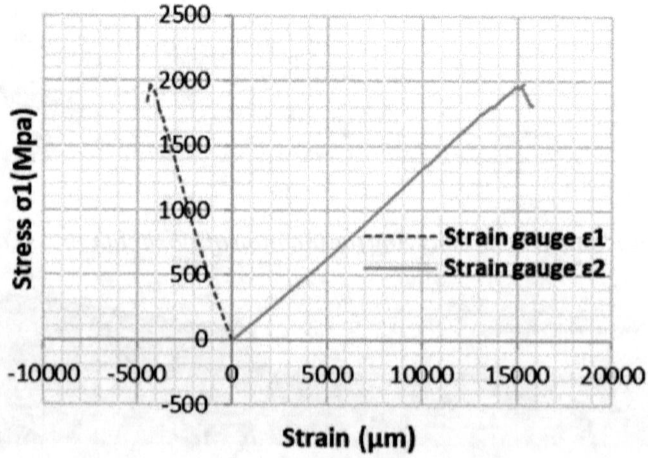

Figure 6. Stress-strain curve for 10° test specimen

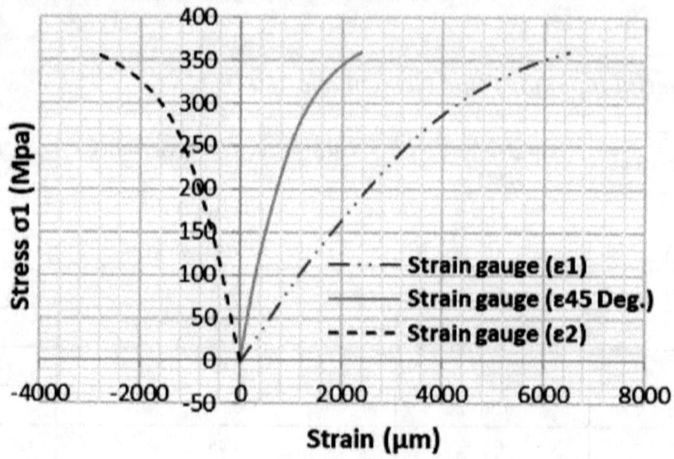

Finite Element Results

After conducting 32 simulations for a full factorial 2-level five-factor design, the normalised stress concentrations were obtained and summarised in Table 3. The design factors were Tab stiffness, Tab thickness, Tab length, Tab taper angle and Adhesive Thickness. The most significant factors were determined via analysis of variance (ANOVA). The P-values for each design factors were determined (See Table 4).

Figure 7. Shear (stress-strain) curve

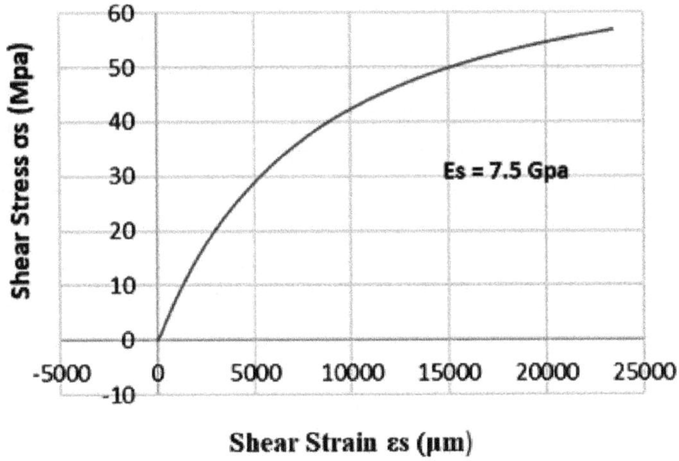

Figure 8. Shear failure of 10° specimen

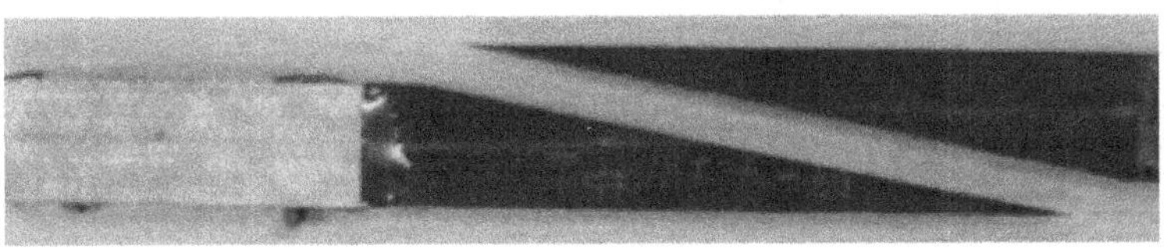

Table 2. Elastic properties of E-glass Non-crimp fabric

Composite	FVF (%) *	Ex (GPa)	Gxy (Gpa)	Vxy
UD-Glass/Epoxy NCF	71	132	7.5	0.307

*Fibre Volume Fraction

The P-values of each factor were determined using ANOVA to observe their significance in minimising stress concentration. The p-value results as summarised in Table 4 shows that the most significant factors that influence stress concentration for bonded tabs are in descending order are tab stiffness > adhesive thickness > tab taper angle> tab thickness > and tab length.

Table 3. 2-level factorial design

Tab Stiffness (Gpa)	Tab Thickness (mm)	Tab Length (mm)	Tap Tapper Angle (degrees)	Adhesive Thickness (mm)	σx_{max} (Normalized)	σy_{max} (Normalized)	τxy_{max} (Normalized)
32.6	0.5	50	90	1.5	1.193	0.070	0.038
32.6	1.5	100	90	0.25	1.394	0.126	0.084
32.6	1.5	100	90	1.5	1.251	0.104	0.057
32.6	1.5	100	5	0.25	1.151	0.045	0.031
32.6	0.5	50	90	0.25	1.297	0.079	0.053
132	1.5	50	90	1.5	1.329	0.133	0.072
132	0.5	100	5	0.25	1.500	0.145	0.096
32.6	0.5	50	5	1.5	1.201	0.082	0.045
32.6	0.5	100	90	0.25	1.285	0.083	0.055
32.6	1.5	50	5	1.5	1.199	0.081	0.044
132	1.5	100	5	1.5	1.339	0.147	0.079
32.6	1.5	50	90	0.25	1.402	0.123	0.082
32.6	1.5	50	90	1.5	1.244	0.096	0.052
132	0.5	50	90	0.25	1.591	0.164	0.108
132	0.5	100	90	0.25	1.596	0.174	0.116
132	1.5	100	90	0.25	1.655	0.198	0.132
32.6	0.5	50	5	0.25	1.151	0.045	0.031
132	1.5	100	90	1.5	1.346	0.145	0.078
32.6	0.5	100	5	1.5	1.195	0.079	0.043
32.6	1.5	50	5	0.25	1.151	0.045	0.031
132	0.5	100	90	1.5	1.313	0.130	0.070
132	0.5	100	5	1.5	1.328	0.142	0.077
32.6	0.5	100	5	0.25	1.151	0.045	0.031
32.6	0.5	100	90	1.5	1.197	0.076	0.042
132	0.5	50	5	1.5	1.338	0.147	0.079
132	1.5	50	5	0.25	1.505	0.149	0.098
132	1.5	50	90	0.25	1.651	0.191	0.127
132	1.5	50	5	1.5	1.342	0.148	0.080
132	0.5	50	5	0.25	1.501	0.148	0.098
32.6	1.5	100	5	1.5	1.198	0.080	0.044
132	1.5	100	5	0.25	1.505	0.149	0.098
132	0.5	50	90	1.5	1.299	0.119	0.064

Table 4. P-values for stress concentrations in bonded tabs

Factor	σx_{max}	σy_{max}	τxy_{max}
Tab Stiffness	0.000	0.000	0.000
Tab Thickness	0.117	0.010	0.020
Tab Length	**0.979**	**0.581**	**0.612**
Tab Taper Angle	0.001	0.000	0.001
Adhesive Thickness	0.000	0.000	0.001

Taguchi Optimisation Results

The Taguchi L8 (2^5) orthogonal array DOE was selected for analysis and shown in Table 6. The stress concentrations σx_{max}, σy_{max} and τxy_{max} were obtained from finite element analysis for all combinations of the design factors using Taguchi approaches. SN ratios were calculated for the optimisation of the factors. The factors and levels for optimisation are shown in Table 5. The resulting Taguchi design with corresponding stress concentration response values are presented in Table 7. Minimising stress concentration at the tab termination region is critical to preventing premature failures which contribute to inaccurate, inconsistent results and a significant reduction in measured tensile strength. The "lower-the-better equation was therefore selected for the computation of the SN ratios.

An SN response table was generated from the analysis of effects of the design factors as shown in Table 8. This Taguchi design table provides the optimal levels of each design parameters. Table 8 shows the values of the SN ratios for observations of the induced stress concentrations. The optimal tab design configuration required to minimise the combined stress concentrations σx_{max}, σy_{max} and τxy_{max} are presented in Tables 9. The highest S/N ratio of the level for the control factor was selected as the optimal level. All optimal

Table 5. Tab design parameters and their levels

Design Factors	Symbol	Level 1	Level 2
Tab stiffness	A	32.6	132
Tab Thickness	B	0.5	1.5
Tab length	C	50	100
Tab taper angle	D	5°	90°
Adhesive thickness	E	0.25	1.5

Table 6. Taguchi orthogonal array design [Taguchi $L_8\,(2^5)$]

Simulation no.	Factor A	Factor B	Factor C	Factor D	Factor E
1	1	1	1	1	1
2	1	1	1	2	2
3	1	2	2	1	1
4	1	2	2	2	2
5	2	1	2	1	2
6	2	1	2	2	1
7	2	2	1	1	2
8	2	2	1	2	1

Table 7. Taguchi DOE with response stress concentration values

Simulation No.	A	B	C	D	E	σx (norm)	σy (norm)	Txy (norm)
1	32.6	0.5	50	5°	0.25	1.201	0.0817	0.0449
2	32.6	0.5	50	90°	1.50	1.193	0.0701	0.0384
3	32.6	1.5	100	5°	0.25	1.198	0.0801	0.0440
4	32.6	1.5	100	90°	1.50	1.251	0.1039	0.0566
5	132	0.5	100	5°	1.50	1.328	0.1417	0.0767
6	132	0.5	100	90°	0.25	1.596	0.1742	0.1157
7	132	1.5	50	5°	1.50	1.342	0.1484	0.0803
8	132	1.5	50	90°	0.25	1.651	0.1908	0.1265

Table 8. The results of simulations and SN ratios values

No.	Control factors					σx_{max}	SN ratio for σx_{max}	σy_{max}	SN ratio for σy_{max}	τxy_{max}	SN ratio for τxy_{max}
	A	B	C	D	E						
1	32.6	0.5	50	5	0.25	1.20146	-1.59417	0.081713	21.7542	0.044865	26.9618
2	32.6	0.5	50	90	1.50	1.19333	-1.53519	0.070129	23.0820	0.038440	28.3043
3	32.6	1.5	100	5	0.25	1.19809	-1.56976	0.080150	21.9220	0.044028	27.1255
4	32.6	1.5	100	90	1.50	1.25070	-1.94305	0.103892	19.6683	0.056558	24.9501
5	132	0.5	100	5	1.50	1.32795	-2.46366	0.141730	16.9708	0.076705	22.3036
6	132	0.5	100	90	0.25	1.59594	-4.06035	0.174220	15.1781	0.115730	18.7311
7	132	1.5	50	5	1.50	1.34246	-2.55800	0.148434	16.5693	0.080278	21.9080
8	132	1.5	50	90	0.25	1.65100	-4.35493	0.190798	14.3885	0.126509	17.9576

values are represented with bold text. The main effect SN ratio plots for all three stress concentration and the global optimal are shown graph forms in Figures 9a -9d.

According to the results, the levels and S/N ratios for the design factors that minimised stress concentration at the tab termination region were specified as factor A (Level 1, S/N = 3.083), factor B (Level 1, S/N = 2.312), factor C (Level 1or Level 2, S/N = 2.212), factor D (Level 1, S/N = 2.679) and factor E (Level 2, S/N = 2.599). Therefore, for this specific material, to minimise the overall stress concentration induced by the bonded tabs during tensile testing, the optimum tab design configuration was obtained with a tab stiffness of 32.6 Gpa, tab thickness of 50mm, Tab length at either 50mm or 100mm, tab taper angle of 5° and adhesive thickness of 1.5mm. From the main effect plots (Figure 9a-d) it is clear that the most influential factors are tab stiffness, tab taper angle and adhesive thickness.

Taguchi–Multiple Response Optimisation Using Desirability Results

The desirability approach to optimisation of the tab design configuration was carried out using Table 7 as the Taguchi DOE. The optimisation parameters with the corresponding weights are shown in Table 10. The calculated optimal design configuration is presented in Table 11 and the composite desirability plot is shown in Figure 10 (optimal values are in red).

Table 9. SN response table for the combined stress concentrations (σx_{max}, σy_{max}, τxy_{max})

Levels	Control factors (σx_{max}, σy_{max}, τxy_{max})				
	A	B	C	D	E
	Tab Stiffness	Tab Thickness	Tab Length	Tab Taper Angle	Adhesive Thickness
Level 1	**3.083**	**2.312**	**2.212**	**2.679**	14
Level 2	1.340	2.111	**2.212**	1.744	**2.599**
Delta	1.743	0.201	0.000	0.935	0.774
Rank	1	4	5	2	3

Bold values show the optimal levels of design factors.

Figure 9. SN main effects plots for (a) $\boldsymbol{\sigma} x_{max}$ *(b)* $\boldsymbol{\sigma} x_{max}$ *(c)* $\boldsymbol{\sigma} x_{max}$ *(d) global main effect*

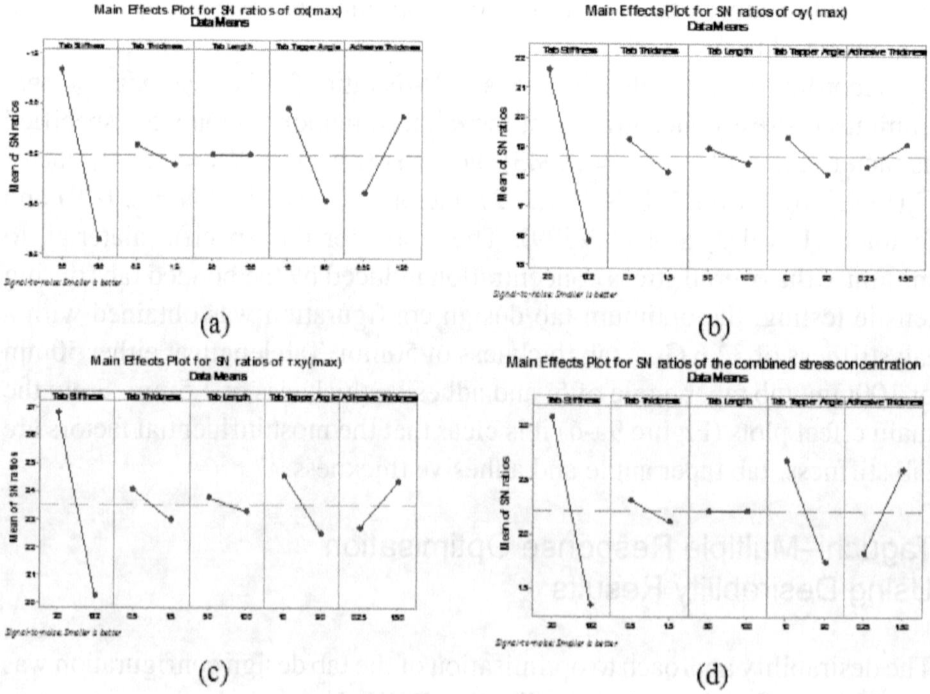

Table 10. Optimization parameters

Response	Goal	Target	Upper	Weight	Importance
τxy (Norm)	Minimum	0.03844	0.12651	1	1
σy (Norm)	Minimum	0.07013	0.19080	1	1
σx (Norm)	Minimum	1.19333	1.65100	1	1

Table 11. Multiple Response Prediction (Optimized configuration)

Variable	Optimal Tab Configuration
Tab Stiffness	32.6 (Gpa)
Tab Thickness	0.5 (mm)
Tab Length	100 (mm)
Tab Taper Angle	5°
Adhesive Thickness	1.5 (mm)

Figure 10. Composite desirability plot

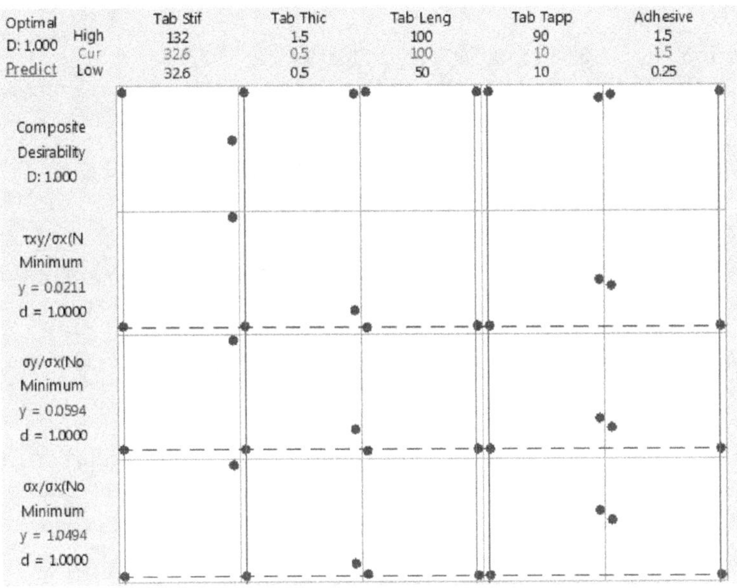

The aim of using the desirability approach for conducting the multiple response optimisation was to obtain a composite desirability close to or equal to 1. To ensure that all factors were of equal importance and weight, a value of 1 was assigned to each of them as observed in Table 11. The goal of the analysis was to minimise the three stress concentrations. From table 12 and, the optimal design configuration for minimising the stress concentration was tab stiffness (32.6 GPa), Tab thickness (0.5mm), tab length (50mm), tab taper angle (5°) and adhesive thickness (1.5mm). The desirability value for all three stress concentrations was 1. Therefore, the composite desirability for the analysis was 1 as shown in Figure 10.

Taguchi–Genetic Algorithm Optimisation Results

The regression equations for the three induced stresses obtained from the Taguchi L_8 (2^5) DOE were used as the objective functions for running a multi-objective optimisation using GA. The formulation of the optimisation problem is presented below:

```
(1) - Tab stiffness
x(2) - Tab thickness
x(3) - Tab length
```

```
x(4) - Tab taper angle
x(5) - Adhesive thickness
Lower bound = [32.6 0.5 50 5⁰ 0.25 1]
Upper bound = [132 1.5 100 90⁰ 1.5 1]
```

$$y\left(1\right) = Objective1 - -equationfor\sigma x\left(Norm\right)minimize$$

$$y\left(1\right) = 1.1678 + 0.001220x\left(1\right) + 0.0309x\left(2\right) - 0.000078x\left(3\right) + 0.001827x\left(4\right) - 0.1064x\left(5\right)$$

$$y\left(2\right) = Objective2 - -equation\ for\ \sigma y\left(Norm\right)minimize$$

$$y\left(2\right) = 0.0583 + 0.000363x\left(1\right) + 0.01387x\left(2\right)0.000045x\left(3\right) + 0.000256x\left(4\right) - 0.01254x\left(5\right)$$

$$y\left(3\right) = Objective3 - -equation\ for\ \tau xy\left(Norm\right)minimize$$

$$y\left(3\right) = 0.0332 + 0.000245x\left(1\right) + 0.00791x\left(2\right) + 0.000015x\left(3\right) + 0.000269x\left(4\right) - 0.01583x\left(5\right)$$

The objective function value at the solution were observed as Func 1 [1.049491143, 0.053284701], Func 2 [0.057215173, 0.059403764] and Func [0.020405058, 0.021134588] as shown in Figure 11a. The average distance described in Figure 11b is 0.00107454444268082, while the average spread shown in Figure 11c is 0.541749461994625. The optimal solution was attained after 105 generations. A summary of the optimal design parameters are presented in Table 12. A comparison of results from the optimisation techniques discussed is summarised in Table 13.

The optimal results were quickly and easily obtained as the problem was linear. The optimal configuration found to be tab stiffness (32.6 GPa), Tab thickness (0.5mm), tab length (50mm or 100mm), tab taper angle (5°) and adhesive thickness (1.5mm) as shown in Table 12.

A comparison of all the three optimisation techniques as shown in Table 13 reveals that the results were similar and in agreement with the P-values obtained from ANOVA. Therefore, in general, to minimise stress concentration induced by bonded tabs, low stiffness, taper angle and high adhesive thickness is recommended (Adams & Adams, 2002). Although a low stiffness value is preferable, it must carefully be selected so not to be too compliant as to

Figure 11. (a) Optimal Objective function (b) Average distance between individuals (c) Average Spread

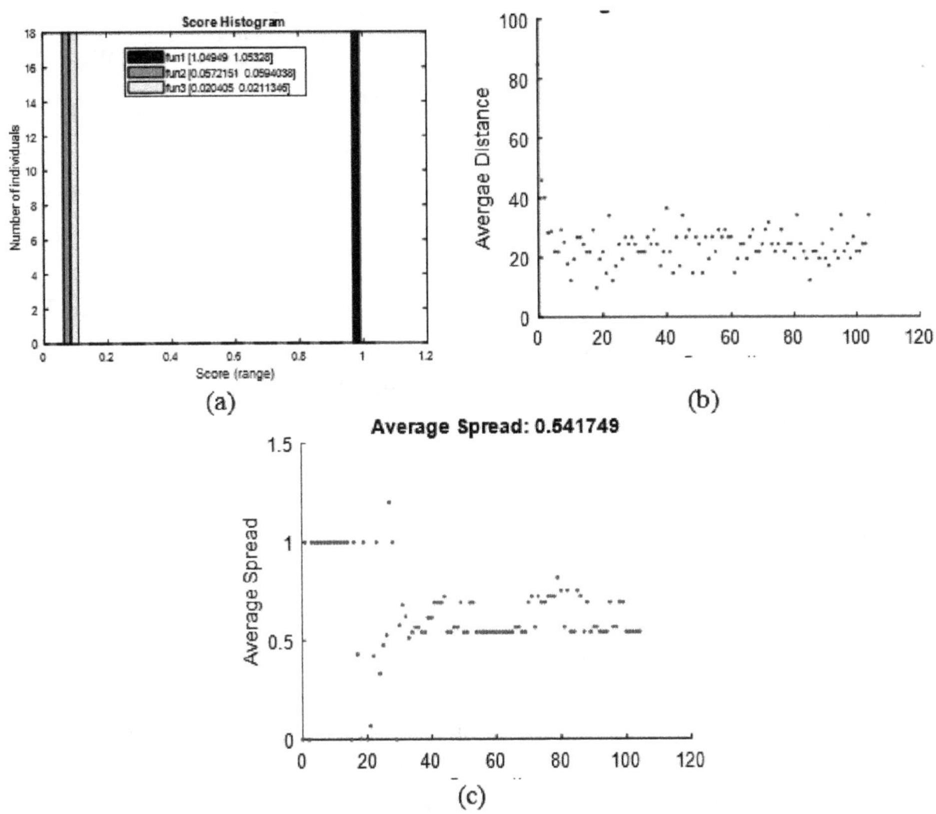

Table 12. Optimal solution for design parameters using Taguchi-GA hybrid approach

Obj. Fun 1	Obj. Fun 2	Obj. Fun 3	Tab Stiffness	Tab Thickness	Tab Length	Tap Tapper Angle	Adhesive Thickness
1.053284	0.057215	0.020405	32.6	0.5	50.004	5	1.5
1.049491	0.059404	0.021135	32.6	0.5	98.639	5	1.5

cause tab failure during tensile testing. G-10 glass-epoxy is very compliant and therefore suitable for use as tabs, it is also stiff enough to prevent tab failure during testing. It is also observed that for the Taguchi and Taguchi-GA approaches both 50mm and 100mm tab lengths were acceptable. This is supported by the p-values for tab length for all three stress concentrations; σx_{max} (P=0.979), σy_{max} (P=0.581) and τxy_{max} (P=0.612). All the p-values were

Table 13. Comparison of all optimization techniques

Optimisation Method	Design Parameters				
	Tab Stiffness	Tab Thickness	Tab Length	Tab Taper Angle	Adhesive Thickness
Taguchi	32.6	0.5	**50/100**	5°	1.5
Taguchi – MRO	32.6	0.5	50	5°	1.5
Taguchi – GA	32.6	0.5	**50/100**	5°	1.5

MRO: Mulit-Response Optimisation

above 0.05 and hence not significant to minimising stress concentration. The same can be implied about tab thickness, especially for $\boldsymbol{\sigma}x_{max}$. The general rule of thumb in practice is to select a tab thickness that is 1 to 4 times the sample (Adams & Adams, 2002; Chamis & Sinclair, 1977)

This study shows that all three optimisation techniques are equally efficient in optimizing the design parameters for bonded tabs. Furthermore, the Taguchi and Taguchi-desirability approaches are the simplest to use while the Taguchi-GA approach can solve both linear and non-linear problems and very efficient. However, although the desirability approach is simple to use, the accuracy of the solution depends on the weight and importance assigned to the factors. The main advantage of implementing the Taguchi DOE was to reduce the number of simulations or experimentation required. For this study 32 simulations were required however, the Taguchi DOE reduced it to only eight (8) simulations that did not affect the outcome of the analysis; this a 75% reduction.

CONCLUSION

Three optimisation techniques namely, Taguchi, Taguchi-Multiple response using desirability and Taguchi-GA were considered in this study to determine the optimal tab design properties required for minimising stress concentration during tensile testing. All three methods showed that the overall induced stress concentration could be reduced when low stiffness and taper angle with a high adhesive thickness is used. Taguchi DOE was utilised to significantly reduce the number of simulations by 75% without compromising the analysis. The Taguchi and Taguchi-Desirability optimisations were the simplest to adopt however, the Taguchi-GA approach is the most versatile as it suitable for both linear and non-linear problem. These methods can be modified for solving many engineering optimisation problems.

REFERENCES

Abarghooei, H., Arabi, H., Seyedein, S. H., & Mirzakhani, B. (2017). Modeling of steady state hot flow behavior of API-X70 microalloyed steel using genetic algorithm and design of experiments. *Applied Soft Computing*, *52*, 471–477. doi:10.1016/j.asoc.2016.10.021

Adams, D. (2011). Tabbing composite test specimens: When and why. *High-Performance Composites, 19*(2).

Adams, D. O., & Adams, D. F. (2002). *Tabbing Guide for Composite Test Specimens*. Retrieved from http://www.dtic.mil/docs/citations/ADA411472

Affenzeller, M., Winkler, S., Wagner, S., & Beham, A. (2009). Genetic Algorithms and Genetic Programming. *Simulation, 20093626*. doi:10.1201/9781420011326

Alfano, M., Furgiuele, F., Rangarajan, R., Lew, A. J., Krull, B., & Patrick, J., … Donald F. Adams. (. (2011). Tabbing Guide for Composite Test Specimens. *Composite Joints and Connections*, *40*(April), 341–362. doi:10.1533/9780857094926.2.341

Ali, A. H. M., Shlaby, M. S., & Elfaki, E. F. (2016). Mechanical properties of the prosthesis limp from PVC glass fiber sandwich. *International Journal of Mechanical And Production Engineering*, *4*(5), 41–45.

Anusavis, K. (2013). Mechanical properties of dental materials. In K. J. Anusavice, C. Shen, & H. R. Rawls (Eds.), *Phillips' science of dental materials* (12th ed.; pp. 48–68). St.Louis: Elsevier Inc.

Asiltürk, I., & Akkuş, H. (2011). Determining the effect of cutting parameters on surface roughness in hard turning using the Taguchi method. *Measurement: Journal of the International Measurement Confederation*, *44*(9), 1697–1704. doi:10.1016/j.measurement.2011.07.003

ASTM D5083 - 17. (n.d.). *ASTM D5083 - 17 Standard Test Method for Tensile Properties of Reinforced Thermosetting Plastics Using Straight-Sided Specimens*. Retrieved from https://www.astm.org/Standards/D5083.htm

ASTM International. (2014). ASTM D3039/D3039M-14 Standard Test Method for Tensile Properties of Polymer Matrix Composite Materials. *Annual Book of ASTM Standards*, 1–13. doi:10.1520/D3039

Balaji, M., Venkata Rao, K., & Rao, M. (2015, August). N., & Murthy, B. S. N. (2018). Optimization of drilling parameters for drilling of TI-6Al-4V based on surface roughness, flank wear and drill vibration. *Measurement: Journal of the International Measurement Confederation*, *114*, 332–339. doi:10.1016/j.measurement.2017.09.051

Belingardi, G., Paolino, D. S., & Koricho, E. G. (2011). Investigation of influence of tab types on tensile strength of E-glass/epoxy fiber reinforced composite materials. Procedia Engineering, 10, 3279–3284. doi:10.1016/j.proeng.2011.04.541

Berry, D. A. (1987). Composite Materials for Orthotics and Prosthetics. *Journal of Prosthetists and Orthotics*.

Bhushan, R. K. (2013). Multiresponse Optimization of Al Alloy-SiC Composite Machining Parameters for Minimum Tool Wear and Maximum Metal Removal Rate. *Journal of Manufacturing Science and Engineering*, *135*(2), 021013. doi:10.1115/1.4023454

Campbell, A. I., Sexton, S., Schaschke, C. J., Kinsman, H., McLaughlin, B., & Boyle, M. (2012). Prosthetic limb sockets from plant-based composite materials. *Prosthetics and Orthotics International*, *36*(2), 181–189. doi:10.1177/0309364611434568 PMID:22307862

Chamis, C. C., & Sinclair, J. H. (1977). Ten-deg Off-axis Test for Shear Properties in Fiber Composites. *Experimental Mechanics*, *17*(9), 339–346. doi:10.1007/BF02326320

Coguill, R. J., & Adams, D. F. (1999). Selection of the proper wedge grip surface for tensile testing composite materials. In *International SAMPE Symposium and Exhibition (Proceedings)* (Vol. 44). Retrieved from http://www.scopus.com/inward/record.url?eid=2-s2.0-0033309663&partnerID=tZOtx3y1

De Baere, I., Van Paepegem, W., & Degrieck, J. (2009). On the design of end tabs for quasi-static and fatigue testing of fibre-reinforced composites. *Polymer Composites*, *30*(4), 381–390. doi:10.1002/pc.20564

Derringer, G., & Suich, R. (1980). Simultaneous-Optimization of Several Response Variables. *Journal of Quality Technology*, *12*(4), 214–219. doi:10.1080/00224065.1980.11980968

Dyer, S. R., Lassila, L. V. J., Jokinen, M., & Vallittu, P. K. (2004). Effect of fiber position and orientation on fracture load of fiber-reinforced composite. *Dental Materials*, *20*(10), 947–955. doi:10.1016/j.dental.2003.12.003 PMID:15501323

Ganzert, C. (2012). *Basalt: An investigation into a new Prosthetic & Orthotic material option.* Academic Press.

Gerschutz, M. J., Haynes, M. L., Nixon, D., & Colvin, J. M. (2012). Strength evaluation of prosthetic check sockets, copolymer sockets, and definitive laminated sockets. *Journal of Rehabilitation Research and Development*, *49*(3), 405. doi:10.1682/JRRD.2011.05.0091 PMID:22773200

Goldberg, D. E. (1989). *Genetic Algorithms in Search, Optimization, and Machine Learning*. Addison Wesley; doi:10.100710589-009-9261-6

Gulsen, M., & Smith, A. (1998). *A Hierarchical Genetic Algorithm for System Identification and Curve Fitting with a Supercomputer Implementation.* Academic Press.

Gupta, A., Singh, H., & Aggarwal, A. (2011). Taguchi-fuzzy multi output optimization (MOO) in high speed CNC turning of AISI P-20 tool steel. *Expert Systems with Applications*, *38*(6), 6822–6828. doi:10.1016/j.eswa.2010.12.057

Hart-Smith, L. (1978). Mechanically-Fastened Joints for Advanced Composites -Phenomenological Consideration and Simple Analyses. In E. M. Lenoe, D. W. Oplinger, & J. J. Burke (Eds.), *Fourth Conference on Fibrous Composites in Structural Design* (pp. 543–574). San Diego, CA: Plenum Press.

Haupt, R. L., & Haupt, S. E. (2004). *Practical Genetic Algorithms* (2nd ed.). Practical Genetic Algorithms. doi:10.1002/0471671746.fmatter

Hodgkinson, J. M. (2000). *Mechanical testing of advanced fibre composites*. CRC Press.

Holland, J. H. (1975). *Adaptation in Natural and Artificial Systems*. University of Michigan Press. doi:10.1137/1018105

ISO 527-1:2012. (n.d.). *ISO 527-1:2012 - Plastics -- Determination of tensile properties -- Part 1: General principles*. Retrieved September 28, 2017, from https://www.iso.org/standard/56045.html

Joyce, P. J., Violette, M. G., & Moon, T. J. (2002). Finite element analysis of unidirectional composite compression test specimens: A parametric study. *Composite Materials: Testing, Design, and Acceptance Criteria, 1416*, 30–68.

Kadhim Oleiwi, J., & Namah Hadi, A. (2016). *Design of Prosthetic Foot from Polymer Materials Reinforced by Carbon Fibers. Engineering & Technology Journal.*

Kanie, T., Fujii, K., Arikawa, H., & Inoue, K. (2000). Flexural properties and impact strength of denture base polymer reinforced with woven glass fibers. *Dental Materials*, *16*(2), 150–158. doi:10.1016/S0109-5641(99)00097-4 PMID:11203537

Kivak, T., Samtaş, G., & Çiçek, A. (2012). Taguchi method based optimisation of drilling parameters in drilling of AISI 316 steel with PVD monolayer and multilayer coated HSS drills. *Measurement: Journal of the International Measurement Confederation*, *45*(6), 1547–1557. doi:10.1016/j.measurement.2012.02.022

Kuo, C., Li, Z., & Wang, C. (2017). Multi-objective optimisation in vibration-assisted drilling of CFRP/Al stacks. *Composite Structures*, *173*, 196–209. doi:10.1016/j.compstruct.2017.04.026

Mandal, N., Doloi, B., Mondal, B., & Das, R. (2011). Optimization of flank wear using Zirconia Toughened Alumina (ZTA) cutting tool: Taguchi method and Regression analysis. *Measurement: Journal of the International Measurement Confederation*, *44*(10), 2149–2155. doi:10.1016/j.measurement.2011.07.022

Maruo, Y., Nishigawa, G., Irie, M., Yoshihara, K., & Minagi, S. (2015). Flexural properties of polyethylene, glass and carbon fiber-reinforced resin composites for prosthetic frameworks. *Acta Odontologica Scandinavica*, *73*(8), 581–587. doi:10.3109/00016357.2014.958875 PMID:25892406

Me, R. C., Ibrahim, R., & Tahir, P. M. (2012). Natural Based Biocomposite Material for Prosthetic Socket Fabrication. *ALAM CIPTA*, *5*(1), 27–34.

Meriç, G., Dahl, J. E., & Ruyter, I. E. (2005). Physicochemical evaluation of silica-glass fiber reinforced polymers for prosthodontic applications. *European Journal of Oral Sciences*, *113*(3), 258–264. doi:10.1111/j.1600-0722.2005.00209.x PMID:15953252

News Medical Life Science. (2017). *World's first split-keel fiberglass foot launched by Freedom Innovations*. Retrieved November 10, 2018, from https://www.news-medical.net/news/20170829/Worlds-first-split-keel-fiberglass-foot-launched-by-Freedom-Innovations.aspx

Palanikumar, K. (2011). Experimental investigation and optimisation in drilling of GFRP composites. *Measurement: Journal of the International Measurement Confederation*, *44*(10), 2138–2148. doi:10.1016/j.measurement.2011.07.023

Phillips, S. L., & Craelius, W. (2005). Material properties of selected prosthetic laminates. *Journal of Prosthetics and Orthotics*, *17*(1), 27–34. doi:10.1097/00008526-200501000-00007

Sivanandam, S. N., & Deepa, S. N. (2008). *Introduction to genetic algorithms*. Introduction to Genetic Algorithms; doi:10.1007/978-3-540-73190-0

Slocumb, W. (2014). *Bamboo Fiber Reinforced Composites for Prosthetics and Orthotics*. Retrieved from https://www.csueastbay.edu/programs/csr/files/docs/2014%2520CSU%2520Award%2520Winner%252 0Summaries/WilliamSlocumb¬2014%2520Summary.pdf

Sumathi, S., & Surekha, P. (2016). *Computational Intelligence Paradigms: Theory andApplications Using MATLAB*. CRC Press, Taylor & Francis Group.

Tabassum, M., & Mathew, K. (2014). *A Genetic Algorithm Analysis towards Optimization solutions. International Journal of Digital Information and Wireless Communications*. doi:10.17781/P001091

Vallittu, P. K. (2007). Effect of 10 years of in vitro aging on the flexural properties of fiber-reinforced resin composites. *The International Journal of Prosthodontics*, *20*(1), 43–45. PMID:17319361

van Heumen, C. C. M., Kreulen, C. M., Bronkhorst, E. M., Lesaffre, E., & Creugers, N. H. J. (2008). Fiber-reinforced dental composites in beam testing. *Dental Materials*, *24*(11), 1435–1443. doi:10.1016/j.dental.2008.06.006 PMID:18692230

Wysk, R. A., Niebel, B. W., Cohen, P. H., & Simpson, T. W. (2000). Taguchi's Robust Design Method. *Manufacturing Processes: Integrated Product and Process Design*, 1–9.

Yeng, Y., Mahfouf, M., & Linkens, D. (2003). Parameter optimization of stress- strainconstitutive equations using genetic algorithm. *Journal of Materials Science and Technology*, *19*, 5–8.

Section 4
Orthotics

Chapter 9
A Review on Materials for Orthotic Devices:
Processing and Characterization

Hridayjit Kalita
BIT Mesra, India

Divya Zindani
National Institute of Technology Silchar, India

ABSTRACT

The recent use of fiber-reinforced composites as bio-material in fabrication of orthoses have accelerated the research in finding the most compatible combinations of bio-polymeric composites. The strength, flexibility, biological compatibility, durability, and fatigue strength can be easily altered considering different combinations of polymers and their reinforced structures. In this chapter, a review of the presently used polymeric composites as orthotic materials, their properties, and their applications based on their availability for common people, for a variety of specialized functions, and for the best quality and compatibility factor were discussed. The common orthotic devices mainly used on patients to support weak joints or limbs, materials used, and processing techniques were discussed. Characterization tests for polyethylene composites performed for material properties like ultimate tensile and bending strength, elastic modulus, thermal degradation properties, and surface resistance were discussed, which validates the usability of polyethylene in orthotic fabrication.

DOI: 10.4018/978-1-5225-8235-9.ch009

INTRODUCTION

Fibre- reinforced composites have gained popularity and is widely used today for its ease of suitably altering the properties to be suited to any body parts in certain ranges of compatibility in stiffness, tensile strength, fatigue strength, surface interaction between body and orthotic, durability and functional needs (sporting purpose, general purpose). Polymer composites can be selected to operate under certain conditions which can be classified based on their surface compatibility and their mechanical compatibility [Ramakrishna S et al., 2001]. Surface compatibility factors include all body/prosthetic interface interactions such as allergic to the material, biological, chemical and physical suitability of the orthotic material to the muscles and bones in contact with it. Mechanical compatibility factors include strength, stiffness, elasticity, impulsive load on the body part by the orthotic [Ramakrishna S et al., 2001; Wintermantel E et al., 2001].

The stress being subjected to the human bones regularly is approximately 4MPa while the tendons and ligaments take about 80MPa or above. The motion of the joints and fingers in body can be calculated in terms of cycles/per day to be 10^6 [Ramakrishna S et al., 2001]. The advancement of polymer technology have facilitated its modification to mimic the mechanical behaviour of a human bone and synchronizing with the functions being transmitted from the body in contact. Metal plates and screws like stainless steel were commonly used as materials for orthotic and prosthetic implants. But metal plates possess few drawbacks. Metal plates are stiffer and stronger than human bone which on using with it makes the bone the weaker member and non resisting to fatigue shocks or surface wear. The surface of the interface between soft bone material and the metal greatly influences the compatibility factor between the two materials. Polymer composites can be a better replacement while considering these compatibility issues. The stiffness and other properties in the orthotic material can be altered and maintained to adjust itself to mimic the bone material property so that necessary rigidity, shocks and load could be provided to the bone joint. The polymer composite holds the ability to get processed in a wide variety of properties and the range of properties for the compatibility with the bone material is easily achieved.

One disadvantage is that, though polymer material (fibreless) can be synchronized well with the bone in the domain of comfort and softness, the stiffness and strength are still very less to hold the necessary weight of the body or any peak load. So the property of the preferred best material lies somewhere in between both the polymer and the metal. Fibre reinforced polymer holds the solution to the above mentioned problem, which is basically a combination of a polymeric matrix reinforced with metallic or non-metallic fibres. The necessary stiffness, hardness and wear resistance is provided by the fibres while the matrix provides the softness, surface finish and cushioning effect to the body [Kumari et al., 2018]. The strength of the orthotic material made of fibre reinforced polymer mainly depends on the relative arrangement of both the constituents or the alignment of the fibres apart from their individual properties [Ramakrishna S et al., 2001, Sen N., 2004]. Replacing polymer composites in place of metal prosthetics or orthotics also enabled visual imaging of injuries or healing process imaging behind the metal plates and screws [Scholz et al., 2011]. In this paper, section 1 is dedicated to classification of different orthotic materials and the significance of using a fibre reinforced thermosetting polymer composite (carbon-epoxy) over a fibre reinforced thermoplastic (glass fibre-nylon) in achieving the best quality orthotics. Section 2 deals in material processing and fabrication techniques involved in production of orthotic devices. Section 3 gives an account of the significance of Polyethylene (PE) as orthotic material and its property characterization.

Bio Materials, Its Classification and Properties

Orthotic application of Biomaterial substitutes the function of a body part and matching with the properties of it. Based on the biological consideration of compatibility, bio materials can be mainly classified into biologically inert material (first generation), bio active and degradable materials and bio resorbable and bio active material (third generation) [Scholz et al., 2011]. First generation materials are widely used in prosthetic applications of joints and bones as plates and bars of materials such as stainless steel, titanium, alumina and ultra high molecular weight polyethylene (UHMWPE). Second generation materials react biologically to form bonds with the bones which supports in transferring loads and shocks to and fro the body. They include certain inorganic compounds like bioceramics having composition of glass ceramic, hydroxyapatite (HA) or crystalline calcium phosphates. They usually possess a low value of fatigue strength and are often used in conjunction with the bio-polymers such as poly methyl methacrylate (PMMA), Poly-ethylene (PE) [Misra et al., 2007]. Third generation biomaterial includes those which can provide the necessary support to the body structure and tune into the material composition to stimulate tissue regeneration. They are 3 Dimensional porous structure which can activate genes and recently these porous structures are also being made out of metals specifically titanium and titanium alloys.

Metals of the first generation bio materials are widely used for prosthetic and orthotic applications but it possess certain drawbacks such as heavy weight, non-resorbable and inability to provide comfort to the wearer. Polymer composites can provide solution to above mentioned all problems by giving enough flexibility to distribute the force throughout the limb and provide comfort. It also attains specific tensile strength about 4 times that of the stainless steel and aluminium [Suresh et al., 2003]. Recent use of carbon fibre composites as orthoses material have recorded a drop in heart rate and oxygen usage by 10% as compared to the condition when metal orthotics were used due to reduction in weight [Hachisuka K et al., 2007].

Natural fibres were commonly used as reinforcements in polymer matrix and posses a few advantageous qualities like easy availability, processibility, affordability, bio degradable and are renewable. It also finds application in automotive and packaging industry. Natural fibres include jute, flax, hemp, sisal, etc which have the property that depends on the species of the derived fibre or matrix, climatic condition, method of fibre preparation, etc. The major drawback in incorporating bio materials in polymers is their tendency to absorb water and deformation or distortion in the material due to drying of it. Biomaterials have also the tendency to exhibit anisotropic nature of their strength, uniformity and arrangements. Experiments were being carried out with both the matrix and reinforced structures as bio material and found to be quite suitable compared to the synthetically made polymer composites. Prajer and Ansell took poly L-lactide acid as matrix and sisal fibre as reinforcements for the experiment purpose and found to have a high stiffness and having flexural modulus and strength as 22GPa and 286MPa [Prajer et al., 2014].

Bio materials such as PALF-derived NanoCellulose embedded polyurethane has been applied in fabricating various prosthetic implants and support and some common applications include surgical gloves, medical bags, medical disposable, non-latex condom and in wound dressing [Cherian et al., 2011, Reddy et al., 2013]. The hydrophilic property of natural fibre is exhibited by their constituent materials such as cellulose and lignin and due to this property of it with contrast to the polymer tendency of being hydrophobic has raised questions on surface compatibility between the two. Few techniques have been adopted for reducing the incompatibility factor of the interfaces and to increase the interlocking quality between the two surfaces. One such technique is by chemical treatment where hydroxyl and carboxyl groups are treated to modify it in the form of easily adhering to the polymer material. Removing of lignin layer from the natural fibre reinforcement using sodium hydroxide is such used technique [Xie et al., 2010]. Polymer composites can be made out in two types which are thermoplastic and thermosetting plastic polymer. Bio composites are a combination of few thermoplastic material matrix such as polypropylene (PP), polyethylene (PE) and polystyrene (PS) or bio material matrix (PLA) and the bio fibres. These materials can be recycled, bio degraded, renewable and are corrosion and fatigue resistant, possess less weight and density and ease of processing [recent advnces in polyethelene, importance of biocomposites]. Thermosetting plastic are non-recyclable and can be melted and formed only once. Some of them include, phenol formaldehyde, epoxy resin, polyester and vinyl ester [Mansor et. al, 2018, importance of biocomposites].

Polymer composites can be classified based on their compatibility with the human body part into avital/avital material and avital/vital material. Avital/avital materials are composed of all non living matrix and fibre. Vital/avital include both living and non-living components. Avital/avital composites can be further classified into resorbable, partially resorbable and fully resorbable type of polymers[Ramakrishna S et al., 2001, Kharazi et al., 2009]. Resorbable composites are those which exhibits favourable structural stiffness and strength as of the human bone material and can be easily synchronized with the functioning and material property of the human bones. In some cases, resorbable matrix is coupled with non resorbable material to enhance stiffness and strength of the orthotics. These composites can be called as partial resorbable composites. Some of the materials included resorbable, partial resorbable and fully resorbable polymers are given in Fig 2 of [Banoriya et al., 2017].

Recent orthotic incorporates highly developed polymer composites such as CF/PEEK which are biologically inert and possess resorbable characteristics such as high strength and fatigue resistance nearly equivalent to the metallic parts at similar plate thickness[Fujihara K et al., 2004]. The only drawback is the processing hurdles of fabricating CF/PEEK which exhibits poor quality [Fujihara K et al., 2004].

As already mentioned, polymer composites are made up of matrix and reinforcements. Matrix provides the necessary protection to the fibres and resists outer adhesion and wear. It also holds the fibres together which gives a cumulative strength to the orthotic structure. Matrix material can be varied between polymers, graphite, carbon and metals, among which polymer can be considered the most feasible choice of utilization. Reinforcements on the other hand can be fibres and fillers and are able to resist bending and axial stresses.

Polymer composites can be thermoplast or thermoset based, of which the thermoset based composite is mostly preferred. It is manufactured by the process of compression moulding which binds the reinforced fibres by curing the dry fabric layers of thermoset at room temperature providing necessary stiffness and strength[Meredith et al., 2015]. Thermoset based composites are moisture and chemical resistive, environmental friendly, insulators of electricity and maintains a good aesthetic appearance. Moreover, the components in thermoset based polymer composites are available in market at a lower price as compared to metallic parts. Thermoplast based composites are generally manufactured by extrusion and injection moulding and does not require curing. The process only consists of heating, shaping and cooling procedures which is quite fast, efficient and repetive. It has similar surface interaction properties as in the thermoset based, but looses in terms of strength and stiffness. Also, thermoplast materials can be manufactured 100 times, repeating the same material which proves to be quite cost effective [Otheguy et al., 2001].

A tribological experimental setup to determine the suitability of the fibre reinforced thermoplast and thermoset composite, based on the effect on wear resistance and coefficient of friction is studied in [Kumari et al., 2018]. For the thermoplast based composites, the matrix and the filler material were taken as nylon and glass respectively while for the thermoset based composite, the material for matrix and the filler were taken as epoxy and carbon. Samples of size $(99 \times 88 \times 4.5)mm^3$ of 6-7 in number has been prepared. The void content was found to be lesser in thermoplast while it was more in case of thermoset based composite. This is because of the production processes applied for fabrication where the thermoplast was manufactured by injection moulding in molten condition while thermoset was produced by compression moulding. Tribological tests were performed using the multi tribo tester and coefficient of friction and specific wear rate were compared between both the samples. It was found that the epoxy-carbon composite sample exhibited much lesser number than the nylon-glass filler composite. This is due to the self lubricating property of the carbon composite and ability to withstand deformation.

Orthotic Components, Material Processing and Fabrication

Orthoses are basically used to provide support externally to the limb, to provide functional assistance and protection to the joint movement and to limit the movement of it. On the other hand, Prostheses or exo-prostheses are generally used to replace limbs and joints completely and provide necessary motion to the leg as desired without causing any pain or inconvenience to the other parts of the body. Transfemoral prostheses are more difficult to manage as the amputee requires time to slowly adjust to the amputations provided because of the different complexities including the knee joint mechanism. Recently, improved and developed transfemoral prostheses involves servo motors, hydraulic drives, etc which eases the functioning of the prostheses and a little force is required to obtain an amplified desired motion. In contrast to it, transtibial prostheses are easier to operate and do not require much effort from the amputee.

For orthotic applications, the materials currently in use are metals, polymer composites, fabric, leather and elastomers. Metals were used extensively for orthotic component production which was rigid. With newer development in material technology, polymers and polymer composites have come to replace the metallic use of orthotics which were made available in a variety of strength and stiffness values and can be distinguished as soft and semi-rigid materials. Some of the commonly used lower limb orthotic components are ankle foot assembly, knee joint, bands and uprights and knee and hip braces.

The lower limb orthoses can be classified into 3 divisions which are ankle foot orthoses, knee ankle foot orthoses and knee orthoses. Detailed description of the knee ankle foot orthoses is described below.

Knee Ankle Foot Orthoses (KAFO)

The KAFO assembly mainly consists of, thigh bands, thigh uprights, knee lock and knee joints [Chung et al.]. Knee joints are of three types. The first type, i.e. straight set knee joints allows rotation only in one axis which facilitates flexion but restricts hyperextension. The second type of knee joint, i.e. polycentric knee joint which is also used as sports knee orthosis allows movement of the femur and tibia in two axes facilitating both flexion and extension. The third type is the posterior offset knee joint which is employed when the patient has weaker knee extensors and hip extensor.

Knee locks are generally employed to assist locking of the knee and allowing smooth lifting of the user from a seated to standing position in small incremental angle. These are mainly available in four types which are the ratchet lock, drop lock, bail lock and dial lock.

Thigh bands are wide straps of moulded plastic or metal which is employed to transfer load from the foot to the upper thighs, supports the orthotic device and distribute the pressure throughout the upper thigh surface for comfort.

Orthoses Fabrication

Orthoses can be manufactured in a number of methods, but in all methods the initial step begins with the casting of a negative model of the limb to be supported and then proceeds with the manufacturing of the positive model. The production of polymer composite orthotic devices is performed in the next phase.

Negative mould involves preparing a plaster mould, the material of which is discussed below [Wong et al., 2019].

- **Gypsum Plaster of Paris (POP):** A plaster of Paris cast is produced which conforms to the shape and size of the limb acting as a positive model. The process starts with wrapping a POP bandage around the limb which is of cotton and contains calcium sulphate hemihydrates on it. It forms the negative model of the limb. The POP paste is then made out of a mixture of POP powder and water which fills in the negative model to obtain the positive model. For large castings, sand filler is also mixed with the POP paste to reduce the cast weight.
- **Fibre Glass Bandage:** Fibre glass bandage is made out of knitting fibres of glass and then soaking it with Polyrethane (PUR) resin. This bandage is then immersed into water for activation and wrapped around the limb to be cast. The formability of a fibre glass cast is not as high as in the case of POP bandage and is mainly used for light supporting limb cast but it has the advantage of getting set in a lesser time.
- **Foam Box Impression:** It is mainly used in substitution to POP bandage which is a closed cell and moisture resistant phenolic foam made out of curing of phenolic resin. It generates the impression of a limb into which liquid plaster is poured to obtain the final positive casting.

- **Alginate:** Alginate is a polysaccharide powder mixed with water to form a gelatinous sticky paste which can imprint minute details of feet, fingers, hands, etc. On curing, it behaves like an elastic.

Once the positive model has been produced, the next is the fabrication of the orthoses using polymer composite either by laminating over the mould or by thermoforming. Positive models can be produced in number of ways apart from the above mentioned casting techniques. Modern CAD/CAM manufacturing employs laser light to scan the desired limb and forming a 3D geometry so that it can be fed to the milling machine for carving directly out of a PUR block. In some cases, the fabrication of the negative model was completely replaced with the laser white and blue light scanning and forming digital 3D map to directly feed to the 3D printers for fabricating with the polymer composites. Apart from the polymer composite and metals a few other materials which are directly used as components in orthotic devices are:

- **Leather:** Leather is derived from animal skin and hides which has the property to easily get formed and stretched. It exhibits good strength and vapour permeability and the properties vary with the type of hides used and the method of tanning. It is mainly employed in making of straps, belts and to provide cover to the edges of the metal parts of the orthotic device as linings.
- **Fabric:** Fabrics are mainly employed in fabrication of straps, lining cover, orthotic socks, upper limb orthoses harnesses and base support for less rigid orthoses. It is made out of blending of cotton, wool, and other synthetic fibres like nylon and acrylics. Nylon can also be used in fabrication of cords and cables for suspension components and power transmission in body operated orthotic devices.
- **Elastomers:** Elastomers are mainly employed as shock absorbers in orthotic shoes and suspension components which utilizes its property of being easily able to regain its original shape and size once deforming load is released. Natural and synthetic rubbers, thermoplastic elastomers, silicone and PUR are some of the materials included in elastomers. [Wong et al., 2019]

The methods for forming of the polymer composites are different for both thermoplast and thermoset type. Thermoforming for thermoplastic polymer and laminating for thermosetting polymer.

In *thermoforming*, the most commonly used method is vacuum drape forming where the thermoplastic polymer is heated to its formability and adhesiveness temperature and is held against the surface layout of the positive mould by activating vacuum between the mould and the plastic sheet. After cooling, the thermoplastic gets solidified, imprinting all details of the positive mould.

After removing the formed polymer from the positive mould, the surfaces of the component is checked thoroughly and any sharp edges and rough cut lines on the surface that could injure the patient or feel inconvenience are smooth out. Any stress raisers that could fatigue fracture the component are also eliminated. The end orthotic component is much flexible and comfortable than that of the thermoset type and can be modified even at the later stages.

In *thermoset laminating technique*, orthotic components are made out of thermosetting plastic which is a mixture of a reinforced fabric and monomer resin. The procedure starts with placing a Polyvinyl Alcohol (PVA) layer or bag over the positive mould and evacuating the air in between the mould and the PVA. Fabric fibres are then wrapped around the mould and another layer of PVA is placed over it which is then fitted to a vacuum generator. For the treatment of the monomer resin, catalyst is added to it to start the chemical reaction which is then poured into the PVA bag. The vacuum created between the resin and the PVA layer pulls the resin to conform to the surface layout of the mould.

Another method named, Pre-impregnated (pre-preg) lamination involves a process where fabric fibre and resin is mixed beforehand, applying over the positive mould and is maintained at a cold temperature to delay the curing so that it is not thermally treated until the heating was applied over the positive mould.

The resin is first activated with catalyst and applied over a fibre cloth using a pregging machine which is then kept in a condition under reduced temperature. Now, to prepare the mould surface, a separating film is layered which prevents sticking of the resin to the mould. After wrapping the resin-fibre cloth around the mould multiple times depending on the required strength, thickness and stiffness, a layer of bleeders were applied over it to remove excess resin and a bagging provision to create vacuum during thermally heating. Prepreg lamination ensures desired selection of the quantity of the fibres to be reinforced with limited resin.

Thermoset lamination technique gives a rigid orthotic structure of desired strength and stiffness.

In *computer aided design and fabrication* of positive mould, laser scanners are used and measurements taken of the layout of the body limb are programmed to built a 3D model on the computer screen which can then be modified in a variety of aspects as in twists, alignment, bending, pressure and load applications and other aesthetic aspects. Merely changing the data or updating the previous data enables the operator to make changes to the surface layout of the positive model in accordance with the convenience and functional requirement of the limb.

The final data produced are fed to the computer aided manufacturing (CAM) for directing the machine tools to carve the PUR block as per the 3D modified model data. After fabricating the positive mould, the rest of the procedural steps of constructing the orthotic component remain the same.

The limitation of this process lies in carving a complex 3D model having complicated cross-sections and undercuts using a 3-axis CAM lathe but is now made possible with the introduction of 7-axis robotic carver.

3D printing or additive manufacturing is another method of production of polymer composite orthotic components which employs direct fabrication of the component from the modified geometry data obtained from laser scanning and measurements. It eliminates the procedure to carve positive moulds using CAM 3-axis and 7-axis and directly proceeding to the production phase of the orthotic component. Thus, enabling the operators to save time and cost. 3D printing is generally available in 7 techniques, out of which powder bed fusion and extrusion can be considered as the only feasible processes for 3D printing of the orthotic components. For both the techniques, the 3D modified model is segmented into a number of layers of slices which is then fed to the designated machine heads. Polymer fabrication takes place layer upon layer from the bottom base to the top of the desired orthotic component.

In extrusion or Fused Deposition Modelling (FDM), the polymer composite is extruded out from a nozzle of fixed diameter and is then spread across to form a layer of slice. After spreading the previous layer, the extruder head is moved up for the next slice to be layered.

Acrylonitrile Butadiene Styrrene (ABS) and polylactic acid (PLA) are a few polymers that are commonly available commercially in the form of filament feedstock. This feedstock is melted to temperature slightly higher than its melting point inside the deposition head by resistive heating which is then dispensed out in a controlled manner through nozzle or orifice. In large scale polymer extrusion operation [Duty et al., 2018], the heated deposition head is replaced by a single screw mechanism which ensures continuous supply of semi-molten polymer with the input of pelletized polymer. ABS nanocomposites with organic modified montmorillonite (OMMT) reinforcements were tested with different proportional combination using single screw extruder [mechanical and thermal properties..]. With 5% weight percentage of OMMT the tensile strength of the ABS nano composite was found to rise by 43% in FDM while, it rises by 28.9% in case of injection moulding.

PLA has been utilised as biopolymer for extrusion with FDM and found to be having better biodegradable property and tensile strength to be applied for production of bio medical and orthotic components [Raj et al., 2018].

In case of powder bed fusion, the powder form of polymer composites are thermally cured layer after layer by impinging laser beam on to it. This forms the complete orthotic structure from bottom to top. The table on to which the powder is layered moves down after curing each layer by the thickness of the digital slice and proportional error in each layering. This process repeats until the entire orthotic product is obtained including the bands and joint heads.

SIGNIFICANCE AND CHARACTERIZATION OF POLYETHYLENE BIO COMPOSITES

Amputations of lower limb orthotics are commonly needed for people residing in developing countries as the labour population is high, accidents are frequent, war outcomes and manual works in coal mines still prevailing. High cost CF/epoxy composites cannot be employed feasibly to suffice such a large middle income population [Marks et al., 2001, Dubois S. et al., 2007] as a result use of low cost composites are highly preferred. Polypropylene plastics and glass fibre/ high density polyethylene (HDPE) plastics can be fabricated at a lower cost with considerations taken to maximize mechanical performance, comfort level, durability and production rate.

Polyethylene belongs to polyolefin family with ethylene as a monomer unit which is basically a combination of two methylene group bonded together. It is widely used in fabrication of a number of thermoplastic composites and has advantageous features and properties like high toughness, high surface wear resistance, low moisture absorption tendency, high chemical inertness, high insulation and low processing cost [Khanam et al., 2015]. It is available in both branched and linear form. Branched PE includes low density polyethylene (LDPE) and linear low density polyethylene (LLDPE) while linear PE includes high density polyethylene (HDPE) and ultra high molecular weight polyethylene (UHMWPE) [The editors of Encyclopaedia Britannica,

2017]. For total knee replacements, attempts have been made to study the wear resistant including UHMWPE polymer as the matrix material with carbon fibre reinforcements, but did not go well due to surface incompatibility of the UHMWPE with the carbon fibres [Ramakrishna S et al., 2001]. In another consideration, UHMWPE fibres were used as reinforcements in UHMWPE matrix which showed no sign of increase in wear resistant but increased levels of strength, creep resistance and stiffness were achieved [Ramakrishna S et al., 2001]. Cross-linked or branched polyethylene has been considered as replacements and is tested for a number of knee joints by [Utzscheneider et al., 2009] of which the report shown exhibited much lower wear rate than the application of UHMWPE. HDPE has been used widely as structural and engineering material due to its high mechanical qualities [].

Techniques involved in Characterization of polyethylene bio composites are performed based on identification of its mechanical, thermal and morphological properties.

Mechanical Tests

Tensile test is performed taking different combinations of matrix and filler materials. Toughness and modulus of elasticity were generally determined using this tests and different PE types reinforced with filler materials exhibits various ranges in properties which could be employed in different applications of orthoses. Tests performed for HDPE/carbon composites revealed increase in strength, hardness and stress level at fracture with increase in the amount of carbon but strain at fracture will decrease [Fouad et al., 2011]. Reinforcing glass fibres also enhances the strength and elasticity of the LDPE, MDPE and HDPE [AlMaadeed et al., 2013]. HDPE/nickel composites tend to increase in its elastic modulus from 606MPa to 1057MPa at 20% level of filler reinforcing. With lesser amount of filler materials below 10%, the elastic modulus tends to decrease in its value. But the condition may reverse (elasticity decreasing) with increasing the filler material above a certain level of proportion.

Flexural tests are performed to study the rigidity changes in composite materials with different proportional combinations of fillers and polymer plastics. The shear stress at fracture is determined which mainly depends on the interface strength due to adhesion, between the fibre and the plastic matrix. Different PE type exhibits increase in surface and bending stress and almost doubling in their levels in some cases of proportional combinations of fillers and matrix. The bending strength of HDPE/ wood flake composite tends to increase in its level upto a limit of 40% flake content, above which the strength begins to decrease [Balasuriya et al., 2001]. The strength of LDPE tends to get doubled with reinforcements of wood palm powder upto a level of 70% [AlMaadeed et al., 2014].

Impact tests are performed to determine the failure strength in PE composites subjected to high impact force caused by pendulum heavy bob which was dropped on a specimen from a fixed height, utilizing the potential energy during that condition. Among all the PE, the LDPE composites exhibit the highest impact strength but it develops its brittleness once the filler content begins to increase above a certain limit. ASTM D-256 method enables determination of brittle-ductile transition in the composite when the temperature of it is reduced to certain range. The composite between the wood filler and PE polymer in presence of MAPE acting as compatibilizer exhibits higher impact strength of upto 60% increment due to enhancing of the adhesivity action [Yuan et al., 2008, Lai et al., 2003].

Thermal Tests

Differential scanning calorimetry is used to determine the thermal effect on the temperatures of melting, crystallization and the proportion of crystallization which is linked to the nucleation sites formed [Zhang et al., 2006] due to addition of fillers into the PE matrix. The sample is kept in a nitrogen atmosphere while being heated to about 200 degree celcius. Then it is bombarded with oxygen gas after which the exothermic oxidation reaction time was noted. The glass temperature of the sample can also be investigated using this device. Fillers can act as triggering element for nucleation site formation. Moreover, the fillers also restrict the movement of the crystallites formed as a result of these nucleation sites, leading to increase in crystallization temperature.

Dynamic mechanical analysis was performed to study the change in mechanical behaviour like young's modulus and dissipation of energy due to constant periodic deformation of the PE composite material and at the same time applying heat to elevate the temperature. The nano composite HDPE/carbon exhibited an increase in stored energy with increase in carbon content and frequency of deformation [Fouad et al., 2011].

Thermo-gravimetric analysis is done to measure the thermal stability of the composites or the degradation of the specimen (loss of mass with respect to the temperature and time). Natural fibres usually display a decreasing trend in thermal stability with increase in fibre load. PE composites exhibit a higher thermal stability **temperature** with synthetic reinforcements used [AlMaadeed et al., 2013]. PTFE shows higher temperature for degradation compared to the PE which again shows higher thermal stability temperature in comparison to Poly-propylene (PP). Addition of glass fibres on un-irradiated blend waste PE/recycled waste rubber powder and maleic anhydride (WPE/RWRP/MA) exhibits an improvement in degradation temperature [Hassan et al., 2014].

Morphological Tests

Scanning electron microscope (SEM) is an equipment to observe surface patterns, adhesion fracture high magnification image, crystalline and grain structures and their changes with different combinations of composites. Electron are bombarded from a tungsten thermionic cathode head and directed to the specimen by two electromagnetic anode lenses which in turn knock out the secondary electrons and X-ray rays. These electrons are collected and the data is turned into an image by employing raster scans to compare the intensity of the secondary and primary electron beam.

HA/HDPE and glass beads/LDPE composites displayed good interfacial bonding and particle dispersion [Li et al., 1998] while UHMWPE/graphene nanosheet exhibits a weak interfacial bonding and reduced adhesion by displaying fibre pull outs on the SEM image [Wang et al., 2013]. Crystallization in the polymer composite can reduce the ultimate strength and integrity between different fibres due to reduced interaction at the interface between fibres and matrix and displaying pull outs in SEM images [AlMaadeed et al., 2013].

Atomic force microscopy (AFM) is another technique to study the surface topographical and morphological conditions on the polymer composite. AFM is capable of identifying the fibre alignment pattern in MWCNT formed by the extruder die [McNally et al., 2005]. The dimension measurement of reduced graphene sheet in PE matrix can also be obtained using this technique [Kuila et al., 2011].

Transmission electron microscope (TEM) operates on the same electron principle as that in the SEM, the difference lies with the technique of detection of the final electron data output which on TEM, the raster scan (on SEM) is replaced with an electron intensity sensor placed below the thin sample to form an image. Electromagnetic lenses which act as anodes and are used to direct the electron beam to meet at a point on the specimen slice. Thinner cross-sectional specimens are used in this technique to observe the microstructure and crystalline/grain behaviour even inside of the composite sample. If the section is not thin enough, electrons may get loose its energy inside the specimen itself and might not form image on the photo sensing sheet placed below. It is mainly employed to study the crystallite areas, morphological structures, spherulite structures and agglomeration [Mohan et al., 2012]. Graphene/LDPE exhibits a homogenous dispersion of the graphene nanosheets in the LLDPE matrix provided by strong interfacial interaction between the two material surfaces [Kuila et al., 2011].

FUTURE SCOPE

Recent developments in polymer composites have enabled the performance of the orthotic and prosthetic devices to be more user friendly and cost effective. With the development of polymer technology, research has been carried out on more porous material that could be used in tissue engineering as well as applications in orthotic components for additional comfort and conformity with the layout of the weakened limb. The elasticity and stiffness can be enhanced by reinforcing with fibres or particles, of which particle, nano fibre or carbon nanotube reinforcing gives a better result [Rockwood DN et al., 2010; Ayres CE et al., 2009, Shi X et al., 2007; Mekael P et al., 2010]. Functional coatings are another development in polymer composites that can be applied to metal prosthetics and orthotics (O &P) to improve their wear resistance and corrosion. These two characteristics can be considered the main cause in knee and hip implants [Wang et al., 2010].

Pneumatically artificial muscles (PAM), which is in the form of grids and fabric consists of elastomeric cylinders exhibiting linear motions which acts as flexible and inextensible entity meshed together. With the development of PAM, a number of options have opened for its applications in orthotic products such as wearable exoskeleton suits which will provide support to joints or limbs by limiting their movement and at the same time providing comfort by uniformly distributing the load throughout the body. The functions of muscles can be easily reproduced using this mechanism.

Orthotic material can be incorporated with piezoelectric fibres to produce a power generating suit which on movement or individual walking or running might charge batteries or cellphones. These principle can be employed in reverse to power the muscles or to stiffen the polymer composite for restricting movements in joints, muscles or limbs.

Development and implications of 3D printing in production of orthotic devices has led to accurate dimensional fabrications with internal developments still in progress in the field of 3D printing to build a cost effective material and production. Due to accurate processing technique and accurate scan data taken for profile building of an orthotic element, numerous variation and optimum designing can be performed for better effectiveness and comfort of the wearer.

CONCLUSION

The use of fibre-reinforced composite in the application of orthotic and prosthetic devices have accelerated the research in the field of material modification and synthesis to process different combinations of constituents to achieve a common function and aesthetics. Polymer composites have replaced metals in the application of orthotic devices for its unique characteristic to change its structural property with different combinations of fibres and matrix. Thermosetting tends to be better contender in polymer composite material, to replace metals as they reach the limits of stiffness and strength of the metals. The use of natural fibres in polymer composites by surface treating of the fibres so that hydrophilic-hydrophobic effect could be eliminated and a strong interfacial bond can be obtained. These bio-composite can be cost effective and easy production but still it cannot be effectively adopted in orthotic applications due to a number of undesirable factors as already discussed in the previous section. The techniques involved in fabrication phase has been discussed in the above sections which includes positive and negative model making, then casting of polymer matrix with reinforced fibre mesh. The traditional technique is now replaced with laser scanning and measurements, CNC machine tools and CAD/CAM integration tools to completely discard the traditional methods of production and even eliminating the need to produce positive and negative models. Additive manufacturing has reduced the fabricating process to mere digitally coded computer data by introducing laser scanning devices for creating 3D image, manipulating the computer data to make necessary changes to the 3D model and producing the final orthotic product by laser curing of composite powder or by extrusion. A few characterization techniques of polyethylene composites for determining the mechanical, thermal and morphological properties are described and how few polyethylene composite exhibits properties in the range of perfect compatibility with the body.

REFERENCES

AlMaadeed, M. A., Nogellova, Z., Mičušík, M., Novák, I., & Krupa, I. (2014). Mechanical, sorption and adhesive properties of composites based on low density polyethylene filled with date palm wood powder. *Materials & Design*, *53*, 29–37. doi:10.1016/j.matdes.2013.05.093

AlMaadeed, M. A., Ouedern, M., & Noorunnisa, K. P. (2013). Effect of chain structure on the properties of glass fibre/polyethylene composites. *Materials & Design*, *47*, 725–730. doi:10.1016/j.matdes.2012.11.063

Ayres, C. E., Jha, B. S., Sell, S. A., Bowlin, G. L., & Simpson, D. G. (2009). Nanotechnology in the design of soft tissue scaffolds: Innovations in structure and function. *Wiley Interdisciplinary Reviews. Nanomedicine and Nanobiotechnology*, *2*(1), 20–34. doi:10.1002/wnan.55 PMID:20049828

Balasuriya, P. W., Ye, L., & Mai, Y. W. (2001). Mechanical properties of wood flake -polyethylene composites. Part I: Effects of processing methods and matrix melt flow behavior. *Composites. Part A, Applied Science and Manufacturing*, *32*(5), 619–629. doi:10.1016/S1359-835X(00)00160-3

Banoriya, D., Purohit, R., & Dwivedi, R. K. (2017). Advanced Application of Polymer based Biomaterials. *Materials Today: Proceedings*, *4*(2), 3534–3541. doi:10.1016/j.matpr.2017.02.244

Cherian, B. M., Lea˜o, A. L., De Souza, S. F., Costa, L. M. M., De Olyveira, G. M., Kottaisamy, M., ... Thomas, S. (2011). Cellulose nanocomposites with nanofibres isolated from pineapple leaf fibers for medical applications. *Carbohydrate Polymers*, *86*(4), 1790–1798. doi:10.1016/j.carbpol.2011.07.009

Dubois, S. (2007). *Mobility for each one*. Retrieved from http://www.icsid.org/ feature/galleria/galleria38.htm

Duty, C., Ajinjeru, C., Kishore, V., Compton, B., Hmeidat, N., Chen, X., ... Kunc, V. (2018). What makes a material printable? Avicoelastic model for extrusion-based 3D printing of polymer. *Journal of Manufacturing Processes*, *35*, 526–537. doi:10.1016/j.jmapro.2018.08.008

Fouad, H., Elleithy, R., Al-Zahrani, S. M., & Ali, M. A. (2011). Characterization and processing of high density polyethylene/carbon nano-composites. *Materials & Design*, *32*(4), 1974–1980. doi:10.1016/j.matdes.2010.11.066

Fujihara, K., Teo, K., Gopal, R., Loh, P. L., Ganesh, V. K., Ramakrishna, S., ... Chew, C. L. (2004). Fibrous composite materials in dentistry and orthopaedics: Review and applications. *Composites Science and Technology*, *64*(6), 775–788. doi:10.1016/j.compscitech.2003.09.012

Hachisuka, K., Makino, K., Wada, F., Saeki, S., & Yoshimoto, N. (2007). Oxygen consumption, oxygen cost and physiological cost index in polio survivors: A comparison of walking without orthosis, with an ordinary or a carbon-fibre reinforced plastic knee-ankle-foot orthosis. *Journal of Rehabilitation Medicine*, *39*(8), 646–650. doi:10.2340/16501977-0105 PMID:17896057

Hassan, M. M., Aly, R. O., Hasanen, J. A., & El Sayed, F. (2014). The effect of gamma irradiation on mechanical, thermal and morphological properties of glass fiber reinforced polyethylene waste/reclaim rubber composites. *Journal of Industrial and Engineering Chemistry*, *20*(3), 947–952. doi:10.1016/j.jiec.2013.06.027

Khanam, P. N., & AlMaadeed, M. A. A. (2015). Processing and characterization of polyethylenebased composites. *Adv. Manufact. Polym. Composit. Sci.*, *1*(2), 63–79. doi:10.1179/2055035915Y.0000000002

Kharazi, A. Z., Fathi, M. H., & Bahmany, F. (2009). Design of a textile composite bone plate using 3D-finite element method. *Materials & Design*, *31*(3), 1468–1474. doi:10.1016/j.matdes.2009.08.043

Kuila, T., Bose, S., Hong, C. E., Uddin, M. E., Khanra, P., Kim, N. H., & Lee, J. H. (2011). Preparation of functionalized graphene/linear low density polyethylene composites by a solution mixing method. *Carbon*, *49*(3), 1033–1037. doi:10.1016/j.carbon.2010.10.031

Kumari, N., Pradhan, S. K., & Kumar, K. (2018). Suitability of composite material for orthotic callipers- Tribological study. *Materials Today: Proceedings*, *5*(2), 5608–5614. doi:10.1016/j.matpr.2017.12.152

Lai, S. M., Yeh, F. C., Wang, Y., Chan, H. C., & Shen, H. F. (2003). Comparative study of maleated polyolefins as compatibilizers for polyethylene/wood flour composites. *Journal of Applied Polymer Science*, *87*(3), 487–496. doi:10.1002/app.11419

Li, R. K. Y., Liang, J. Z., & Tjong, S. C. (1998). Morphology and dynamic mechanical properties of glass beads filled low density polyethylene composites. *Journal of Materials Processing Technology*, *79*(1), 59–65. doi:10.1016/S0924-0136(97)00319-1

Mansor, Mustafa, Hajar, Fadzullah, Omar, Salim, & Akop. (2018). *Recent advances in polyethylene-based Biocomposites*. Woodhead Publishing Series in Composites Science and Engineering.

Marks, L. J., & Michael, J. W. (2001). Artificial limbs. *BMJ (Clinical Research Ed.)*, *323*(7315), 732–735. doi:10.1136/bmj.323.7315.732 PMID:11576982

McNally, T., Pötschke, P., Halley, P., Murphy, M., Martin, D., Bell, S. E. J., ... Quinn, J. P. (2005). Polyethylene multiwalled carbon nanotube composites. *Polymer*, *46*(19), 8222–8232. doi:10.1016/j.polymer.2005.06.094

Mekael, P., Basu, J., Syam, N., Laurencin, C., & Carter, C. B. (2010). Characterization of carbon nanotube reinforced polymer scaffold for bone tissue engineering. *Microscopy and Microanalysis*, *16*(Suppl. 2), 1032–1033. doi:10.1017/S1431927610060745

Meredith, J., Bilson, E., & Powe, R. (2015). A performance versus cost analysis of prepeg carbon epoxy energy absorption structures. Composite Structures, 124, 206-213.

Misra, S. K., & Boccaccini, A. R. (2007). Biodegradable and bioactive polymer/ceramic composite scaffolds. *Woodhead Publishing Series in Biomaterials*, 72–92.

Mohan, T.P., & Kanny, K. (2012). Effect of nanoclay in HDPE_glass fiber composites on processing, structure, and properties. *Adv. Composit. Mater.*, 315-331.

Otheguy, M.E. Gibson, A.G., Robinson, M., Findon, E., Cripps, B. Ochoa, A., … Castro, A. (2001). Recycling of end-of-life thermoplastic composite boats. *Composites Structures*, 21-42.

Prajer, M., & Ansell, M. P. (2014). Bio-composites for structural applications: poly-L-lactide reinforced with long sisal fiber bundles. *Journal of Applied Polymer Science*, *131*(21), 1–13. doi:10.1002/app.40999

Raj, S. A., Muthukumaran, E. K. J., & Jayakrishna, K. (2018). A Case Study of 3D Printed PLA and Its Mechanical Properties. *Materials Today: Proceedings*, *5*(5), 11219–11226. doi:10.1016/j.matpr.2018.01.146

Ramakrishna, S., Mayer, J., Wintermantel, E., & Leong, K. W. (2001). Biomedical applications of polymer-composite materials: A review. *Composites Science and Technology*, *61*(9), 1189–1224. doi:10.1016/S0266-3538(00)00241-4

Reddy, M. M., Vivekanandhan, S., Misra, M., Bhatia, S. K., & Mohanty, A. K. (2013). Biobased plastics and bionanocomposites: Current status and future opportunities. *Progress in Polymer Science*, *38*(10-11), 1653–1689. doi:10.1016/j.progpolymsci.2013.05.006

Rockwood, D. N., Gil, E. S., Park, S.-H., Kluge, J. A., Grayson, W., Bhumiratana, S., ... Kaplan, D. L. (2010). In growth of human mesenchymal stem cells into porous silk particle reinforced silk composite scaffolds: An in vitro study. *Acta Biomaterialia*, *7*(1), 144–151. doi:10.1016/j.actbio.2010.07.020 PMID:20656075

Scholz, M.-S., Blanchfield, J. P., Bloom, L. D., Coburn, B. H., Elkington, M., Fuller, J. D., ... Bond, I. P. (2011). The use of composite materials in modern orthopaedic medicine and prosthetic devices: A review. *Composites Science and Technology*, *71*(16), 1791–1803. doi:10.1016/j.compscitech.2011.08.017

Sen, N. (2004). Composites: Use in saucepan handles, artificial limbs and the AGNI missile. *Current Science*, *86*(3), 372–375.

Shi, X., Sitharaman, B., Pham, Q. P., Liang, F., Wu, K., Edward Billups, W., ... Mikos, A. G. (2007). Fabrication of porous ultra-short single-walled carbon nanotube nanocomposite scaffolds for bone tissue engineering. *Biomaterials*, *28*(28), 4078–4090. doi:10.1016/j.biomaterials.2007.05.033 PMID:17576009

Suresh, K. R., Niranjan, H. B., Martin Jebaraj, P., & Chowdiah, M. P. (2003). Tensile and wear properties of Aluminum composites. *Wear*, *255*(1-6), 638–642. doi:10.1016/S0043-1648(03)00292-8

Utzschneider, S., Harrasser, N., Schroeder, C., Mazoochian, F., & Jansson, V. (2009). Wear of contemporary total knee replacements – a knee simulator study of six current designs. *Clinical Biomechanics (Bristol, Avon)*, *24*(7), 583–588. doi:10.1016/j.clinbiomech.2009.04.007 PMID:19450910

Wang, B., Li, H., Li, L., Chen, P., Wang, Z., & Gu, Q. (2013). Electrostatic adsorption method for preparing electrically conducting ultrahigh molecular weight polyethylene/graphene nanosheets composites with a segregated network. *Composites Science and Technology*, *89*, 180–185. doi:10.1016/j.compscitech.2013.10.002

Wang, G., & Zreiqat, H. (2010). Functional coatings or films for hard-tissue applications. *Materials (Basel)*, *3*(7), 3994–4050. doi:10.3390/ma3073994 PMID:28883319

Wintermantel, E. (2001). Composites for biomedical applications. In *Encyclopedia of materials: science and technology* (pp. 1371–1376). Oxford, UK: Elsevier. doi:10.1016/B0-08-043152-6/00255-2

Wong, Beygi, & Zheng. (2019). Materials for Exoskeletal Orthotic and Prosthetic Systems. *Encyclopaedia of Biomedical Engineering*, 352-367.

Xie, Y., Hill, C. A. S., Xiao, Z., Militz, H., & Mai, C. (2010). Silane coupling agents used for natural fiber/polymer composites: A review. *Composites. Part A, Applied Science and Manufacturing*, *41*(7), 806–819. doi:10.1016/j.compositesa.2010.03.005

Yuan, Q., Wu, D., Gotama, J., & Bateman, S. (2008). Wood fiber reinforced polyethylene and polypropylene composites with high modulus and impact strength. *J. Thermoplastic Composit. Mater.*, *21*(3), 195–208. doi:10.1177/0892705708089472

Zhang, Q., Rastogi, S., Chen, D., Lippits, D., & Lemstra, P. J. (2006). Low percolation threshold in single-walled carbon nanotube/high density polyethylene composites prepared by melt processing technique. *Carbon*, *44*(4), 778–785. doi:10.1016/j.carbon.2005.09.039

Chapter 10 Modeling and Numerical Analysis of Advanced Machining for Orthotic Components

Pankaj Charan Jena
https://orcid.org/0000-0002-3837-7626
Veer Surendra Sai University of Technology, India

Barsarani Pradhan
Veer Surendra Sai University of Technology, India

D. Dhupal
Veer Surendra Sai University of Technology, India

ABSTRACT

Electrochemical micromachining plays a vital role in the advanced machining domain. Particularly, it helps the medical industry in machining micro-level devices in hardened materials. Though it is maintaining a very small inter-electrode gap during machining, it is required to understand suitable machining parameters before machining. These parameters can be achieved by proper modeling and simulation. In this chapter, a model for flow analysis of electrolytes in inter-electrode gaps is designed to obtain optimal process parameters for machining. The geometric model used in this simulation consists of cylindrical workpiece, an inlet allowing the flow of sodium nitrate

DOI: 10.4018/978-1-5225-8235-9.ch010

solution as electrolyte to the machining zone, and a cylindrical tool with a flat end. Electrolytic flow simulation is incorporated using computational fluid dynamics by ANSYS–CFX 15.0 for finding pressure variation, streamline velocity pattern, turbulent energy, and temperature contour in IEG. According to the CFD analysis, the passivation effect, stagnation effect, pressure, and temperature zone are studied.

INTRODUCTION

Electrochemical micro machining plays a vital role in advanced machining domain. Particularly it helps to medical industry to machining in micro level devices in harden materials. Currently Biomedical instruments are more micro in size and high accuracy. Manufacturing and selecting suitable machining process of such instruments are a challenge for present researchers. Electrochemical process is one of the advanced machining processes and can be possible to manufacture micro sized medical instruments like nozzles, tubes, etc.

Though it is maintaining a very small inter electrode gap during machining therefore it is required to understand a suitable machining parameters before to machining. These parameters can be achieved by proper modeling and simulation. In present research a model for flow analysis of electrolyte in inter electrode gap is designed to obtain optimal process parameter for machining.

Material removal of the dimension ranging between 1.0 micrometers to 999.0 micrometers comes under micromachining. Using conventional micromachining for producing these shapes has its own share of limitations, which include high tool wear rate, thermal stress, and imperfect surface finish. To overcome these limitations, researchers are exploring new non-conventional micromachining technique. One such technique is Electrochemical micromachining (ECMM) having advantages like tool having no wear, stress-free surfaces, machining electrically conductive material regardless of physical as well as chemical property, bright surface finish. ECMM is workedon anodic suspension at atomic level in electrolyte. This problem can be modeled and simulated by studying the flow pattern of electrolyte. This information in turn will help to avoid the passivation, which is one of the major problems in ECMM related to complex shape machining. Another problem, which is associated with ECMM, is generation of hydrogen gas at cathode. As electrolyte passes through cathode, it absorbs hydrogen gas generated at cathode. Due to this absorption, electrical conductivity of electrolyte decreases. As MRR and surface finish in ECMM is directly dependent on the electrical conductivity of the electrolyte, a decrease in it will hamper the machining rate and surface finish of work piece. In order to avoid all these, we need to know the source, effects, & pattern of hydrogen bubble generation. How it affect various critical parameters and overall machining performance.

LITERATURE REVIEW

Ghoshal et al. (2015) in the report more emphasis has given to the scan feed rate calculation at different machining parameters. Scan feed rate plays an important role in microchannel formation for reduction of overcut. The author has observed the taper angle formed by the straight micro tool at different level of concentration of electrolyte and has used MATLAB to solve the mathematical model. Liu et al. (2017) have discussed about the effect of retracted tip tool in electrochemical micromachining process. Aluminum had taken as the work piece and 304 stainless steel had taken as the electrode. To avoid the refracted tip of the tool a mathematical model has developed.

Table 1. Major machining characteristics of ECMM

Major Machining Characteristics of ECMM	
Voltage	< 10
Current	< 1 A
Current Density	75-100 A/ cm^2
Power supply -DC	Pulsed
Frequency	KHz-MHz range
Electrolyte flow	< 3 m/s
Electrolyte temperature	37- 50^0C
Electrolyte type	Natural salt or dilute acid/alkaline solution
Electrolyte concentration	< 20 g/l
Size of the tool	Micro
Inter-electrode gap	5-50μm
Operation	Mask/maskless
Machining rate	5μm/min
Side gap	< 10μm

Kumar et al. (2016) have investigated and ECMM process for finding the effect of machining parameters on diametrical overcut. Simulation has performed by considering the optimum machining parameters in COMSOL MultiphysicsV4.2a software for validating the experiment result.

Kamaraj et al. (2016) have investigated the function of brain through the use of penetrating microelectrode. They have used silicon based material as work material and the fabrication has done by tungsten penetrating microelectrode (10µm). Roughness range was 300nm-500nm with high aspect ratio 400. They have applied FEM for bulking analysis and to determine the machined hole diameter. Singh et al. (2016) have fabricated a complex circuit on printed circuit board (PCB) by using mask electrochemical micromachining (ECMM). Water insoluble glue Araldite mask (50µm) has bonded on a PCB (35×35mm cross-section). With the combination of experiments and numerical simulation by FEM, the optimum conditions for ECMM parameters and the formulation of electrolyte have achieved. Xiaolong et al. (2016) Found that in wire electrochemical micromachining rotary helical electrode is enhanced machining accuracy with faster feed rate and minimizing inter electrode gap. They have considered platinum wire (diameter: 10µm) as electrode and stainless steel as cathode (plate thickness: 100µm) for experiment with electrode gap: 5µm and feed rate: 0.1 µm/s. They have performed numerical calculation by FEM via COMSOL version 5.0. Jiang et al. (2014) havedescribed initial stress on the surface micromachining of silicon nitride, pressure sensor at given temperature and pressure (250C and 101 kPa). They have used FEM with ANSYS software to obtain pressure-displacement curve. Sun et al. (2014) havereported that FEM could use for the measurement of ultra-high strength steel Cr12Ni5MoCo14 at crack tip under applied stress. Qian et al. (2010) have produced micro dimple arrays on surface of friction pairs using modified through mask electrochemical micromachining (ECMM) wherein micro dimples was created on anode by dissolution of its surface with electrolyte by using insulation-coated cathode when voltage was applied. They have used FEM to analyze the electric field and to calculate the distribution of current density on anode surface exposed in the electrolyte. Li et al. (2017) Used ECMM to fabricate micro dimple array. They used inert metal mask closely attached to anode and matrix-hole in the mask, which has machined by CNC. Electrolyte has allowed flowing through at a high speed between cathode and mask and machining has done by dissolution of anodic material by electrolyte. They were analyzed current density distribution by using FEM. Liu et al. (2017) have investigated different method of microelectrode like chemical etching, electric discharge and micromachining. Less than

10μm micro hole has formed by stainless steel in different work piece then analysis of current density and simulation done by FEM method. Jin et al. (2017) have machined micro size-hole on invar alloy film 30-μm (Fe-64% and Ni-36%) with stainless steel 304 tool. They have used Finite element method (FEM) to verify the influence of each parameters of invar alloy. They have machined by using the mask and a part of the photolithography etching process. Lee et al. (2008) have conducted micro machining on bipolar metallic plate for producing fuel cells. SS316 stainless steel sheets (50mm width×0.6mm depth) taken as work piece for drilling 200×500μm micro hole. They have used finite element analysis (FEA) to check rigidity of machine tool platform.Zou et al. (2017) have developed a hybrid system that is Levenberg and simulated annealing by using an artificial neutral network for optimizing the process parameters of electrochemical micro machining. This system results in deciding optimum process parameters for minimum overcut and taper angle.Samanta et al. (2011)haveoptimized heat-affected zone, radial overcut, material removal rate, tool wear rate of electrochemical micromachining process, electrochemical machine, electro discharge machine by using artificial bee colony algorithm and then compared with each other. Singh et al. (2016) haveused firefly algorithm to optimize the material removal rate, heat affected zone, radial overcut of electrochemical micromachining and electrochemical discharge machining process. The better machining process has selected by comparing the both. It has found that fire fly algorithm gives better result for complex numerical problem. IT can be conclude from the report the single optimization values for fire fly algorithm gives better result. Geethapriyan et al. (2016) have done multi objective optimization of Inconel 718 material using taguchi based grey rational analysis in electrochemical micro machining process. In this report two types of electrolyte has used that is NaCl and NaNO3 for finding the optimum result. Optimum parameters has established from the experimental result and optimization.

Nayak et al. (2016) have investigated the model of electrochemical machining process I-shaped tool on the work piece material Inconel-825. Experimental investigation as well as CFD modelling was done in this report. CFD modelling was done for analysis the flow characteristic of the electrolyte within the inter electrode gap. Simulation result give an idea about the formation of pressure profile, velocity profile, turbulence profile from the counter plots which is helpful in designing tool profile. Optimization of experimental data has completed using grey rational analysis (GRA) and the output of the GRA has taken as input for ANOVA analysis for finding the optimized result for material removal rate, overcut and surface roughness.

In this experiment electrolyte concentration, feed rate, voltage has given as input in three level. Rath et al. (2013) have analyzed two-phase flow in electrochemical machining considering models of L-shaped tool using ANSYS-CFX. Computational fluid dynamics flow analysis of three different model has completed for deciding the best model among the three from the simulation result. The effect of formation of hydrogen bubble, stagnation effect, and the effect of passivation has analyzed within the inter electrode gap. The best model after the analysis has selected.

Objective

It is observed that past researchers have discussed various approaches to understand MRR as well as current density distribution in ECMM. They have used different tool geometry for these analyses. In case, complicated micro tool geometryand work pieces, it is very difficult to know the machining variables within the IEG as it is in micro level. However, there is a need to understand about those parameters, the impact of their variation in the IEG as well as in different materials by proper simulation process. Once it is known, then it will be easy to perform real experiment. In this simulation various process parameters at different level for copper tool has considered on Nimonic-75 work piece material. The simulation is first done for steady state and then considering the result of steady state and two transient state analyses is obtained. In this work a total of nine steady state and transient analysis is done.

The following parameters are considered in numerical analysis using ANSYS-CFX:

- Current density
- Velocity profile
- Temperature pattern
- Turbulence kinetic energy
- Pressure profile
- Turbulence eddy dissipation

The outcome of the flow analysis gives an idea about the effect of passivation, stagnation effect, stray current effect within the small inter electrode gap.

MODELLING AND SIMULATION

A Need Towards Modeling and Simulation of ECMM

This sectionis briefing the procedure of the modeling and simulationby utilizing ANSYS CFX (Figure 1). ECMM process comprises of a work piece, tool and an electrolyte solution. W/P ought to be electrically conductive in nature and the device could conceivably be. Commonly utilized electrolyte for ECMM process is $NaNO_3$. As the device shape influences the MRR and to get a required geometry and size in work piece,a tool ought to be planned effectively. Most importantly, this simulation helped in the selection of effective process parameter for achieving the best output.

Overview of ANSYS-CFX

1. **Design Modeler:** It defines geometrical dimensions for the required model using various sketching icons. Naming the faces of the solid body (e.g. Inlet, outlet, wall and symmetry) is done.

Figure 1. Sketch showing overview of ANSYS-CFX

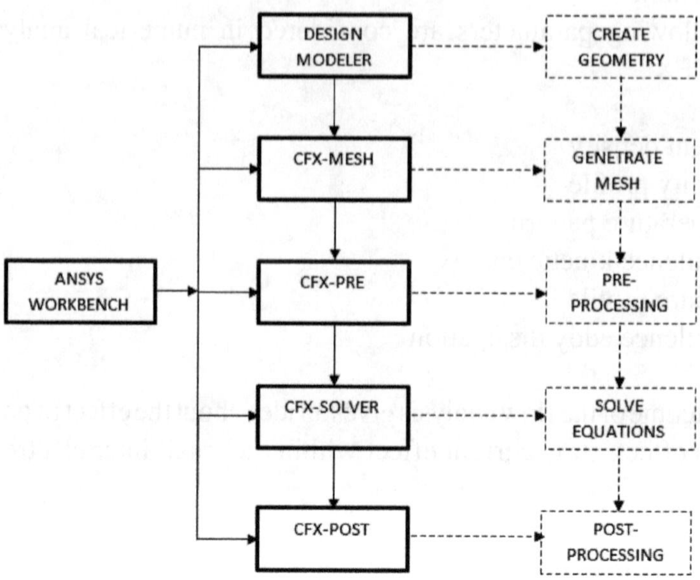

2. **CFx-MESH:** It specifies mesh properties like mesh spacing, inflated boundary thickness. CFx-Mesh provides automated mesh created from the surface mesh generation which depends onSkewness, aspect ratio and element quality.
    a. **Skewness:** It defines as the measure of quality of mesh. The following method is based on the equilateral volume deviation that determines Skewness, which is generally applied for triangles and tetrahedral. The value of Skewness varies from 0-1 and with gradual increase towards 1; it gives an imperfect result.

$$\textbf{Skewness} = \frac{\textit{optimal cell size} - \textit{actual cell size}}{\textit{optimal cell size}}$$

    b. **Aspect Ratio:** Aspect ratio for generic triangles and quads is a function of the ratio of longest side to the shortest side of the reconstructed quadrangles. It needs high quality mesh to overcome numerical diffusion. Several mesh quality metrics are involved in order to quality; however, the Skewness is the primary metric. The aspect ratio and cell size changed mesh metrics are also very important.
    c. **Element Quality:** Various element types for the CFX-Solver include tetrahedral, prism (wedges), pyramids and hexes.
3. **CFX-Pre:** It specifies the type of fluid (water or air), properties of fluid (e.g. density, viscosity etc.), type of turbulence model (e.g. k-ϵ model, wall function etc.), boundary conditions (e.g. speed, length scale, turbulence intensity, fluid speed/mass flow rate/pressure at inlet and outlet), convergence criterions (e.g. number of iteration, residual target etc.).
4. **CFX-Solver:** It solves system of partial differential equations.
5. **CFX-Post:** It analyzes results and creates plots.

Selection of Material and Corresponding Element

Selection of work-piece material, tool material and electrolyte ispresented in Table 2

Table 2. Material and Element type for simulation

SerialNo.	Component	Material	Physical state
1	Work-piece	Nimonic-75	solid
2	Tool	Copper	solid
3	Electrolyte	Sodium nitrate	fluid

Geometrical Modeling of Tool and Work-Piece

The cylindrical work piece is modeled for diameter of 1.0 cm and thickness 0. 15 cm. The cylindrical shaped work piece is having flat end body. The tool is a cylindrical shaped flat end body for 260-micrometer diameter and height 2 mm. The geometrical model for simulation is in Figure2.

Problem Statement

Case: 1

Keeping the potential difference as 6V and the inlet velocity of the electrolyte flow as 1.5m/s, we are varying the Inter Electrode Gap between the anode and the cathode and obtaining the optimized model:

1. 20 micro meter
2. 15 micro meter
3. 10 micro meter

Case: 2

Keeping the optimized Inter Electrode Gap and inlet velocity of the electrolyte flow as 1.5m/s, we are varying the potential difference between the tool and the work piece and getting the optimized model:

1. 3V
2. 6V
3. 9V

Case: 3

Keeping the optimized Inter Electrode Gap and the potential difference between the tool and the work piece as constant, we are varying the inlet velocity of the electrolyte that flows from the tool top over the tool towards the work piece.

1. 0.5m/s
2. 1.5m/s
3. 2.5m

MESHING OF TOOL AND WORKPIECE

Meshing is the process of dividing the Solid/Fluid part into number of infinitesimally small, but non-zero elements. The modeled geometry is meshed in the ANSYS Workbench Mesh module. The solver preference was set as CFX for the model to be meshed. The relevance has maintained at 50 to get acceptable number of elements for the simulation to be carried out. A finer mesh has maintained near the area that is to be machined. The face sizing is used on the area to be given finer mesh. The total number of elements obtained is 350000 and the Skewness is maintained at 0.86, which is acceptable.

The meshed model is shown in the Figure3.

Physics preference selected for the analysis is CFD for flow analysis. Solver preference selected for the meshing is CFX; the output of the mesh structure will be saved. On proximity and curvature, advanced sizing method has enabled for better mesh in curvature and smaller inter electrode gap region. Automatic meshing is used for meshing these geometries with elements having minimum edge length of 6.28e-04 micron. A tetrahedral element generally provides solution that is more automatic with ability to add mesh controls to improve accuracy in central region. Hexahedral meshes give result that is more accurate but it is very difficult to generate. Program controlled automatic inflation method is enabled for meshing.

Mesh methods included in ANSYS are either patch conforming and patch independent methods. As no methods for meshing is selected there is no need for selecting patch conforming or patch independence. Face sizing method is adopted for the better mesh near the inter electrode gap of element size

8e-07micron. The detail specification of the independent model is given in the Table 3.

From the sectional view of the meshed model it can be said that mesh near the inter electrode gap is finer and smaller. Reason for the finer mesh structure near the inter electrode gap is to predicting correct flow pattern near the gap.

Finer the mesh structure will give better result than coarser mesh structure. Mesh structure is set in the relevance standards. When relevance is selected coarse, the mesh structure will be coarser one with element size lesser than finer mesh. The geometric view and the meshed structure by the ANSYS software are as follows:

Name selections in the model are specified below:

Table 3. Meshing details of the present geometrical model

Nodes	Elements	Skewness	Orthogonal quality	relevance
1554841	8191763	0.877	0.9976	fine

Figure 2. IEG between tool and work piece

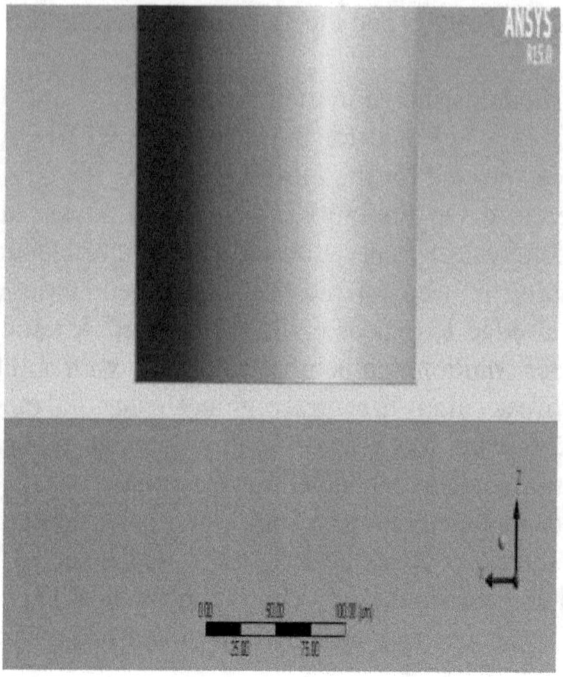

Figure 3. Meshed model

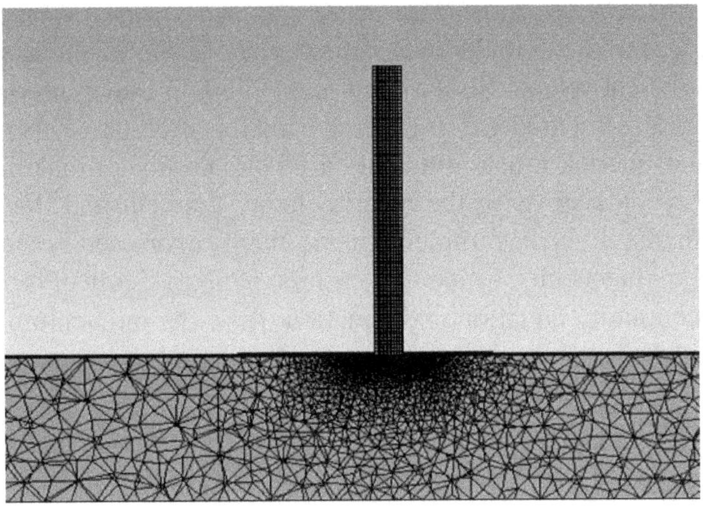

1. Tool
    a. Tool Top-Top face surface of tool.
    b. Tool Bottom-Bottom face surface of tool.
    c. Tool Outer-Outer surface of tool.
2. Work piece
    a. Work Top-Top face surface of work piece.
    b. Work Bottom-Bottom face surface of work piece.
    c. Work Outer-Outer surface of work piece.
3. Brine (Electrolyte)
    a. Velocity Inlet-Starting region of electrolyte.
    b. Pressure Outlet-The portion which electrolyte is flowing out.
    c. Brine groove-the inner surface of the electrolyte in contact with tool
    d. Brine bottom-Bottom face of brine which contacts top surface of work piece.

GOVERNING EQUATIONS FOR ECMM

Simulations in for ECMM are based on governing equations. It is of two types. First one is Computational Fluid Dynamics model equations which are predefined in the software ANSYS and the second one is the user defined equations.

Equations for CFD Model Generated By ANSYS

In this the Reynolds no at the inlet is more than 4000, this means the flow is in the turbulent region. So we want to enable a turbulent model for this simulation. Here k-ϵ model is used for solving this problem. This model is a two equations model. It uses gradient based hypothesis for making relation between Reynolds stress to the mean velocity gradient and the turbulent viscosity. In that 'k' is the turbulent kinetic energy expressed as the variance of fluctuations in velocity. Unit of K is in m^2/s^2.Unit of 'ϵ' is in m^2/s^3. Equation (1) is the continuity equation and equation (4) is the momentum equation for this model.

$$\frac{\partial Á}{\partial t}+\frac{\partial}{\partial x_j}\left(Áu_j\right)=0 \tag{1}$$

$$\frac{\partial \rho U_i}{\rho t}+\frac{\partial}{\partial x_j}(\rho_{u_i u_j})=\frac{\partial P'}{\partial x_i}+\frac{\partial}{\partial x_i}\left(\mu_{eff}\left[\frac{\partial U_i}{\partial x_j}+\frac{\partial U_j}{\partial x_i}\right]\right)+S_m \tag{2}$$

$$\mu_{eff}=\mu+\mu_t \tag{3}$$

In k-ϵ model it is assumed that the turbulence viscosity depends on turbulent kinetic energy and dissipation. The relation is shown in equation (4).

$$\mu_t=C\mu\rho\frac{k^2}{\in} \tag{4}$$

K and ϵ values are coming directly from the differential equations for turbulent kinetic energy and dissipation rate. Those equations are given in equation (5) and (6).

$$\frac{\partial(\rho k)}{\partial t}+\frac{\partial}{\partial x_j}\left(\rho u_{jk}\right)=\frac{\partial}{\partial x_j}\left[\left(\mu+\frac{\mu_t}{\sigma_k}\right)\frac{\partial k}{\partial x_j}\right]+P_k-\rho_\varepsilon+P_{kb} \tag{5}$$

$$\frac{\partial(\rho\varepsilon)}{\partial t}+\frac{\partial}{\partial x_j}\left(\rho u_j\varepsilon\right)=\frac{\partial}{\partial x_j}\left[\left(\mu+\frac{\mu_t}{\sigma_\varepsilon}\right)\frac{\partial\varepsilon}{\partial x_j}\right]+\frac{\varepsilon}{k}\left[C_{\varepsilon1}P_kC_{\varepsilon2}\rho_\varepsilon+C_{\varepsilon1}P_{\varepsilon b}\right] \tag{6}$$

Value for P_k is getting from the relation given in equation (7)

$$P_k = \mu_t \left(\frac{\partial u_i}{\partial x_j} + \frac{\partial u_j}{\partial x_i} \right) \frac{\partial u_i}{\partial x_j} \tag{7}$$

It consists of one more term but in our problem effect of that term is less. Therefore it can neglect that term because for incompressible flow ($\frac{\partial u_k}{\partial x_k}$) having less effect. It has effect in compressible flow with high velocity divergence. For making heat transfer model constructed the solid domains as conjugate heat transfer (CHT) domains. In CFX, boundaries between domains that model heat transfer have temperatures and thermal fluxes calculated automatically and should not have to specify the thermal boundary conditions. Source of thermal energy and radiation can also be added to a CHT domain. ANSYS-CFX allow to create solid regions in which the equations for heat transfer are solved, but without flow. This is known as conjugate heat transfer. Inside the solid domains conservation of energy equation is simplified since there is no flow inside the solid, thus conduction is the only mode of heat transfer. The heat conduction through the solid has transport equations as like shown in equation (8).

$$\frac{\partial \rho C_p T}{\partial t} = \nabla . \left(k . \nabla T \right) + S_E \tag{8}$$

To find out the velocity we have to know the volume flow rate range for the electrolyte. Using equation of continuity given in the equation (9) the inlet velocity within that range can be calculated. The inlet velocity taken here is 2.5 m/s and is kept constant throughout the analysis.

$$Q = av \tag{9}$$

Total duration for analysis taken is 120s with a total time steps of 240 are taken time step having pulse duration of 0.5s for each time step. The material removal rate can be expressed by the given equation (10) and (11).

$$d_i = \frac{J_i \varepsilon A}{F \rho z} \tag{10}$$

$$\varepsilon = \frac{mzF}{ItA} \tag{11}$$

For an anodic reaction the limiting current density is controlled by convective mass transport. The anodic limiting current density (J_L) also changes according to the change in conductivity of the electrolyte and is calculated from the equation (12).

$$J_L = \frac{zFDC_{ast}}{\delta} \tag{12}$$

The current density depends upon thermal conductivity (k). Thermal conductivity is proportional to the temperature as shown in the equation (13).

$$k = k_0(1 + \propto (T_b - T) \tag{13}$$

MATERIAL PROPERTIES OF SOLID AND FLUID DOMAIN:

Materials used for making the simulation are NIMONIC 75 as work piece, copper as tool and 20% brine (Sodium Nitrate) as electrolyte. The required properties for the simulation are given the following Table 4.

Analysis

The analysis is done in ANSYS CFX-15.0 software because it is simpler than FLUENT and MHD option can easily enable within this software. For doing this analysis firstly we need to set the analysis in steady state and then initialize the results of the steady state simulation to the transient case. In such a case the end of the steady state will be the starting point for the transient simulation.

Table 4. Material properties used for analysis

PROPERTIES	BRINE	COPPER	NIMONIC 75	AIR
Molar Mass(Kg/Kmol)	0.084995	63.55	53.74	-
Density(Kg/m^3)	2260	8933	8.37	-
Specific Heat(J/KgK)	1094.75	385	461	-
Dynamic Viscosity (Pa s)	0.001	-	-	-
Thermal Conductivity(W/mK)	0.48	401	11.7	-
Electrical Conductivity(S/m)	20.4 (20g/l)	5.96E+07	0.9E+06	-
Convection Coefficient(W/m^2K)	1000	-	-	100

Assumption

As like every simulation for this simulation also assuming some assumptions. Those assumptions are

1. The inter electrode gap is constant.
2. Material property of the tool and work-piece never change throughout the analysis.
3. Tool and work piece material are homogeneous.
4. Heat generation is due to Joule's heating.
5. The electrolyte is in liquid state and no H2 gas is evolved
6. Material removal only depends on current density

Boundary Conditions

The computational domains should specify first before specifying the boundary conditions. In these simulation four domains i.e. three solid domains and a fluid domainare used, where the tool, work piece and insulator is the solid domain and electrolyte is the fluid domain. Solid domain materials are in the material group conjugate heat transfer solids and consider as pure solids. Morphology of material is given as continuous solid and reference temperature is given 300K. Electric potential model with automatic value is chosen from Electromagnetic model. Fluid domain is constructed for electrolyte. Morphology for fluid domain is taken as continuous fluid. Material properties are given in the Table. Only the conductivity of electrolyte is varying with respect to temperature according to the equation other values are kept constant. This equation is written as CEL expression and directly assigned it as material property. α- value is taken as 0.02 for brine and boiling temperature for brine is taken as 653.2K. In this simulation NIMONIC 75 is used as work piece material, copper is used as tool material and brine solution is used as electrolyte.

Boundary conditions used for these simulations are given below:

1. Inlet

Mass and Momentum = Normal speed = 0.5, 1.5 and 2.5 m/s
Flow regime = Subsonic
Turbulence = Medium Intensity (5%)
Heat transfer static temperature = 300K
Electric field = 0 flux

2. Outlet

Mass and Momentum = Opening pressure and direction = 101.325 kPa and flow normal to the boundary.
Flow regime = Subsonic
Turbulence = Medium Intensity (5%)

3. Tool
   a. Tool Top

Heat transfer = Convection
Convection heat transfer coefficient = 100W/m2 K
Electrical potential = Voltage= 0 V

   b. Tool Outer

Heat transfer = Convection
Convection heat transfer coefficient = 100W/m2 K

4. Work piece
   c. Work Bottom

Heat transfer = Convection
Convection heat transfer coefficient = 15W/m2 K
Electric field = Voltage = 3V,6V,9V

d. Work Outer

Heat transfer = Convection
Convection heat transfer coefficient = 15W/m2 K

5. Interface
    e. Brine Tool

It is the interface between brine top and tool bottom. Type of interaction used = Fluid-Solid.
Heat transfer = Thin material
Heat transfer in Copper = 0.00000002 m.
GGI type mesh connection is used to connect meshes.

f. Brine Work

It is the interface between brine bottom and work piece top.
Heat transfer = Thin material
Heat transfer in NIMONIC 75 = 0.00000002 m
GGI type mesh connection is used to connect meshes.

After the boundary condition set up we need to manage the solver control. High resolution is taken for advection scheme and turbulence numeric. 1 and 240 are given as minimum and maximum time step respectively. Fluid time scale control is set as physical time scale, in that time scale value is given as 0.5 s and in that time step value this simulation is done as an iterative process. So at first it is required to set convergence criteria. The root mean square (RMS) value is 1×10^{-5} is set as convergence criteria. Run mode is selected as HP MPI distributed parallel.

After completion of this analysis, took out the value of current density of work piece at each node in the csv format for calculating the deformation. Deformation at each and every node (d_i, where it denotes the deformation at i^{th} node) within the work piece is calculated using the equation 12. By deducing this value from material removal value and calling back the result file in to CFD post; it is possible to get the deformed or final shape of the work piece.

RESULT AND DISCUSSION

This section contains the simulation result done by ANSYS-CFX 15.0 as per discussed in section-3. Flow pattern analysis in terms of contour plots is described below. Contour plots for optimized result has also described.

Effect of Current Density

Case 1. With Change in IEG

From the above contour plots Figure 4, Figure 5 and Figure 6 for the current density, It can be understand that as the Inter Electrode Gap (IEG) increase from 10 micron to 20 micron, there is an increase the current density. Current density is maximum at the edge of the tool bottom because current is higher at sharper edges. It was observed that the machining is taking place only at the bottom of the tool. From the above contour plots it can be said that the model having the larger Inter Electrode Gap (IEG) has better machining parameters with increase in the current density. So the optimized IEG is 20μm for Case1.Here the current density profile are plotted in the range of 1.175e-05 to 1.645e+06

Effect of Pressure

Case 1. With Change in the Inter Electrode Gap

From the above pressure contour plot Figure 7 and Figure 8, it can be observed that there is an increase in the electrolyte pressure with decrease in the Inter Electrode Gap (IEG). Since pressure increased at the outlet, there is increase in the flow of electrolyte in the work-piece, which helps in reducing the stagnation of flow. It is observed from the contour plots that pressure near the edges is little higher and less pressure is observed near the center region, because of formation of hydrogen bubbles at the outer boundaries.

Figure 4. Current density with case 1(b) for 15 micron IEG

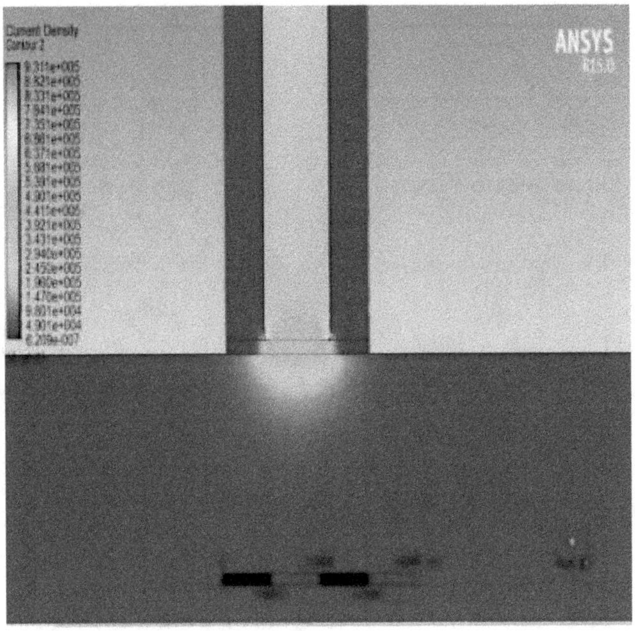

Figure 5. Current density with case 1(a) for 10 micron IEG

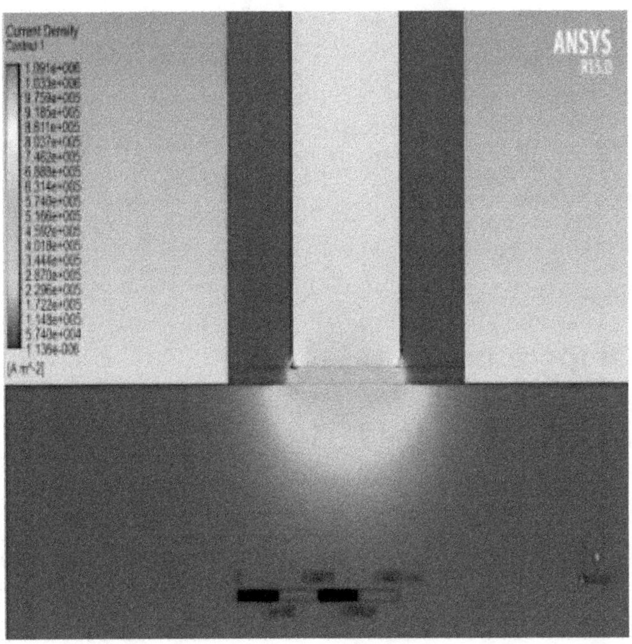

Figure 6. Current density for case 1(c) for 20 micron IEG

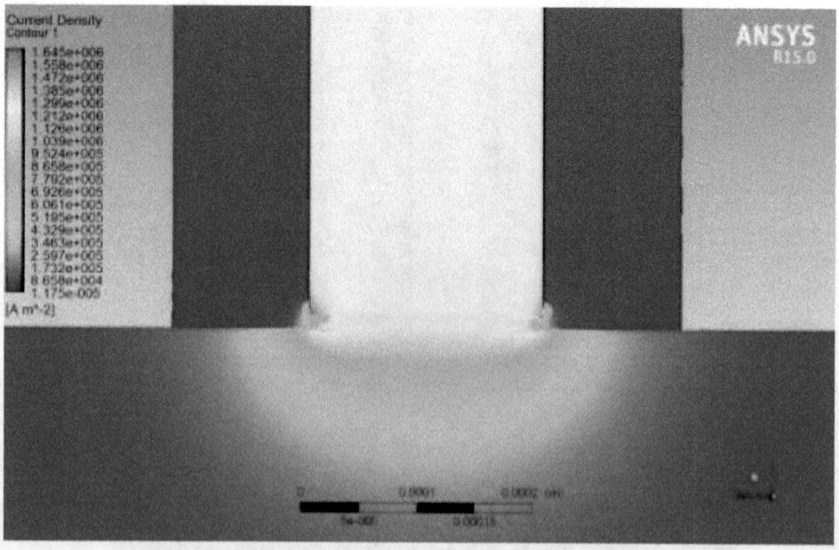

Figure 7. Pressure contour for Case 1: (a) 10µm IEG and (b) 15µm IEG

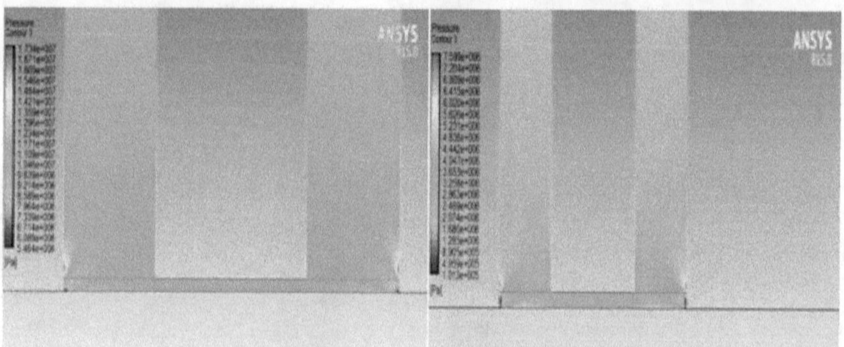

Effect of Temperature

Case 1. With Change in the IEG

For the experimention12; the simulation imagesare shown in Figure 18 and Figure 19.

From the above contour plots Figure 11 and Figure 12, it was infer that the temperature distribution on the surface of the work piece is less in 10µm IEG compared to the work piece having higher IEG.

Figure 8. Pressure contour for Case 1 (c) 20μm IEG

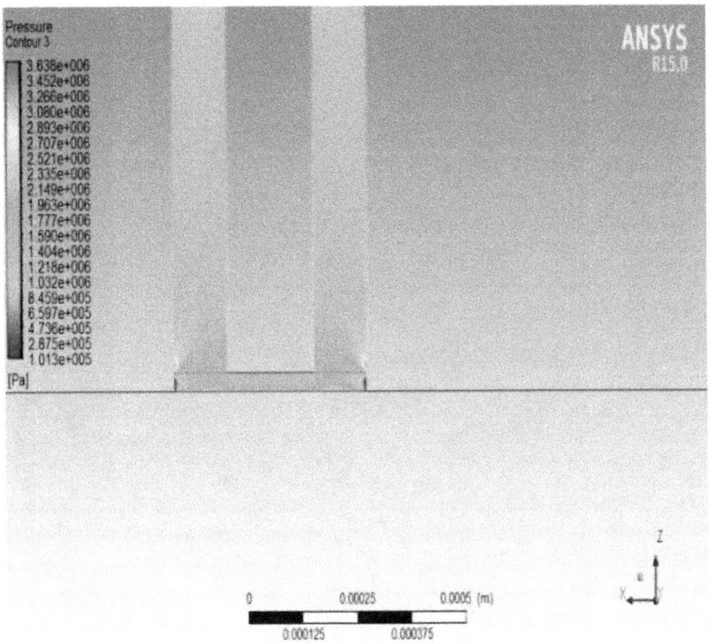

Flow Behavior of the Electrolyte

From the above Figure 13, Figure 14 and Figure 15streamline plots, it is observed that there is no change in the flow pattern of the electrolyte, as we are not changing the geometry.But we can note that with change in the Inter Electrode gap between the tool and the work piece there is an increase in the outlet velocity with increase in IEG.

Effect of Turbulent Eddy Dissipation

From the above contour plots, we can observe that with increase in the IEG gap, the turbulent eddy dissipation is reduced. This is because as the electrolyte flows towards the outlet, the area between the tool and the work piece is reduced as the IEG is reduced. This causes the turbulence in the region.

Figure 9. Mid plane temperature contour on work-piece for 20 micron IEG

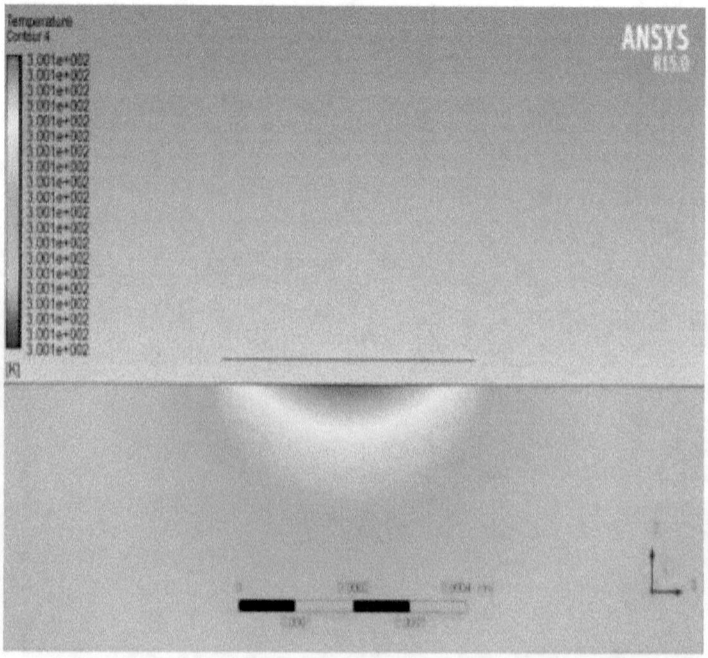

Figure 10. Top surface temperature contour on work-piece for 20 micron IEG

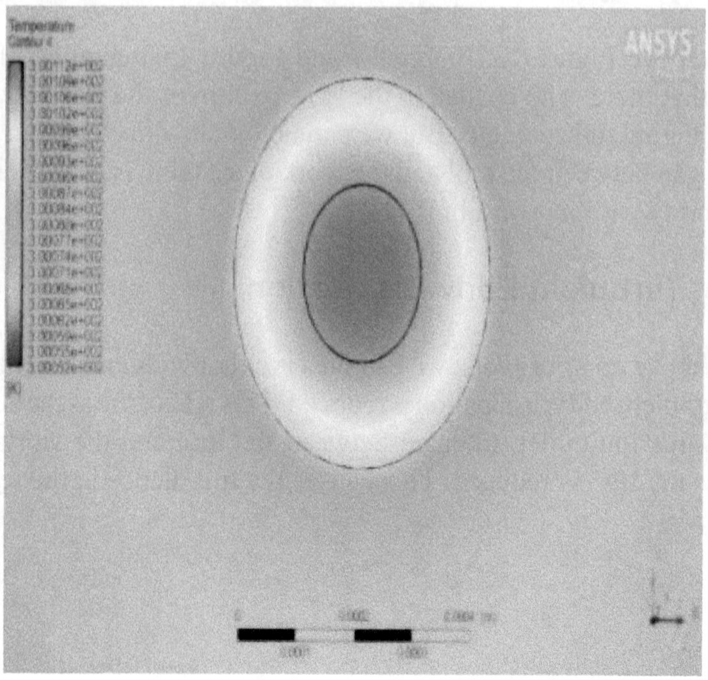

Figure 11. Top surface temperature contour on work-piece for 10 micron IEG

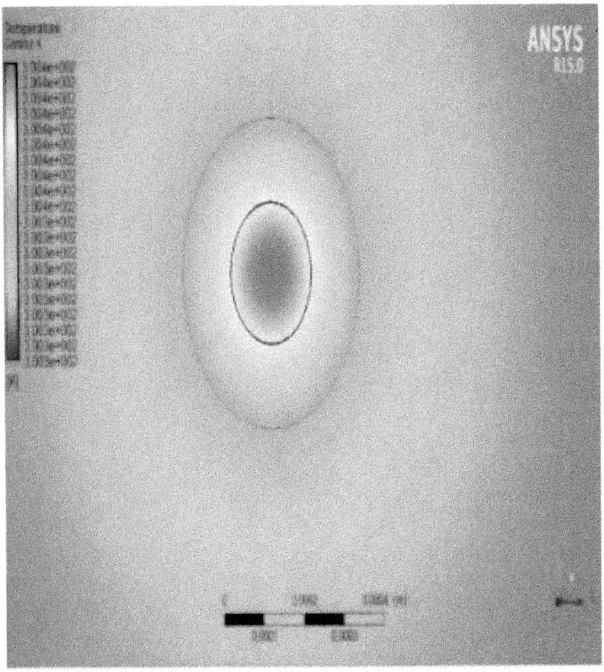

Figure 12. Mid plane temperature contour on work-piece for 10 micron IEG

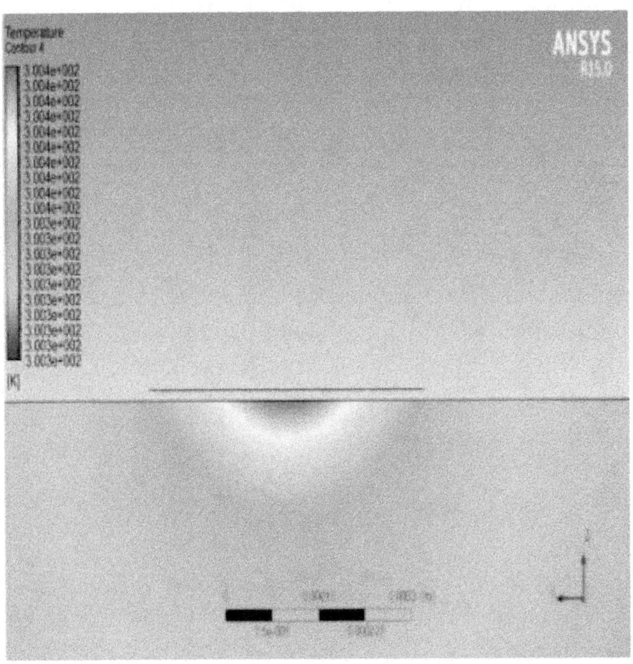

Figure 13. Velocity streamlines of electrolyte with 15μm IEG

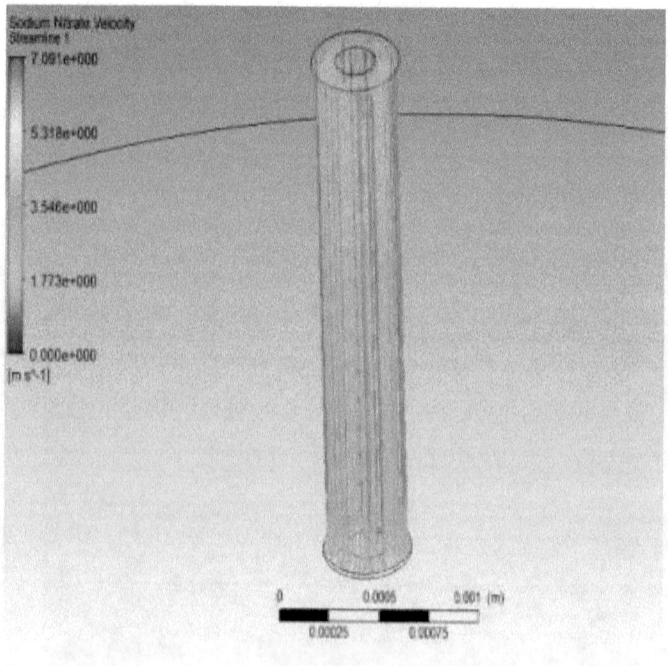

Figure 14. Velocity streamlines of Electrolyte with 20μm IEG

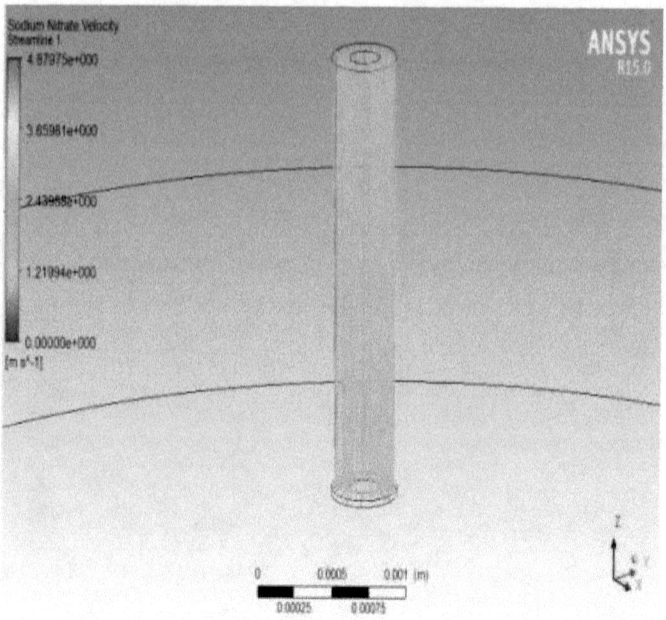

Figure 15. Velocity streamlines of electrolyte with 10μm IEG

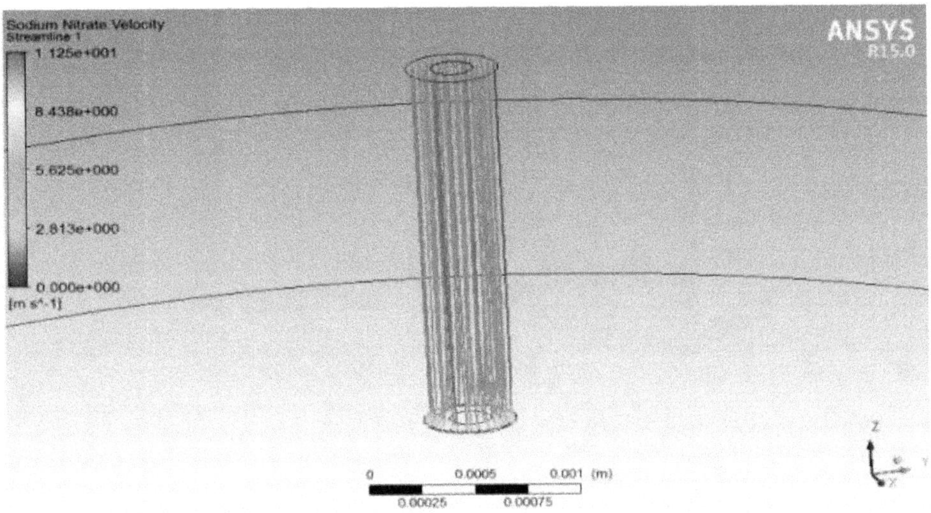

Figure 16. Turbulent Eddy Dissipation of electrolyte with 10μm

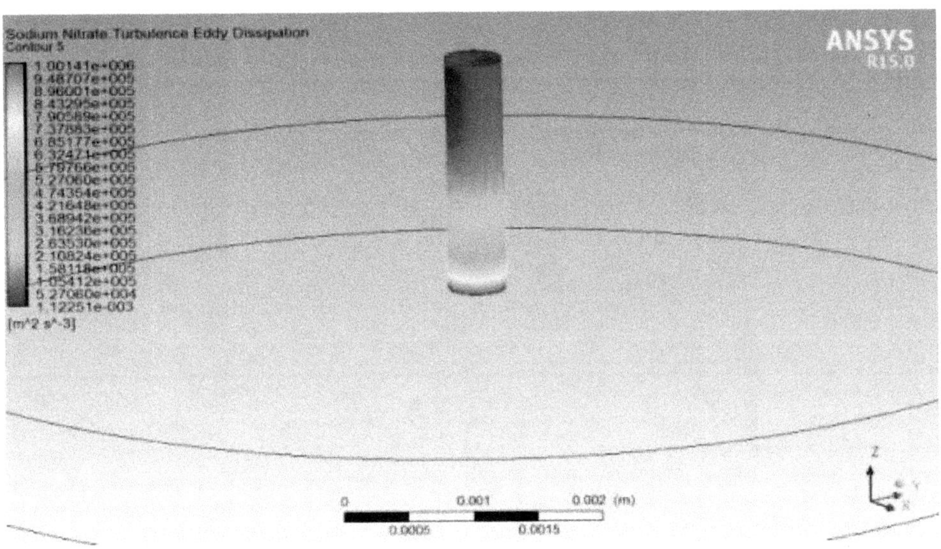

Figure 17. Turbulent Eddy Dissipation of electrolyte with 20μm IEG

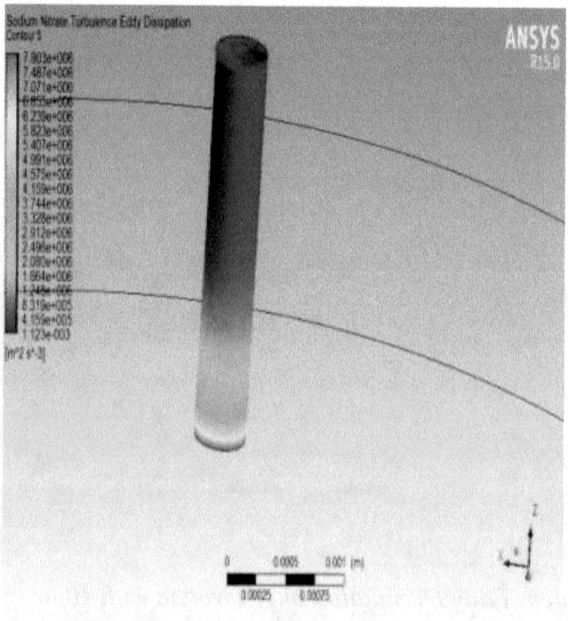

Figure 18. Turbulent Eddy Dissipation of electrolyte with 15μm IEG

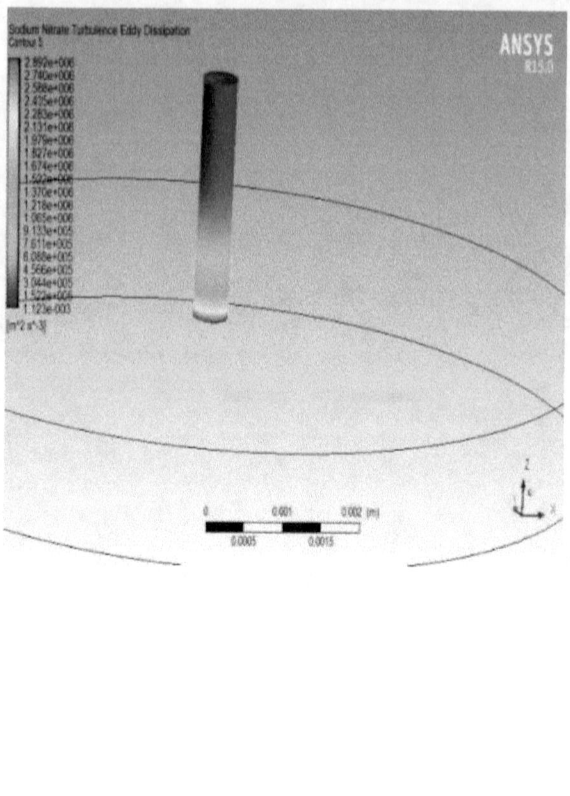

Final Shape of Work Piece

The Figure 19 is showing the final shape of the micro hole from the simulated result.

Case 2. With Change in Potential Difference (Voltage)

In Case 2, by keeping the optimized Inter Electrode gap from Case 1 that is 10μm and varying the potential difference it is observed that there is an increase in the current density with increase in the voltage. The voltage is varied from 3V-9V and we observe that 9V has better machining parameters compared to the 3V(Figure 20 and Figure 21).From this it can be said that increase in voltage gives us better machining parameter with respect to current density.

Final Shape of the Work Piece

Case 3. With Change in the Inlet Velocity

In the case 3, 20μm Inter Electrode Gap (IEG) and 9V potential difference as constant and varying the inlet velocity of the brine for 0.5m/s,1.5m/s and 2.5m/s is kept respectively. Thus, it can be concluded that with higher inlet velocity there is a presence of little improved machining parameters, which is verified from the experiment. The From the experiment it was found that in velocity 0.5 m/s and velocity 1.5 m/s machining is not going on properly because of the slurry within the IEG was not flushing away properly(Figure 25and Figure 26).

Effect of Pressure

From the above contour plot (Figure 25 and Figure 26)it can be observed that with increase in the velocity at the inlet there is increase in the pressure at the outlet. With increase in pressure, there is no stagnation of electrolyte towards the area to be machined.

Figure 19. Final shape of the work piece with 20µm IEG

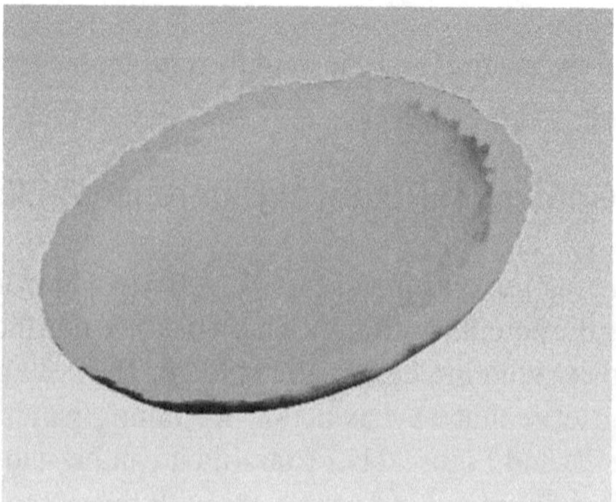

Figure 20. Current density for Case2(a) with 3V potential difference

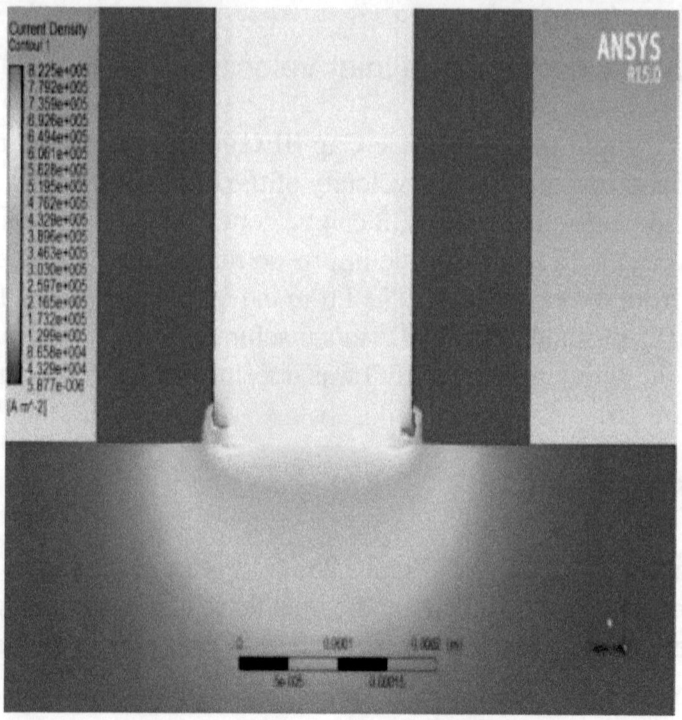

Figure 21. Current density for Case2(c) with 9V potential difference

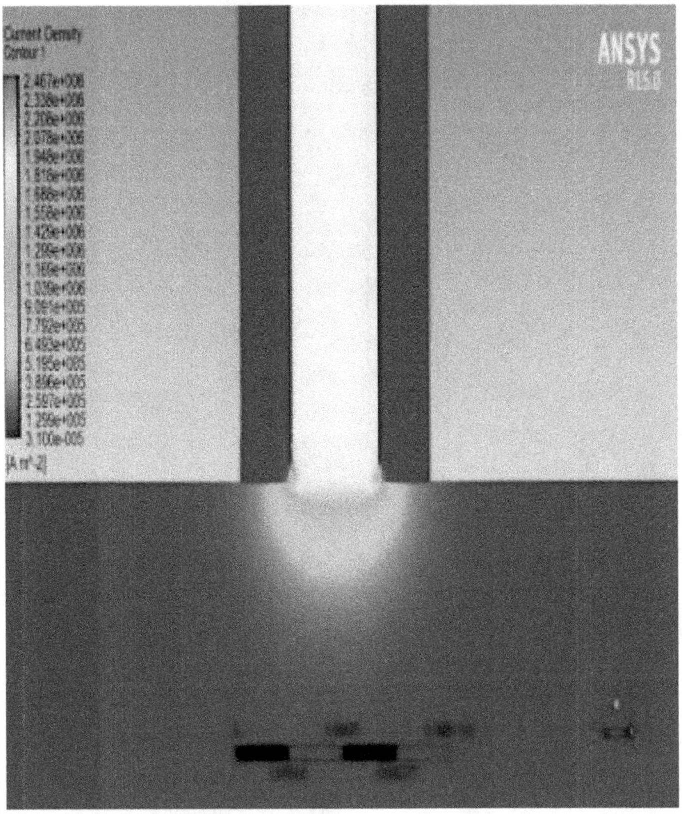

Figure 22. Final shape of the work piece at 9v potential difference

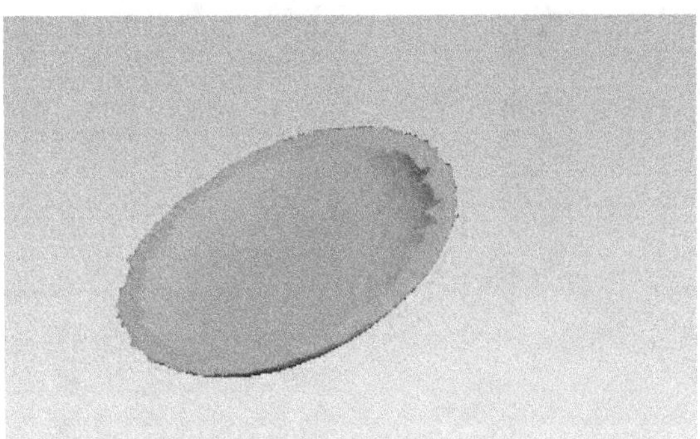

Figure 23. Current density for Case 3(c) with 2.5m/s inlet velocity

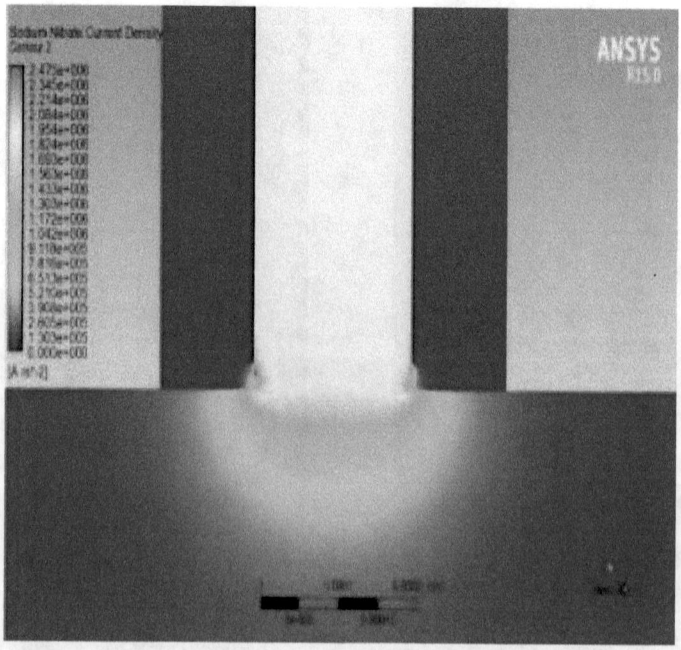

Figure 24. Current density for Case 3(a) with 0.5m/s inlet velocity

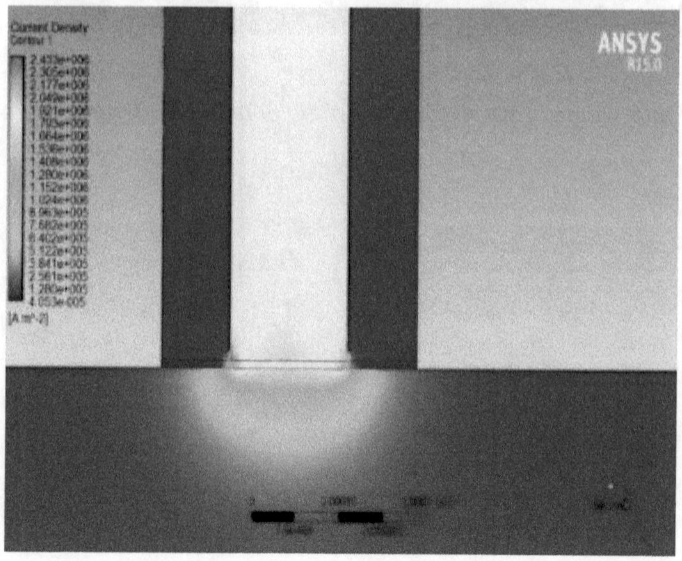

Figure 25. Pressure contour of electrolyte with 0.5 m/s velocity

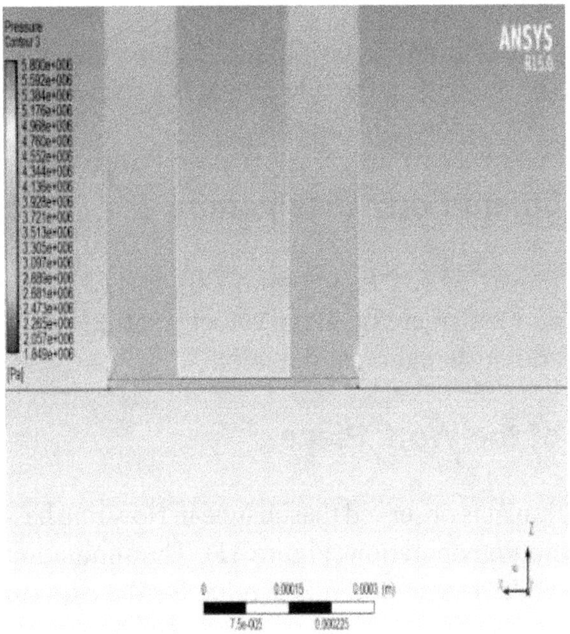

Figure 26. Pressure contour plot of electrolyte with 2.5m/s

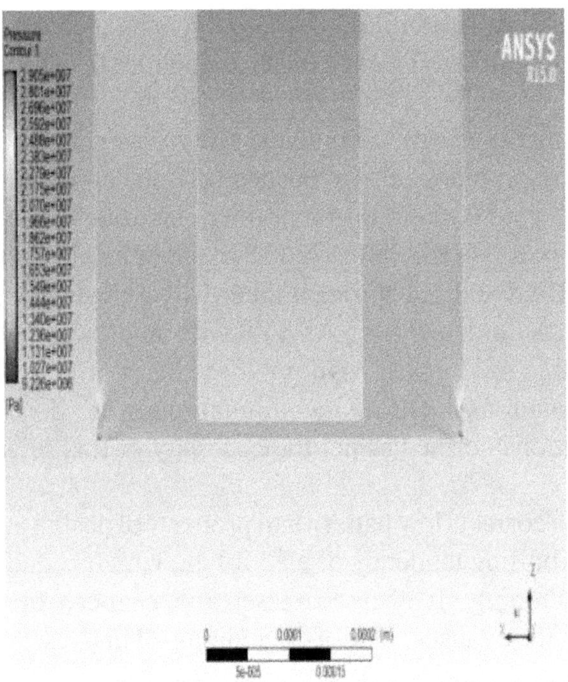

Flow Behavior of Electrolyte

From the above streamlines(Figure 27 and Figure 28), it is observed that with increase in the velocity at the inlet, there is a subsequent increase in the velocity towards the region to be machined.

Effect of Turbulent Eddy Dissipation

From the above plots(Figure 29 and Figure 30), it is observed that for 10μm IEG as constant and with increase in the velocity at the inlet, there is increase in the turbulent eddy dissipation at the inlet.

Final Shape of the Work Piece

From the simulation, it is observed that change in flow rate has very negligible effect on the machining operation (Figure 31). The simulation result for flow rate2.5m/scan be taken as an optimized value for the experimentation.

CONCLUSION

This work is based on machining of micro holes by electro-chemical micro machine with a cylindrical flat end tool, is giving idea of effect on distribution of velocity, pressure pattern, variation of profile of temperature, distribution of turbulence kinetic-energy, turbulence eddy dissipation, current density distribution. It also provides a clue about need of transient state analysis (Pulsed DC) over steady state (DC) in different inter electrode gap. In this analysis, work-piece material is NIMONIC-75 nickel super alloy, Cupper is taken as the tool material and Sodium Nitrate is taken as the electrolyte. The complete geometrical part is modeled using ANSYS with an orthogonal quality of 0.9, which ensures this model will have good results. For convergence criteria RMS value is taken as 1×10^5. Nine simulations were done with different boundary conditions defined as per the necessity of this research.

1. Predicting a correct flow pattern and proper tool design are important for preventing boiling tendency of electrolyte, which is due to overheating during machining. It also decreases the chances of passivation of electrolyte that causes a poor machining. This research work is an

Figure 27. Velocity streamlines of electrolyte for 2.5m/s

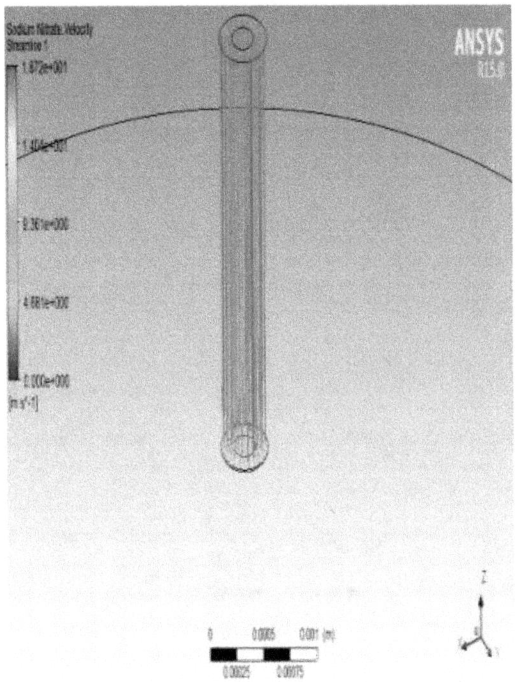

Figure 28. Velocity streamlines of the electrolyte for 0.5 m/s

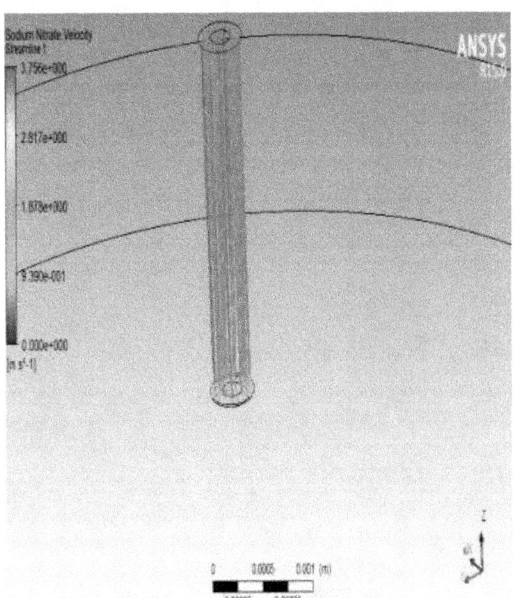

Figure 29. Turbulent Eddy Dissipation contour for 0.5m/sec

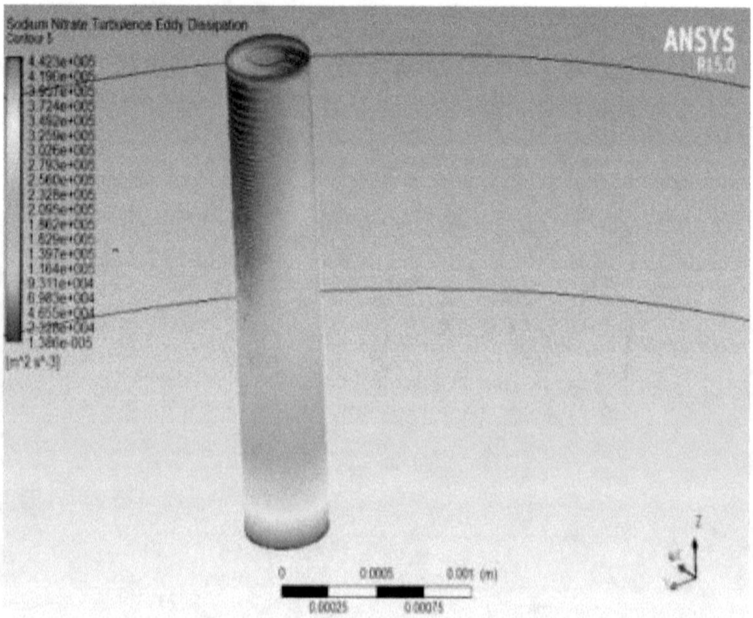

Figure 30. Turbulent Eddy Dissipation contour plot for 2.5m/sec

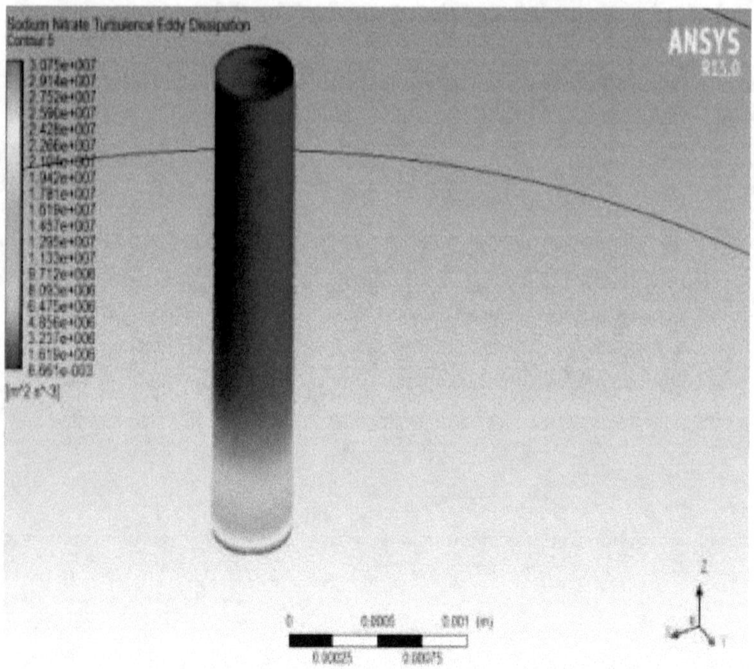

Figure 31. Final shape of the work piece with 2.5m/s

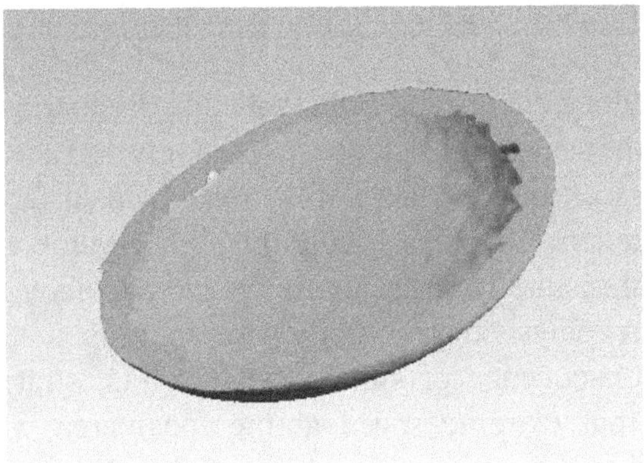

endeavor to optimize the design of tool, which ensures a sufficient flow of electrolyte.

2. Transient analysis or a state of pulsed DC used for machining process provides a more efficient ECMM process as compared to a steady state analysis. With pulsed DC improves the accuracy of the work piece. It is seen a uniformity in current density and temperature distribution throughout the work piece with a smooth variation in this case.
3. It can be concluded that the rise in temperature of electrolyte at the inlet speeds up the simulation process. This leads to an enhancement of current density on the surface area to be machined and as well as MRR. From the above discussions, it is clearly understood that with the increase in inlet temperature, there is almost a same value of temperature rise at the machining zone in steady state, but large variation in current density is seen for different input parameters for machining. For steady state, the temperature-increasing tendency is more rapid with the machining duration, which may go beyond the boiling temperature of electrolyte resulting in reduction in its conductivity and leads to an invalid result.
4. It can be concluded from above discussion that, a more concentrated electrolyte gives better MRR as well as surface finish as it offers a low resistance to flow of machining current through it for the specific operating voltage.
5. The maximum range of velocity is same for all steady state provided the same pattern for the flow of electrolyte. However, for transient states the range of maximum velocity is more as compared to steady state as after entering into the chamber one component of electrolyte velocity defined

as the function of other component of velocity to give a combined effect of velocity, for getting a good impulse action of electrolyte on the work piece.

6. Turbulent kinetic energy and turbulent eddy dissipation determines the energy and the scale of turbulence respectively and a less value of these means the lesser the roughness of the machined surface.
7. The simulated result gives a slightly higher value than that of the experimental result. The surface finish and accuracy is better in case of a transient analysis than a steady state analysis.
8. From the consequence of simulation by CFD, strategy it has been discovered that extreme speed at the focal area with consistently appropriated speed over the periphery of tool. Lesser speed saw close to the sharp edges of tool, which prompts slurry formation.
9. Pressure counter at the minimum at the central region that leads to turbulence and eddy formation. At the outlet, the pressure is more than the central region, which might leads to slurry formation.
10. Depth of the machined hole increases with increase in voltage, feed rate, concentration, whereas pulse on/off ratio and inter electrode gap has less effect on the machining deep hole.
11. Material removal rate increases with the increase in voltage and feed rate but decreases with increase concentration, inter electrode gap, and pulse on/off ratio.
12. Overcut of the hole increases with increase in voltage, molar concentration of electrolyte and feed rate whereas decreases with increasing pulse on /off ratio and inter electrode gap.
13. The optimum conditions with voltage 9V, 10gm/l and 17.1717 micrometer inter electrode gap, 2.5 pulse on /off ratio (pulse on time 5 millisecond and pulse off time-2 millisecond) and 2.7374 *12 micron/min for best output, which will give maximum depth, minimum overcut and maximum material removal rate.

REFERENCES

Geethapriyan, T., Kalaichelvan, K., & Muthuramalingam, T. (2016). Multi performance optimization of electrochemical micro-machining process surface related parameters on machining Inconel 718 using Taguchi-grey relational analysis. *La Metallurgia Italiana*, *4*, 13–19.

Ghoshal, B., & Bhattacharyya, B. (2015). Investigation on profile of microchannel generated by electrochemical micromachining. *Journal of Materials Processing Technology*, *222*, 410–421. doi:10.1016/j.jmatprotec.2015.03.025

Jiang, H., Cao, G., Xu, C., Zhang, Z., & Liu, S. (2014, August). Effects of residual stress in the membrane on the performance of surface micromachining silicon nitride pressure sensor, In *Electronic Packaging Technology (ICEPT), 2014 15th International Conference on* (pp. 664-670). IEEE. 10.1109/ICEPT.2014.6922742

Jin, D. S., Chun, K. H., & Lee, E. S. (2017). Analysis of the current density characteristics in through-mask electrochemical micromachining (TMECMM) for fabrication of micro-hole arrays on invar alloy film. *Chinese Journal of Aeronautics*, *30*(3), 1231–1241. doi:10.1016/j.cja.2016.10.021

Kamaraj, A. B., Sundaram, M. M., & Mathew, R. (2013). Ultra high aspect ratio penetrating metal microelectrodes for biomedical applications. *Microsystem Technologies*, *19*(2), 179–186. doi:10.100700542-012-1653-3

Kumar, M. P., Prakasan, K., & Kalaichelvan, K. (2016). Experimental investigation and multiphysics simulation on the influence of micro tools with various end profiles on diametrical overcut of holes machined using electrochemical micromachining for a predetermined optimum combination of process parameters. *Russian Journal of Electrochemistry*, *52*(10), 943–954. doi:10.1134/S1023193516100104

Lee, S. J., Lee, C. Y., Yang, K. T., Kuan, F. H., & Lai, P. H. (2008). Simulation and fabrication of micro-scaled flow channels for metallic bipolar plates by the electrochemical micro-machining process. *Journal of Power Sources*, *185*(2), 1115–1121. doi:10.1016/j.jpowsour.2008.07.087

Li, D., Zhu, D., & Li, H. (2011). Microstructure of electrochemical micromachining using inert metal mask. *International Journal of Advanced Manufacturing Technology*, *55*(1-4), 189–194. doi:10.100700170-010-3025-4

Liu, W., Ao, S., Li, Y., Liu, Z., Luo, Z., Wang, Z., & Song, R. (2017). Modeling and fabrication of micro hole by electrochemical micromachining using retracted tip tool. *Precision Engineering*, *50*, 77–84. doi:10.1016/j.precisioneng.2017.04.015

Liu, Y., Zhu, D., Zeng, Y., & Yu, H. (2011). Development of microelectrodes for electrochemical micromachining. *International Journal of Advanced Manufacturing Technology*, *55*(1-4), 195–203. doi:10.100700170-010-3035-2

Nayak, A. A., Gangopadhyay, S., & Sahoo, D. K. (2016). Modelling, simulation and experimental investigation for generating 'I'shaped contour on Inconel 825 using electro chemical machining. *Journal of Manufacturing Processes*, *23*, 269–277. doi:10.1016/j.jmapro.2016.05.001

Qian, S., Zhu, D., Qu, N., Li, H., & Yan, D. (2010). Generating micro-dimples array on the hard chrome-coated surface by modified through mask electrochemical micromachining. *International Journal of Advanced Manufacturing Technology*, *47*(9-12), 1121–1127. doi:10.100700170-009-2246-x

Rath, U. 2013, *Two phase flow analysis in electrochemical machining for l-shaped tool: A CFD APPROACH* (Doctoral dissertation).

Samanta, S., & Chakraborty, S. (2011). Parametric optimization of some non-traditional machining processes using artificial bee colony algorithm. *Engineering Applications of Artificial Intelligence*, *24*(6), 946–957. doi:10.1016/j.engappai.2011.03.009

Singh, D., & Shukla, R. S. (2016). Optimization of electrochemical micromachining and electrochemical discharge machining process parameters using firefly algorithm. *International Journal of Mechatronics and Manufacturing Systems*, *9*(2), 137–159. doi:10.1504/IJMMS.2016.076169

Singh, J., Jain, V. K., & Ramkumar, J. (2016). Fabrication of complex circuit on printed circuit board (PCB) using electrochemical micro-machining. *International Journal of Advanced Manufacturing Technology*, *85*(9-12), 2073–2081. doi:10.100700170-015-7817-4

Sun, M., Xiao, K., Dong, C., Li, X., & Zhong, P. (2014). Effect of stress on electrochemical characteristics of pre-cracked ultrahigh strength stainless steel in acid sodium sulphate solution. *Corrosion Science*, *89*, 137–145. doi:10.1016/j.corsci.2014.08.023

Xiaolong, F., Xianghe, Z., Pengfei, Z., Yongbin, Z., & Ningsong, Q. (2016). Improving machining accuracy in wire electrochemical micromachining using a rotary helical electrode. *International Journal of Advanced Manufacturing Technology*, *84*(5-8), 929–939.

Zou, P., Rajora, M., Ma, M., Chen, H., Wu, W., & Liang, S. Y. (2017). January. Electrochemical Micro-Machining Process Parameter Optimization Using a Neural Network-Genetic Algorithm Based Approach. *Proceedings of the International Conference on Manufacturing Technologies,* 19-21.

APPENDIX

Table 5. List of abbreviations

Abbreviation	Description
CEL	CFX Expression Language
CFD	Computational Fluid Dynamics
CHT	Conjugate Heat Transfer
ECM	Electro Chemical Machining
ECMM	Electrochemical Micro Machining
FEM	Finite Element Method
GGI	General Grid Interface
IEG	Inter Electrode Gap
MRR	Material Removal Rate
W/P	Workpiece

Table 6. List of symbols

Symbols	Nomenclature	Units (MKS)
A	Area at the inlet	m^2
A	Area of element	m^2
A_i	Atomic weight	Kg
A_t	Area of the tool	m^2
C_p	Specific heat capacity	J
t_s	Total time step	s
ε	Current efficiency	-
F	Faraday's constant	-
I	Current	A
J	Current density	A/m^2
k	Thermal conductivity of electrolyte	W/mK
k_o	Initial thermal conductivity of electrolyte	W/mK
l	Edge length of tetrahedron	m
m	Weight of metal dissolves or deposited	kg
μ_{eff}	Effective viscosity of turbulence	m^2/s
μ_t	Turbulence viscosity	m^2/s
d_i	Material removed at i^{th} node	g/min
P'	Modified pressure	Pa
P_K	Turbulence production due to viscous force	N/m
P_{kb}&$P_{\varepsilon b}$	Influence of buoyancy force	
Q	Volume flow rate	m^3/s
t	Total machining time	s
r	Specific resistance	Ohm
T_b	Boiling temperature of electrolyte	K
v_i	Velocity at inlet	m/s
i	Inter electrode gap	m
z	Valance	-
C_{pe}	Average specific heat of electrolyte	J
ρ_ε	Density of electrolyte	kg/m^3
D	Effective diffusion coefficient	m^2/s
d	Pulse on/pulse off ratio	-
f	Feed rate	m/s
v	Voltage	V
c	Concentration of electrolyte	gm/Lt
α	Thermal diffusivity	m^2/s

Compilation of References

(2013). Science and society: Experts warn against bans on 3D printing. *Science, 342*(6157), 439. PMID:24163835

Abarghooei, H., Arabi, H., Seyedein, S. H., & Mirzakhani, B. (2017). Modeling of steady state hot flow behavior of API-X70 microalloyed steel using genetic algorithm and design of experiments. *Applied Soft Computing, 52*, 471–477. doi:10.1016/j.asoc.2016.10.021

Adams, D. (2011). Tabbing composite test specimens: When and why. *High-Performance Composites, 19*(2).

Adams, D. O., & Adams, D. F. (2002). *Tabbing Guide for Composite Test Specimens*. Retrieved from http://www.dtic.mil/docs/citations/ADA411472

Affenzeller, M., Winkler, S., Wagner, S., & Beham, A. (2009). Genetic Algorithms and Genetic Programming. *Simulation, 20093626*. doi:10.1201/9781420011326

Alan, F.J. (2015). Bioprinting of human pluripotent stem cells and their directed differentiation into hepatocyte-like cells for the generation of minilivers in 3D. *Biofabrication, 7*(4), 044102.

Albrektsson, T., & Johansson, C. (2001). Osteoinduction, osteoconduction and osseointegration. *European Spine Journal, 10*(Suppl 2), S96–S101. doi:10.1007005860100282 PMID:11716023

Alfano, M., Furgiuele, F., Rangarajan, R., Lew, A. J., Krull, B., & Patrick, J., … Donald F. Adams. (. (2011). Tabbing Guide for Composite Test Specimens. *Composite Joints and Connections, 40*(April), 341–362. doi:10.1533/9780857094926.2.341

Ali, A. H. M., Shlaby, M. S., & Elfaki, E. F. (2016). Mechanical properties of the prosthesis limp from PVC glass fiber sandwich. *International Journal of Mechanical And Production Engineering, 4*(5), 41–45.

AlMaadeed, M. A., Nogellova, Z., Mičušík, M., Novák, I., & Krupa, I. (2014). Mechanical, sorption and adhesive properties of composites based on low density polyethylene filled with date palm wood powder. *Materials & Design, 53*, 29–37. doi:10.1016/j.matdes.2013.05.093

AlMaadeed, M. A., Ouedern, M., & Noorunnisa, K. P. (2013). Effect of chain structure on the properties of glass fibre/polyethylene composites. *Materials & Design, 47*, 725–730. doi:10.1016/j.matdes.2012.11.063

Almeida, J. I., Javier, J. J., Mackay, E., Bautista, C., & Proebstle, T. M. (2013). First human use of cyanoacrylate adhesive for treatment of saphenous vein incompetence. *Journal of Vascular Surgery. Venous and Lymphatic Disorders*, *1*(2), 174–180. doi:10.1016/j.jvsv.2012.09.010 PMID:26992340

Amaral, M., Lopes, M. A., Silva, R. F., & Santos, J. D. (2002). Densification route and mechanical properties of Si3N4-bioglass biocomposites. *Biomaterials*, *23*(3), 857–862. doi:10.1016/S0142-9612(01)00194-6 PMID:11771704

Anandhan, S., De, P. P., De, S. K., Bandyopadhyay, S., & Bhowmick, A. K. (2003). Mapping of Thermoplastic Elastomeric Nitrile Rubber / Poly (Styrene-Co-Acrylonitrile) Blends Using Tapping Mode Atomic Force Microscopy. *Journal of Materials Science*, *8*(13), 2793–2801. doi:10.1023/A:1024416031172

Anasane, S. S., & Bhattacharyya, B. (2017). Electrochemical Micromachining of Titanium and Its Alloys. In Non-traditional Micromachining Processes (pp. 337–365). Cham: Springer. doi:10.1007/978-3-319-52009-4_9

Anasane, S. S., & Bhattacharyya, B. (2017). Experimental investigation into micromilling of microgrooves on titanium by electrochemical micromachining. *Journal of Manufacturing Processes*, *28*, 285–294. doi:10.1016/j.jmapro.2017.06.016

Anusavis, K. (2013). Mechanical properties of dental materials. In K. J. Anusavice, C. Shen, & H. R. Rawls (Eds.), *Phillips' science of dental materials* (12th ed.; pp. 48–68). St.Louis: Elsevier Inc.

Ashman, O., & Phillips, A. M. (2013). Treatment of non-unions with bone defects: Which option and why? *Injury*, *44*(1), 43–45. doi:10.1016/S0020-1383(13)70010-X PMID:23351870

Asiltürk, I., & Akkuş, H. (2011). Determining the effect of cutting parameters on surface roughness in hard turning using the Taguchi method. *Measurement: Journal of the International Measurement Confederation*, *44*(9), 1697–1704. doi:10.1016/j.measurement.2011.07.003

ASTM D5083 - 17. (n.d.). *ASTM D5083 - 17 Standard Test Method for Tensile Properties of Reinforced Thermosetting Plastics Using Straight-Sided Specimens*. Retrieved from https://www.astm.org/Standards/D5083.htm

ASTM F2792–10 Standard Terminology for Additive Manufacturing Technologies.

ASTM International. (2014). ASTM D3039/D3039M-14 Standard Test Method for Tensile Properties of Polymer Matrix Composite Materials. *Annual Book of ASTM Standards*, 1–13. doi:10.1520/D3039

Astorino, M., Gerbeau, J. F., Pantz, O., & Traor, K. F. (2008). Fluid-Structure Interaction and Multi-Body Contact Application to Aortic Valves. *8th.World Congress on Computational Mechanics (WCCM8).*

Auricchio, Ferrara, & Morganti. (2012). Comparison and critical analysis of invariant-based models with respect to their ability in fitting human aortic valve data. In *Annals of Solid and Structural Mechanics*. Springer.

Ayres, C. E., Jha, B. S., Sell, S. A., Bowlin, G. L., & Simpson, D. G. (2009). Nanotechnology in the design of soft tissue scaffolds: Innovations in structure and function. *Wiley Interdisciplinary Reviews. Nanomedicine and Nanobiotechnology*, *2*(1), 20–34. doi:10.1002/wnan.55 PMID:20049828

Bagga, C. S., Erbe, E. M., Murphy, J. P., Freid, J. M., & Pomrink, G. J. (2017). *U.S. Patent No. 9,629,728*. Washington, DC: U.S. Patent and Trademark Office.

Bakhshayesh, P., Boutefnouchet, T., & Tötterman, A. (2016). Effectiveness of non invasive external pelvic compression: A systematic review of the literature. *Scandinavian Journal of Trauma, Resuscitation and Emergency Medicine*, *1824*(1), 73. doi:10.118613049-016-0259-7 PMID:27193135

Balaji, M., Venkata Rao, K., & Rao, M. (2015, August). N., & Murthy, B. S. N. (2018). Optimization of drilling parameters for drilling of TI-6Al-4V based on surface roughness, flank wear and drill vibration. *Measurement: Journal of the International Measurement Confederation*, *114*, 332–339. doi:10.1016/j.measurement.2017.09.051

Balasuriya, P. W., Ye, L., & Mai, Y. W. (2001). Mechanical properties of wood flake -polyethylene composites. Part I: Effects of processing methods and matrix melt flow behavior. *Composites. Part A, Applied Science and Manufacturing*, *32*(5), 619–629. doi:10.1016/S1359-835X(00)00160-3

Bandyopadhyay, S. (2008). Applications of Atomic Force Microscope (AFM) in the Field of Nanomaterials and Nanocomposites. In S. Seal (Ed.), *Functional Nanostructures Processing, Characterization, and Applications* (pp. 504–568). New York, NY: Springer-Verlag. doi:10.1007/978-0-387-48805-9_9

Banks, J. (2013). Adding value in additive manufacturing: Researchers in the United Kingdom and Europe look to 3D printing for customization. *IEEE Pulse*, *4*(6), 22–26. doi:10.1109/MPUL.2013.2279617 PMID:24233187

Banoriya, D., Purohit, R., & Dwivedi, R. K. (2017). Advanced Application of Polymer based Biomaterials. *Materials Today: Proceedings*, *4*(2), 3534–3541. doi:10.1016/j.matpr.2017.02.244

Bar-Cohen, Y. (2005). *Biomimetics—Biologically Inspired Technologies*. Boca Raton, FL: CRC Press. doi:10.1201/9780849331633

Bar-Cohen, Y. (2006). Biomimetics—using nature to inspire human innovation. *Bioinspiration & Biomimetics*, *1*(1), 1–12. doi:10.1088/1748-3182/1/1/P01 PMID:17671297

Barrere, F., Mahmood, T. A., de Groot, K., & van Blitterswijk, C. A. (2008). Advanced biomaterials for skeletal tissue regeneration: Instructive and smart functions, Mater. Sci. Eng. *R Rep.*, *59*(1), 38–71. doi:10.1016/j.mser.2007.12.001

Barriobero-Vila, P., Gussone, J., Haubrich, J., Sandlöbes, S., Da Silva, J. C., Cloetens, P., ... Requena, G. (2017). Inducing stable α+ β microstructures during selective laser melting of Ti-6Al-4V using intensified intrinsic heat treatments. *Materials (Basel)*, *10*(3), 268. doi:10.3390/ma10030268 PMID:28772630

Behrsin, J. F., & Briggs, C. A. (1988). Ligaments of the lumbar spine: A review. *Surgical and Radiologic Anatomy*, *10*(3), 211–219. doi:10.1007/BF02115239 PMID:3147534

Belingardi, G., Paolino, D. S., & Koricho, E. G. (2011). Investigation of influence of tab types on tensile strength of E-glass/epoxy fiber reinforced composite materials. Procedia Engineering, 10, 3279–3284. doi:10.1016/j.proeng.2011.04.541

Bellini, H., Moyano, J., Gil, J., & Puigdollers, A. (2016). Comparison of the superelasticity of different nickel–titanium orthodontic archwires and the loss of their properties by heat treatment. *Journal of Materials Science. Materials in Medicine*, *27*(10), 158. doi:10.100710856-016-5767-5 PMID:27623709

Benyus, J. M. (2009). *Biomimcry. Innovation Inspired by Nature*. Harper Collins Publishers.

Berry, D. A. (1987). Composite Materials for Orthotics and Prosthetics. *Journal of Prosthetists and Orthotics*.

Bhattacharyya, B., Malapati, M., & Munda, J. (2005). Experimental study on electrochemical micromachining. *Journal of Materials Processing Technology*, *169*(3), 485–492. doi:10.1016/j.jmatprotec.2005.04.074

Bhattacharyya, B., & Munda, J. (2003). Experimental investigation into electrochemical micromachining (ECMM) process. *Journal of Materials Processing Technology*, *140*(1-3), 287–291. doi:10.1016/S0924-0136(03)00722-2

Bhattacharyya, B., & Munda, J. (2003). Experimental investigation on the influence of electrochemical machining parameters of machining rate and accuracy in micromachining domain. *International Journal of Machine Tools & Manufacture*, *43*(13), 1301–1310. doi:10.1016/S0890-6955(03)00161-5

Bhisitkul, R. B., & Keller, C. G. (2005). Development of Microelectromechanical Systems (MEMS) forceps for intraocular surgery. *Journal of Ophthalmology*, *89*, 1586–1588. PMID:16299136

Bhushan, R. K. (2013). Multiresponse Optimization of Al Alloy-SiC Composite Machining Parameters for Minimum Tool Wear and Maximum Metal Removal Rate. *Journal of Manufacturing Science and Engineering*, *135*(2), 021013. doi:10.1115/1.4023454

Bhuyan, D. (2018). Designing of a Twin Tube Shock Absorber: A Study in Reverse Engineering. In Design and Optimization of Mechanical Engineering Products (pp. 83 – 104). Hershey, PA: IGI Global. doi:10.4018/978-1-5225-3401-3.ch005

Bhuyan, D., & Kumar, K. (2017). *Indian Patent application no. 1319/KOL/2015*. Kolkata: India Indian Patent.

Black, J., & Hastings, G. (1998). *Handbook of Biomaterial Properties*. Chapman & Hall. doi:10.1007/978-1-4615-5801-9

Boanini, E., Gazzano, M., & Bigi, A. (2010). Ionic substitutions in calcium phosphates synthesized at low temperature. *Acta Biomaterialia*, *6*(6), 1882–1894. doi:10.1016/j.actbio.2009.12.041 PMID:20040384

Boccaccio, A., Ballini, A., Pappalettere, C., Tullo, D., Cantore, S., & Desiate, A. (2011). Finite element method (FEM), mechanobiology and biomimetic scaffolds in bone tissue engineering. *International Journal of Biological Sciences*, *7*(1), 112–132. doi:10.7150/ijbs.7.112 PMID:21278921

Bohner, M. (2000). Calcium orthophosphates in medicine: From ceramics to calcium phosphate cements. *Injury*, *31*, D37–D47. doi:10.1016/S0020-1383(00)80022-4 PMID:11270080

Bonanomi, G., Rebello, K., Lebouitz, K., Riviere, C., Di Martino, E., Vorp, D., & Zenati, M. A. (2003). Microelectromechanical systems for endoscopic cardiac surgery. *The Journal of Thoracic and Cardiovascular Surgery*, *126*(3), 851–852. doi:10.1016/S0022-5223(03)00393-3 PMID:14502165

Bose, S., Roy, M., & Bandyopadhyay, A. (2012). Recent advances in bone tissue engineering scaffolds. *Trends in Biotechnology*, *30*(10), 546–554. doi:10.1016/j.tibtech.2012.07.005 PMID:22939815

Bowen, W. R., & Doneva, T. A. (2000). Artefacts in AFM Studies of Membranes: Correcting Pore Images Using Fast Fourier Transform Filtering. *Journal of Membrane Science*, *171*(1), 141–147. doi:10.1016/S0376-7388(00)00297-0

Boyce, E. (2009). Simulating the Fluid Dynamics of Natural and Prosthetic Heart Valves using the Immersed Boundary Method. *International Journal of Applied Mechanics*, *1*(1), 137–177. doi:10.1142/S1758825109000113

Breuls, R. G. M., Jiya, T. U., & Smit, T. H. (2008). Scaffold stiffness influences cell behavior: Opportunities for skeletal tissue engineering. *The Open Orthopaedics Journal*, *2*(2), 103–109. doi:10.2174/1874325000802010103 PMID:19478934

Broggini, N., McManus, L. M., Hermann, J. S., Medina, R., Schenk, R. K., Buser, D., & Cochran, D. L. (2006). Peri-implant inflammation defined by the implant-abutment interface. *Journal of Dental Research*, *85*(5), 473–478. doi:10.1177/154405910608500515 PMID:16632764

Brydone, A. S., Meek, D., & Maclaine, S. (2010). Bone grafting, orthopaedic biomaterials, and the clinical need for bone engineering. *Proceedings of the Institution of Mechanical Engineers. Part H, Journal of Engineering in Medicine*, *224*(12), 1329–1343. doi:10.1243/09544119JEIM770 PMID:21287823

Buchko, C. J., Kozloff, K. M., & Martin, D. C. (2001). Surface Characterization of Porous, Biocompatible Protein Polymer Thin Films. *Biomaterials Biomaterials*, *22*(11), 1289–1300. doi:10.1016/S0142-9612(00)00281-7 PMID:11336301

Byambaa, B., Annabi, N., Yue, K., Trujillo-de Santiago, G., Alvarez, M. M., Jia, W., ... Khademhosseini, A. (2017). Bioprinted osteogenic and vasculogenic patterns for engineering 3D bone tissue. *Advanced Healthcare Materials*, *6*(16), 1700015. doi:10.1002/adhm.201700015 PMID:28524375

Campbell, A. I., Sexton, S., Schaschke, C. J., Kinsman, H., McLaughlin, B., & Boyle, M. (2012). Prosthetic limb sockets from plant-based composite materials. *Prosthetics and Orthotics International*, *36*(2), 181–189. doi:10.1177/0309364611434568 PMID:22307862

Campbell, J. W., & Childs, C. W. (1980). The S.A.F.E. Foot. *Orthotics and Prosthetics*, *34*(3), 3–16.

Cao, X., & Chen, D. (2005). The BMP signaling and in vivo bone formation. *Gene*, *357*(1), 1–8. doi:10.1016/j.gene.2005.06.017 PMID:16125875

Cappiello, M., Luongo, R., Di Iorio, D., Bugea, C., Cocchetto, R., & Celletti, R. (2008). Evaluation of peri-implant bone loss around platform-switched implants. *International Journal of Periodontics & Restorative Dentistry*, *28*(4). PMID:18717373

Chamis, C. C., & Sinclair, J. H. (1977). Ten-deg Off-axis Test for Shear Properties in Fiber Composites. *Experimental Mechanics*, *17*(9), 339–346. doi:10.1007/BF02326320

Chang, W. C., Hawkes, E. A., Kliot, M., & Sretavan, D. W. (2007). In Vivo Use of aNanoknife for Axon Microsurgery. *Neurosurgery*, *61*(4), 683–692. doi:10.1227/01.NEU.0000298896.31355.80 PMID:17986929

Cheah, C.M., Chua, C.K., Tan, K.H., & Teo, C.K. (2003). Integration of laser surface digitizing with CAD/CAM techniques for developing facial prostheses. Part 1: Design and fabrication of prosthesis replicas. *Int J Prosthodont Jul 1, 16*(4).

Chen, G., Dong, C., Yang, L., & Lv, Y. (2015). 3D scaffolds with different stiffness but the same microstructure for bone tissue engineering. *ACS Applied Materials & Interfaces*, *7*(29), 15790–15802. doi:10.1021/acsami.5b02662 PMID:26151287

Chen, Q., Zhu, C., & Thouas, G. A. (2012). Progress and challenges in biomaterials used for bone tissue engineering: Bioactive glasses and elastomeric composites. *Prog. Biomater.*, *1*(1), 2. doi:10.1186/2194-0517-1-2 PMID:29470743

Chen, Y., Xu, Z., Smith, C., & Sankar, J. (2014). Recent advances on the development of magnesium alloys for biodegradable implants. *Acta Biomaterialia*, *10*(11), 4561–4573. doi:10.1016/j.actbio.2014.07.005 PMID:25034646

Cherian, B. M., Lea˜o, A. L., De Souza, S. F., Costa, L. M. M., De Olyveira, G. M., Kottaisamy, M., ... Thomas, S. (2011). Cellulose nanocomposites with nanofibres isolated from pineapple leaf fibers for medical applications. *Carbohydrate Polymers*, *86*(4), 1790–1798. doi:10.1016/j.carbpol.2011.07.009

Chiellini, E., & Solaro, R. (1996). Biodegradable polymeric materials. *Advanced Materials*, *8*(4), 305–313. doi:10.1002/adma.19960080406

Childress, D. S. (1985). Historical Aspects of Powered Limb Prostheses. *Clinical Prosthetics & Orthotics*, *9*(1), 2–13.

Christina, A. (2004). Degenerative mechanics of the lumbar spine. *The Spine Journal*, *4*(6), 202–208. doi:10.1016/j.spinee.2004.07.013 PMID:15016399

Clements, I. P. (2008). *How Prosthetic Limbs Work*. Retrieved 16 April 2016 from http://science.howstuffworks.com/prosthetic-limb.htm

Coguill, R. J., & Adams, D. F. (1999). Selection of the proper wedge grip surface for tensile testing composite materials. In *International SAMPE Symposium and Exhibition (Proceedings)* (Vol. 44). Retrieved from http://www.scopus.com/inward/record.url?eid=2-s2.0-0033309663&partnerID=tZOtx3y1

Cole, K. M., Kirk, D. W., Singh, C. V., & Thorpe, S. J. (2017). Optimizing electrochemical micromachining parameters for Zr-based bulk metallic glass. *Journal of Manufacturing Processes*, *25*, 227–234. doi:10.1016/j.jmapro.2016.11.015

Colnot, C. (2011). Cell sources for bone tissue engineering: Insights from basic science. *Tissue Engineering. Part B, Reviews*, *17*(6), 449–457. doi:10.1089/ten.teb.2011.0243 PMID:21902612

Condie, D. N. (2008). The modern era of orthotics. *Prosthetics and Orthotics International*, *32*(3), 313–323. doi:10.1080/03093640802113006 PMID:18825575

Coombs, D. J., Laz, P. J., Rao, M., Smith, S. D., Bushelow, M., & Rullkoetter, P. J. (2012). Stepwise Validated Finite Element Model of the Human Lumbar Spine. *SIMULIA Customer Conference.*

Cui, X., & ... . (2012). Thermal inkjet printing in tissue engineering and regenerative medicine, Recent Pat. drug Deliv. *Formulation*, *6*(2), 149–155. PMID:22436025

Daniels, A. U., Chang, M. K., Andriano, K. P., & Heller, J. (1990). Mechanical properties of biodegradable polymers and composites proposed for internal fixation of bone. *Journal of Applied Biomaterials*, *1*(1), 57–78. doi:10.1002/jab.770010109 PMID:10148987

Das, A., Baruah, J., & Bhuyan, D. (2018). The Anatomy of the Foot-Ankle Complex and The Mechanics of Walking: A Brief Review. *Asian Journal of Convergence in Technology, 4*(1).

Datta, S., Sarkar, R., Vyas, V., Bhutoria, S., Barui, A., Roy Chowdhury, A., & Datta, P. (2018). Alginate-honey bioinks with improved cell responses for applicationsas bioprinted tissue engineered constructs. *Journal of Materials Research*, 1–11.

David, C., De Kesel, C., Lefebvre, F., & Weiland, M. (1994). The biodegradation of polymers: Recent results. *Die Angewandte Makromolekulare Chemie: Applied Macromolecular Chemistry and Physics*, *216*(1), 21–35. doi:10.1002/apmc.1994.052160102

De Baere, I., Van Paepegem, W., & Degrieck, J. (2009). On the design of end tabs for quasi-static and fatigue testing of fibre-reinforced composites. *Polymer Composites*, *30*(4), 381–390. doi:10.1002/pc.20564 de Groot, K. (1993). Clinical applications of calcium phosphate biomaterials: A review. *Ceramics International, 19*(5), 363–366. doi:10.1016/0272-8842(93)90050-2

De Hart. (2002). *Fluid-Structure Interaction in the Aortic Heart Valve-a three-dimensional computational analysis* (PhD thesis). Eindhoven University of Technology.

De Hart, J., Cacciola, G., Schreurs, P. J. G., & Peters, G. W. M. (1998). A three-dimensional analysis of a fibre-reinforced aortic valve prosthesis. *Journal of Biomechanics, 31*(7), 629–638. doi:10.1016/S0021-9290(98)00063-3 PMID:9796685

de Jager, M. (1993). Mathematical Modelling of the Human Cervical Spine: A Survey of the Literature. *Proceedings of the 1993 International IRCOBI Conference on the Biomechanics of Impact.*

DeAngelis, N. A., Wixted, J. J., Drew, J., Eskander, M. S., Eskander, J. P., & French, B. G. (2008). Use of the trauma pelvic orthotic device (TPOD) for provisional stabilisation of anterior–posterior compression type pelvic fractures: A cadaveric study. *Injury, 39*(8), 903–906. doi:10.1016/j.injury.2007.12.008 PMID:18586248

Dehghani, F. N., & Annabi, N. (2011). Engineering porous scaffolds using gas-based techniques. *Current Opinion in Biotechnology, 22*(5), 661–666. doi:10.1016/j.copbio.2011.04.005 PMID:21546240

Dellon, B., & Matsuoka, Y. (2007, March). Prosthetics, Exoskeletons, and Rehabilitation: Now and for the Future. *IEEE Robotics & Automation Magazine*, 30–34. doi:10.1109/MRA.2007.339622

Derringer, G., & Suich, R. (1980). Simultaneous-Optimization of Several Response Variables. *Journal of Quality Technology, 12*(4), 214–219. doi:10.1080/00224065.1980.11980968

Dimitriou, R., Tsiridis, E., & Giannoudis, P. V. (2005). Current concepts of molecular aspects of bone healing. *Injury, 36*(12), 1392–1404. doi:10.1016/j.injury.2005.07.019 PMID:16102764

Diniz Dos Santos, N. M. (2007). *Numerical methods for fluid-structure interaction problems with valves* (PhD thesis). University of Parie and Marie Curie.

Dixon, J. C. (2007). *The Shock Absorber Handbook* (2nd ed.). John Wiley and Sons Ltd. doi:10.1002/9780470516430

Do, A. V., Khorsand, B., Geary, S. M., & Salem, A. K. (2015). 3D printing of scaffolds for tissue regeneration applications. *Advanced Healthcare Materials, 4*(12), 1742–1762. doi:10.1002/adhm.201500168 PMID:26097108

Douglas, B. (2006). *Generation of 3-D parametric solid model of human spine using anthropomorphic parameters* (MS Thesis). Ohio University.

Dubois, S. (2007). *Mobility for each one*. Retrieved from http://www.icsid.org/ feature/galleria/galleria38.htm

Dupes, B. (n.d.). *Prosthetic Knee Systems*. Retrieved 19 April 2016 from http://www.amputee-coalition.org/military-instep/knees.html

Duty, C., Ajinjeru, C., Kishore, V., Compton, B., Hmeidat, N., Chen, X., ... Kunc, V. (2018). What makes a material printable? Avicoelastic model for extrusion-based 3D printing of polymer. *Journal of Manufacturing Processes*, *35*, 526–537. doi:10.1016/j.jmapro.2018.08.008

Dyer, S. R., Lassila, L. V. J., Jokinen, M., & Vallittu, P. K. (2004). Effect of fiber position and orientation on fracture load of fiber-reinforced composite. *Dental Materials*, *20*(10), 947–955. doi:10.1016/j.dental.2003.12.003 PMID:15501323

Eaton, P., & West, P. (2010). *Atomic Force Microscopy*. New York, NY: Oxford University Press Inc. doi:10.1093/acprof:oso/9780199570454.001.0001

El Sayed, T., Mota, A., Fraternali, F., & Ortiz, M. (2008). Biomechanics of traumatic brain injury. *Computer Methods in Applied Mechanics and Engineering*, *197*(51-52), 4692–4701. doi:10.1016/j.cma.2008.06.006

Eli, J. (2010). On the multiscale modeling of heart valve biomechanics in health and disease. *Biomechanics and Modeling in Mechanobiology*, *9*(4), 373–387. doi:10.100710237-009-0181-2 PMID:20066464

Erdemir, A., McLean, S., Herzog, W., & van den Bogert, A. J. (2007). Model-based estimation of muscle forces exerted during movements. *Clinical Biomechanics (Bristol, Avon)*, *22*(2), 131–154. doi:10.1016/j.clinbiomech.2006.09.005 PMID:17070969

Faulkner-Jones, A., Greenhough, S., A King, J., Gardner, J., Courtney, A., & Shu, W. (2013). Development of a valve-based cell printer for the bformation of human embryonic stem cell spheroid aggregates. *Biofabrication*, *5*(1), 15–13. doi:10.1088/1758-5082/5/1/015013 PMID:23380571

Fennema, E., Rivron, N., Rouwkema, J., van Blitterswijk, C., & de Boer, J. (2013). Spheroid culture as a tool for creating 3D complex tissues. *Trends in Biotechnology*, *31*(2), 108–115. doi:10.1016/j.tibtech.2012.12.003 PMID:23336996

Fouad, H., Elleithy, R., Al-Zahrani, S. M., & Ali, M. A. (2011). Characterization and processing of high density polyethylene/carbon nano-composites. *Materials & Design*, *32*(4), 1974–1980. doi:10.1016/j.matdes.2010.11.066

Freivalds. (2004). *Biomechanics of the upper limbs- Mechanics, modeling and musculoskeletal injuries*. CRC Press.

Fujihara, K., Teo, K., Gopal, R., Loh, P. L., Ganesh, V. K., Ramakrishna, S., ... Chew, C. L. (2004). Fibrous composite materials in dentistry and orthopaedics: Review and applications. *Composites Science and Technology*, *64*(6), 775–788. doi:10.1016/j.compscitech.2003.09.012

Ganzert, C. (2012). *Basalt: An investigation into a new Prosthetic & Orthotic material option.* Academic Press.

Gao, X., & Nie, J. F. (2007). Characterization of strengthening precipitate phases in a Mg–Zn alloy. *Scripta Materialia, 56*(8), 645–648. doi:10.1016/j.scriptamat.2007.01.006

Garbacz, H., Wieciński, P., Adamczyk-Cieślak, B., Mizera, J., & Kurzydłowski, J. K. (2010). Studies of Aluminium Coatings Deposited by Vacuum Evaporation and Magnetron Sputtering. *Journal of Microscopy, 237*(3), 475–480. doi:10.1111/j.1365-2818.2009.03297.x PMID:20500421

Gasser & Holzapfel. (2007). Finite element modeling of balloon angioplasty by considering overstretch of remnant non-diseased tissues in lesions. *Computational Mechanics, 40*, 47–60.

Gbureck, U., Hölzel, T., Klammert, U., Würzler, K., Müller, F. A., & Barralet, J. E. (2007). Resorbable dicalcium phosphate bone substitutes prepared by 3D powder printing. *Advanced Functional Materials, 17*(18), 3940–3945. doi:10.1002/adfm.200700019

Geethapriyan, T., Kalaichelvan, K., & Muthuramalingam, T. (2016). Multi performance optimization of electrochemical micro-machining process surface related parameters on machining Inconel 718 using Taguchi-grey relational analysis. *La Metallurgia Italiana, 4*, 13–19.

Gepreel, M. A. H., & Niinomi, M. (2013). Biocompatibility of Ti-alloys for long-term implantation. *Journal of the Mechanical Behavior of Biomedical Materials, 20*, 407–415. doi:10.1016/j.jmbbm.2012.11.014 PMID:23507261

Gerschutz, M. J., Haynes, M. L., Nixon, D., & Colvin, J. M. (2012). Strength evaluation of prosthetic check sockets, copolymer sockets, and definitive laminated sockets. *Journal of Rehabilitation Research and Development, 49*(3), 405. doi:10.1682/JRRD.2011.05.0091 PMID:22773200

Ghoshal, B., & Bhattacharyya, B. (2015). Investigation on profile of microchannel generated by electrochemical micromachining. *Journal of Materials Processing Technology, 222*, 410–421. doi:10.1016/j.jmatprotec.2015.03.025

Ghoshal, B., & Bhattacharyya, B. (2015). Vibration assisted electrochemical micromachining of high aspect ratio micro features. *Precision Engineering, 42*, 231–241. doi:10.1016/j.precisioneng.2015.05.005

Ghoshal, B., & Bhattacharyya, B. (2016). Electrochemical micromachining of microchannel using optimum scan feed rate. *Journal of Manufacturing Processes, 23*, 258–268. doi:10.1016/j.jmapro.2016.05.003

Glier, M. W., McAdams, D. A., & Linsey, J. S. (2011). Concepts in Biomimetic Design: Methods and Tools to Incorporate Into a Biomimetic Design Course. *Proceedings of the ASME 2011 Design Engineering Technical Conferences & Computers and Information in Engineering Conference, 7.*

Goldberg, D. E. (1989). *Genetic Algorithms in Search, Optimization, and Machine Learning*. Addison Wesley; doi:10.100710589-009-9261-6

Gołek, F., Mazur, P., Ryszka, Z., & Zuber, S. (2014). AFM Image Artifacts. *Applied Surface Science, 304*, 11–19. doi:10.1016/j.apsusc.2014.01.149

Gravlee, J. R., & Van Durme, D. J. (2007). Braces and Splints for Musculoskeletal Conditions. *American Family Physician*, *75*, 342–348. PMID:17304865

Gu, Zhao, & Froemming. (2012). Arterial Wall Mechanics and Clinical Implications after Coronary Stenting: Comparisons of Three Stent Designs. *International Journal of Applied Mechanics*, *4*(2), 1–12.

Guise, Mezghani, Aissaoui, & Hagemeister. (2011). New comprehensive methods for the biomechanical analysis of knee osteoarthritis. Understanding Osteoarthritis from Bench to Bedside, 85-102.

Gulsen, M., & Smith, A. (1998). *A Hierarchical Genetic Algorithm for System Identification and Curve Fitting with a Supercomputer Implementation*. Academic Press.

Gunatillake, P. A., & Adhikari, R. (2003). Biodegradable synthetic polymers for tissue engineering. *European Cells & Materials*, *5*(1), 1–16. doi:10.22203/eCM.v005a01 PMID:14562275

Guo, R., Merkel, A. R., Sterling, J. A., Davidson, J. M., & Guelcher, S. A. (2015). Substrate modulus of 3D-printed scaffolds regulates the regenerative response in subcutaneous implants through the macrophage phenotype and Wnt signaling. *Biomaterials*, *73*, 85–95. doi:10.1016/j.biomaterials.2015.09.005 PMID:26406449

Gupta, A., Singh, H., & Aggarwal, A. (2011). Taguchi-fuzzy multi output optimization (MOO) in high speed CNC turning of AISI P-20 tool steel. *Expert Systems with Applications*, *38*(6), 6822–6828. doi:10.1016/j.eswa.2010.12.057

Gurkan, U. A., El Assal, R., Yildiz, S. E., Sung, Y., Trachtenberg, A. J., Kuo, W. P., & Demirci, U. (2014). Engineering anisotropic biomimetic fibrocartilage microenvironment by bioprinting mesenchymal stem cells in nanoliter gel droplets. *Molecular Pharmaceutics*, *11*(7), 2151–2159. doi:10.1021/mp400573g PMID:24495169

Gu, X. N., & Zheng, Y. F. (2010). A review on magnesium alloys as biodegradable materials. *Frontiers of Materials Science in China*, *4*(2), 111–115. doi:10.100711706-010-0024-1

Habibovic, P., Yuan, H., van der Valk, C. M., Meijer, G., van Blitterswijk, C. A., & de Groot, K. (2005). 3D microenvironment as essential element for osteoinduction by biomaterials. *Biomaterials*, *26*(17), 3565–3575. doi:10.1016/j.biomaterials.2004.09.056 PMID:15621247

Hachisuka, K., Makino, K., Wada, F., Saeki, S., & Yoshimoto, N. (2007). Oxygen consumption, oxygen cost and physiological cost index in polio survivors: A comparison of walking without orthosis, with an ordinary or a carbon-fibre reinforced plastic knee-ankle-foot orthosis. *Journal of Rehabilitation Medicine*, *39*(8), 646–650. doi:10.2340/16501977-0105 PMID:17896057

Hall, S. J. (2011). *Basic Biomechanics* (6th ed.). McGraw Hill.

Handschel, J. G. K. (2007). Prospects of micromass culture technology in tissue engineering. *Head & Face Medicine*, 3. PMID:17212823

Hart-Smith, L. (1978). Mechanically-Fastened Joints for Advanced Composites -Phenomenological Consideration and Simple Analyses. In E. M. Lenoe, D. W. Oplinger, & J. J. Burke (Eds.), *Fourth Conference on Fibrous Composites in Structural Design* (pp. 543–574). San Diego, CA: Plenum Press.

Hassan, M. M., Aly, R. O., Hasanen, J. A., & El Sayed, F. (2014). The effect of gamma irradiation on mechanical, thermal and morphological properties of glass fiber reinforced polyethylene waste/ reclaim rubber composites. *Journal of Industrial and Engineering Chemistry*, *20*(3), 947–952. doi:10.1016/j.jiec.2013.06.027

Haupt, R. L., & Haupt, S. E. (2004). *Practical Genetic Algorithms* (2nd ed.). Practical Genetic Algorithms. doi:10.1002/0471671746.fmatter

He, C., Bin, S., Wu, P., Gao, C., Feng, P., Yang, Y., ... Shuai, C. (2017). Microstructure evolution and biodegradation behavior of laser rapid solidified Mg–Al–Zn alloy. *Metals*, *7*(3), 105. doi:10.3390/met7030105

Hertel, J. (2002). Functional Anatomy, Pathomechanics, and Pathophysiology of Lateral Ankle Instability. *Journal of Athletic Training*, *37*(4), 364–375. PMID:12937557

He, Y., Tao, H., Zhang, Y., Jiang, Y., Zhang, S., Zhao, C., ... Zhang, X. (2009). Biocompatibility of bio-Mg-Zn alloy within bone with heart, liver, kidney and spleen. *Chinese Science Bulletin*, *54*(3), 484–491.

Hing, K. A., Best, S. M., Tanner, K. E., Bonfield, W., & Revell, P. A. (2004). Mediation of bone ingrowth in porous hydroxyapatite bone graft substitutes. *Journal of Biomedical Materials Research. Part A*, *68*(1), 187–200. doi:10.1002/jbm.a.10050 PMID:14661264

Hodgkinson, J. M. (2000). *Mechanical testing of advanced fibre composites*. CRC Press.

Hofstad C.J., van der Linde H., van Limbeek J. & Postema, K. (2004). Prescription of Prosthetic Ankle-Foot Mechanisms after Lower Limb Amputation. *Cochrane Database of Systematic Reviews, 1*.

Hofstad, C. J., van der Linde, H., van Limbeek, J., & Postema, K. (2004). Prescription of Prosthetic Ankle-Foot Mechanisms after Lower Limb Amputation. *Cochrane Database of Systematic Reviews*, (1): CD003978. doi:10.1002/14651858.CD003978.pub2 PMID:14974050

Hofstetter, J., Becker, M., Martinelli, E., Weinberg, A. M., Mingler, B., Kilian, H., ... Löffler, J. F. (2014). High-strength low-alloy (HSLA) Mg–Zn–Ca alloys with excellent biodegradation performance. *JOM*, *66*(4), 566–572. doi:10.100711837-014-0875-5

Hofstetter, J., Martinelli, E., Weinberg, A. M., Becker, M., Mingler, B., Uggowitzer, P. J., & Löffler, J. F. (2015). Assessing the degradation performance of ultrahigh-purity magnesium in vitro and in vivo. *Corrosion Science*, *91*, 29–36. doi:10.1016/j.corsci.2014.09.008

Holland, J. H. (1975). *Adaptation in Natural and Artificial Systems*. University of Michigan Press. doi:10.1137/1018105

Hollinger, J. O., & Battistone, G. C. (1985). *Biodegradable bone repair materials: synthetic polymers and ceramics*. Army Inst of Dental Research.

Hollister, S. J. (2005). Porous scaffold design for tissue engineering. *Nature Materials*, *4*(7), 518–524. doi:10.1038/nmat1421 PMID:16003400

Holzapfel. (2004). Computational Biomechanics of Soft Biological Tissue. In Encyclopedia of Computational Mechanics. John Wiley & Sons.

Holzapfel, G. A., Gasser, T. C., & Ogden, R. W. (2000). A New Constitutive Framework for Arterial Wall Mechanics and a Comparative Study of Material Models. *Journal of Elasticity*, *61*(1/3), 1–48. doi:10.1023/A:1010835316564

Holzapfel, G. A., & Ogden, R. W. (2010). Constitutive modeling of arteries. *Proceedings of Royal Society*, *466*(2118), 1551–1597. doi:10.1098/rspa.2010.0058

Holzapfel, G. A., Stadler, M., & Gasser, T. C. (2005). Changes in the Mechanical Environment of Stenotic Arteries during interaction with Stents: Computational Assessment of Parametric Stent Designs. *Transactions of the ASME*, 127, 167-180. 10.1115/1.1835362

Horgan, T. J., & Gilchrist, M. D. (2003). The creation of three-dimensional finite element models for simulating head impact biomechanics. *International Journal of Crash*, *8*(4), 353–366. doi:10.1533/ijcr.2003.0243

Hornbeck, L. J. (1997). Digital light processing for high-brightnesshigh-resolution applications. In *Proceedings of Electronic Imaging'97*. International Society for Optics and Photonics.

Houdaille, M. (1908). *Improvements in or Relating To Shock-Absorbing or Dash-Pot Apparatus for Motor Vehicles and the Like.* France Patent number FR394081-A.

Houdaille, M. (1909). *Shock-absorbing apparatus*. United States Patent Number US933076 A.

Hou, S.-M., Hsu, C.-C., Wang, J.-L., Chao, C.-K., & Lin, J. (2004). Mechanical tests and finite element models for bone holding power of tibial locking screws. *Clinical Biomechanics (Bristol, Avon)*, *19*(7), 738–745. doi:10.1016/j.clinbiomech.2004.04.012 PMID:15288461

Howk, D., & Chu, T. M. (2006). Design variables for mechanical properties of bone tissue scaffolds. *Biomedical Sciences Instrumentation*, *42*, 278–283. PMID:16817621

Huang, Y., Van Dessel, J., Martens, W., Lambrichts, I., Zhong, W. J., Ma, G. W., ... Jacobs, R. (2015). Sensory innervation around immediately vs. delayed loaded implants: A pilot study. *International Journal of Oral Science*, *7*(1), 49–55. doi:10.1038/ijos.2014.53 PMID:25214361

Huang, Z. M., Zhang, Y.-Z., Kotaki, M., & Ramakrishna, S. (2003). A review on polymer nanofibers by electrospinning and their applications in nanocomposites. *Composites Science and Technology*, *63*(15), 2223–2253. doi:10.1016/S0266-3538(03)00178-7

Huelke, D. F., & Nusholtz, G. S. (1986). Cervical Spine Biomechanics: A Review of the Literature. *Journal of Orthopedics Research*, *4*(2). PMID:3519910

Human Biomechanics and Control Lab. (2007). *Dynamic Elastic Response Foot* [Electronic image]. Retrieved January 2016. From http://www-personal.umich.edu/~artkuo/Lab/2008/06/elastic-preload-energy-storage-in.html

Humphrey, J. D. (1995). Mechanics of arterial wall: Review and directions. *Critical Reviews in Biomedical Engineering, 23*(1-2), 1–162. doi:10.1615/CritRevBiomedEng.v23.i1-2.10 PMID:8665806

Humphrey, J. D., & Delange, S. L. (2003). *An introduction to Biomechanics- Solids and Fluids, Analysis & Design*. Springer.

Hunter, G. (2005). *Creation of Oxidized Zirconium Orthopaedic Implants*. Academic Press.

Hussain, D., Khurshid, A., Jianmin, S., & Hui, X. (2017). Advances in the Atomic Force Microscopy for Critical Dimension Metrology. *Measurement Science & Technology, 28*(1), 012001. doi:10.1088/0957-0233/28/1/012001

Hutmacher, D. W. (2000). Scaffolds in tissue engineering bone and cartilage. *Biomaterials, 21*(24), 2. doi:10.1016/S0142-9612(00)00121-6 PMID:11071603

Hutmacher, D. W., Schantz, J. T., Lam, C. X. F., Tan, K. C., & Lim, T. C. (2007). State of the art and future directions of scaffoldbased bone engineering from a biomaterials perspective. *Journal of Tissue Engineering and Regenerative Medicine, 1*(4), 245–260. doi:10.1002/term.24 PMID:18038415

Illich, D. J., Demir, N., Stojković, M., Scheer, M., Rothamel, D., Neugebauer, J., ... Zöller, J. E. (2011). Concise review: induced pluripotent stem cells and lineage reprogramming: prospects for bone regeneration. *Stem Cells (Dayton, Ohio), 29*(4), 555–563. doi:10.1002tem.611 PMID:21308867

ISO 527-1:2012. (n.d.). *ISO 527-1:2012 - Plastics -- Determination of tensile properties -- Part 1: General principles*. Retrieved September 28, 2017, from https://www.iso.org/standard/56045.html

Jacobs, T. D. B., Junge, T., & Lars, P. (2017). Quantitative Characterization of Surface Topography Using Spectral Analysis. *Surface Topography: Metrology and Properties, 5*(1), 13001.

Jagadamma. (2010). *The biomechanical optimisation (tuning) of The Ankle Foot Orthosis - Footwear Combination (AFO-FC) of children with Cerebral Palsy - the effects on sagittal gait characteristics, muscle and joint characteristics and quality of life* (PhD Thesis). Queen Margret University.

Jakus, A.E. (2016). Hyperelastic "bone": A highly versatile, growth factorefree, osteoregenerative, scalable, and surgically friendly biomaterial. *Sci. Transl. Med., 8*(358).

Jang, T. H., & Ekwaro-Osire, S. (2010). *Stochastic Finite Element Approach in Low Cervical Spine For Increasing Analysis Reliability*. Society for Design and Process Science.

Jiang, H., Cao, G., Xu, C., Zhang, Z., & Liu, S. (2014, August). Effects of residual stress in the membrane on the performance of surface micromachining silicon nitride pressure sensor, In *Electronic Packaging Technology (ICEPT), 2014 15th International Conference on* (pp. 664-670). IEEE. 10.1109/ICEPT.2014.6922742

Jin, D. S., Chun, K. H., & Lee, E. S. (2017). Analysis of the current density characteristics in through-mask electrochemical micromachining (TMECMM) for fabrication of micro-hole arrays on invar alloy film. *Chinese Journal of Aeronautics*, *30*(3), 1231–1241. doi:10.1016/j.cja.2016.10.021

Jones, D. B., Broeckmann, E., Pohl, T., & Smith, E. L. (2003). Development of a Mechanical Testing and Loading System for Trabecular Bone Studies for Long Term Culture. *European Cells & Materials*, *5*, 48–60. doi:10.22203/eCM.v005a05 PMID:14562272

Joshi, Mehta, Vresilovic, Karduna, & Marcolongo. (2005). Nucleus Implant Parameters Significantly Change the Compressive Stiffness of the Human Lumbar Intervertebral Disc. *Transactions of the ASME,* 127.

Joshi, A. (2006). *Functional compressive mechanics of a PVA/PVP nucleus pulposus replacement* (Vol. 27). Biomaterials.

Joyce, P. J., Violette, M. G., & Moon, T. J. (2002). Finite element analysis of unidirectional composite compression test specimens: A parametric study. *Composite Materials: Testing, Design, and Acceptance Criteria, 1416*, 30–68.

Kadhim Oleiwi, J., & Namah Hadi, A. (2016). *Design of Prosthetic Foot from Polymer Materials Reinforced by Carbon Fibers. Engineering & Technology Journal.*

Kahle, M. (2010). Embryonic stem cells induce ectopic bone formation in rats. *Bio-Medical Materials and Engineering*, *20*(6), 371–380. PMID:21263183

Kaigler, D., Wang, Z., Horger, K., Mooney, D. J., & Krebsbach, P. H. (2006). VEGF scaffolds enhance angiogenesis and bone regeneration in irradiated osseous defects. *Journal of Bone and Mineral Research*, *21*(5), 735–744. doi:10.1359/jbmr.060120 PMID:16734388

Kamaraj, A. B., Sundaram, M. M., & Mathew, R. (2013). Ultra high aspect ratio penetrating metal microelectrodes for biomedical applications. *Microsystem Technologies*, *19*(2), 179–186. doi:10.100700542-012-1653-3

Kanie, T., Fujii, K., Arikawa, H., & Inoue, K. (2000). Flexural properties and impact strength of denture base polymer reinforced with woven glass fibers. *Dental Materials*, *16*(2), 150–158. doi:10.1016/S0109-5641(99)00097-4 PMID:11203537

Karadogan & Williams. (2012). Three-Dimensional Static Modeling of the Lumbar Spine. *Journal of Biomechanical Engineering*, *134*. PMID:22938364

Karst, D., & Yang, Y. (2006). Molecular modeling study of the resistance of PLA to hydrolysis based on the blending of PLLA and PDLA. *Polymer*, *47*(13), 4845–4850. doi:10.1016/j.polymer.2006.05.002

Kelly, D. J., & Prendergast, P. J. (2006). Prediction of the optimal mechanical properties for a scaffold used in osteochondral defect repair. *Tissue Engineering*, *12*(9), 2509–2519. doi:10.1089/ten.2006.12.2509 PMID:16995784

Keriquel, V., Oliveira, H., Rémy, M., Ziane, S., Delmond, S., Rousseau, B., ... Fricain, J.-C. (2017). In situ printing of mesenchymal stromal cells, by laserassisted bioprinting, for in vivo bone regeneration applications. *Scientific Reports*, *7*(1), 1778. doi:10.103841598-017-01914-x PMID:28496103

Khanam, P. N., & AlMaadeed, M. A. A. (2015). Processing and characterization of polyethylenebased composites. *Adv. Manufact. Polym. Composit. Sci.*, *1*(2), 63–79. doi:10.1179/2055035915Y.0000000002

Kharazi, A. Z., Fathi, M. H., & Bahmany, F. (2009). Design of a textile composite bone plate using 3D-finite element method. *Materials & Design*, *31*(3), 1468–1474. doi:10.1016/j.matdes.2009.08.043

Khatib, O., & Demircan, E. (2005). *Robotics-based Synthesis of Human Motion*. Academic Press.

Kim, K., Yeatts, A., Dean, D., & Fisher, J. P. (2010). Stereolithographic bone scaffold design parameters: Osteogenic differentiation and signal expression. *Tissue Engineering. Part B, Reviews*, *16*(5), 523–539. doi:10.1089/ten.teb.2010.0171 PMID:20504065

Kiousis, D. E. (2008). *Biomechanical and Computational Modeling of Atherosclerotic Arteries-Insights into Plaque Vulnerability and Vascular Stenting* (Vol. 4). Computation in Engineering and Science.

Kivak, T. (2014). Optimization of Surface Roughness and Flank Wear Using the Taguchi Method in Milling of Hadfield Steel with PVD and CVD Coated Inserts. *Measurement: Journal of the International Measurement Confederation*, *50*(1), 19–28. doi:10.1016/j.measurement.2013.12.017

Kivak, T., Samtaş, G., & Çiçek, A. (2012). Taguchi method based optimisation of drilling parameters in drilling of AISI 316 steel with PVD monolayer and multilayer coated HSS drills. *Measurement: Journal of the International Measurement Confederation*, *45*(6), 1547–1557. doi:10.1016/j.measurement.2012.02.022

Klein, M. O., Schiegnitz, E., & Al-Nawas, B. (2014). Systematic review on success of narrow-diameter dental implants. *International Journal of Oral & Maxillofacial Implants*, 29. PMID:24660189

Kleiven. (2002). *Finite Element Modeling of the Human Head* (PhD thesis). Royal Institute of Technology.

Knaack, D., Goad, M. E. P., Aiolova, M., Rey, C., Tofighi, A., Chakravarthy, P., & Lee, D. D. (1998). Resorbable calcium phosphate bone substitute. *Journal of Biomedical Materials Research*, *43*(4), 399–409. doi:10.1002/(SICI)1097-4636(199824)43:4<399::AID-JBM7>3.0.CO;2-J PMID:9855198

Knudson, D. (2007). *Fundamentals of Biomechanics* (2nd ed.). Springer.

Kokubo, T., Kim, H. M., & Kawashita, M. (2003). Novel bioactive materials with different mechanical properties. *Biomaterials*, *24*(13), 2161–2175. doi:10.1016/S0142-9612(03)00044-9 PMID:12699652

Kolesky, D. B., Homan, K. A., Skylar-Scott, M. A., & Lewis, J. A. (2016). Three-dimensional bioprinting of thick vascularized tissues. *Proceedings of the National Academy of Sciences of the United States of America*, *113*(12), 3179–3184. doi:10.1073/pnas.1521342113 PMID:26951646

Kopova, I., Stráský, J., Harcuba, P., Landa, M., Janeček, M., & Bačáková, L. (2016). Newly developed Ti–Nb–Zr–Ta–Si–Fe biomedical beta titanium alloys with increased strength and enhanced biocompatibility. *Materials Science and Engineering C*, *60*, 230–238. doi:10.1016/j.msec.2015.11.043 PMID:26706526

Kuboki, Y., Jin, Q., & Takita, H. (2001). Geometry of carriers controlling phenotypic expression in BMP-induced osteogenesis and chondrogenesis. *J. Bone Jt. Surg. Am.*, *83-A*(2), 105–115. PMID:11314788

Kuila, T., Bose, S., Hong, C. E., Uddin, M. E., Khanra, P., Kim, N. H., & Lee, J. H. (2011). Preparation of functionalized graphene/linear low density polyethylene composites by a solution mixing method. *Carbon*, *49*(3), 1033–1037. doi:10.1016/j.carbon.2010.10.031

Kumari, N., Pradhan, S. K., & Kumar, K. (2018). Suitability of composite material for orthotic callipers- Tribological study. *Materials Today: Proceedings*, *5*(2), 5608–5614. doi:10.1016/j.matpr.2017.12.152

Kumar, M. P., Prakasan, K., & Kalaichelvan, K. (2016). Experimental investigation and multiphysics simulation on the influence of micro tools with various end profiles on diametrical overcut of holes machined using electrochemical micromachining for a predetermined optimum combination of process parameters. *Russian Journal of Electrochemistry*, *52*(10), 943–954. doi:10.1134/S1023193516100104

Kuo, Hu, Lin, Huang, Lin, Zhong, & Hsei. (2010). Bio-mechanical analysis of the lumbar spine on facet joint force and intra-discal pressure - a Finite element study. *BMC Musculoskeletal Disorders*.

Kuo, C., Li, Z., & Wang, C. (2017). Multi-objective optimisation in vibration-assisted drilling of CFRP/Al stacks. *Composite Structures*, *173*, 196–209. doi:10.1016/j.compstruct.2017.04.026

Kurutz & Fornet. (2006). Experimental And Numerical Biomechanical Analysis of the Human Lumbar Spine. *Journal of Computational and Applied Mechanics*, *7*(1), 23–39.

Kwasniak, P., Garbacz, H., & Kurzydlowski, K. J. (2016). Solid solution strengthening of hexagonal titanium alloys: Restoring forces and stacking faults calculated from first principles. *Acta Materialia*, *102*, 304–314. doi:10.1016/j.actamat.2015.09.041

Lai, S. M., Yeh, F. C., Wang, Y., Chan, H. C., & Shen, H. F. (2003). Comparative study of maleated polyolefins as compatibilizers for polyethylene/wood flour composites. *Journal of Applied Polymer Science*, *87*(3), 487–496. doi:10.1002/app.11419

Leardini, A., O'Connor, J. J., & Giannini, S. (2014). Biomechanics of the natural, arthritic and replaced human replaced human ankle joint. *Journal of Foot and Ankle Research*, *7*(1), 8. doi:10.1186/1757-1146-7-8 PMID:24499639

Leblanc, E., Trensz, F., Haroun, S., Drouin, G., Bergeron, É., Penton, C. M., ... Grenier, G. (2011). BMP-9-induced muscle heterotopic ossification require changes to the skeletal muscle microenvironment. *Journal of Bone and Mineral Research*, *26*(6), 1166–1177. doi:10.1002/jbmr.311 PMID:21611960

Lee, R.-M., & Chiu, H.-L. (2011). Mathematical Model of Interactive Respiration/Cardiovascular Composite System. *International Conference on Trends in Mechanical and Industrial Engineering (ICTMIE'2011)*, 136-139.

Lee. (2008). *Biomechanical Modeling and Control of the Human Body for Computer Animation* (PhD Thesis). University of California, Los Angeles, CA.

Lee. (2009). Comprehensive Biomechanical Modeling and Simulation of the Upper Body. Academic Press.

Lee, J. W., Han, H. S., Han, K. J., Park, J., Jeon, H., Ok, M. R., ... Yang, S. J. (2016). Long-term clinical study and multiscale analysis of in vivo biodegradation mechanism of Mg alloy. *Proceedings of the National Academy of Sciences of the United States of America*, *113*(3), 716–721. doi:10.1073/pnas.1518238113 PMID:26729859

Lee, S. J., Lee, C. Y., Yang, K. T., Kuan, F. H., & Lai, P. H. (2008). Simulation and fabrication of micro-scaled flow channels for metallic bipolar plates by the electrochemical micro-machining process. *Journal of Power Sources*, *185*(2), 1115–1121. doi:10.1016/j.jpowsour.2008.07.087

LeGeros, R. Z., Lin, S., Rohanizadeh, R., Mijares, D., & LeGeros, J. P. (2003). Biphasic calcium phosphate bioceramics: Preparation, properties and applications. *Journal of Materials Science. Materials in Medicine*, *14*(3), 201–209. doi:10.1023/A:1022872421333 PMID:15348465

Lester. (2009). *The Biomechanical Analysis Of The Hand In Rheumatoid Arthritis Patients with McpArthroplasty* (PhD Thesis). University of Birmingham.

Liao, C. J., Chen, C.-F., Chen, J.-H., Chiang, S.-F., Lin, Y.-J., & Chang, K.-Y. (2002). Fabrication of porous biodegradable polymer scaffolds using a solvent merging/particulate leaching method. *Journal of Biomedical Materials Research*, *59*(4), 676–681. doi:10.1002/jbm.10030 PMID:11774329

Li, C., Vepari, C., Jin, H.-J., Kim, H. J., & Kaplan, D. L. (2006). Electrospun silk-BMP-2 scaffolds for bone tissue engineering. *Biomaterials*, *27*(16), 3115–3124. doi:10.1016/j.biomaterials.2006.01.022 PMID:16458961

Li, D., Zhu, D., & Li, H. (2011). Microstructure of electrochemical micromachining using inert metal mask. *International Journal of Advanced Manufacturing Technology*, *55*(1-4), 189–194. doi:10.100700170-010-3025-4

Li, N., & Zheng, Y. (2013). Novel magnesium alloys developed for biomedical application: A review. *Journal of Materials Science and Technology*, *29*(6), 489–502. doi:10.1016/j.jmst.2013.02.005

Li, R. K. Y., Liang, J. Z., & Tjong, S. C. (1998). Morphology and dynamic mechanical properties of glass beads filled low density polyethylene composites. *Journal of Materials Processing Technology*, *79*(1), 59–65. doi:10.1016/S0924-0136(97)00319-1

Liu, G., Li, Y., Kong, Q., & Tong, H. (2017). Research on ECM process of micro holes with internal features. *Precision Engineering*, *47*, 508–515. doi:10.1016/j.precisioneng.2016.10.006

Liu, W., Ao, S., Li, Y., Liu, Z., Luo, Z., Wang, Z., & Song, R. (2017). Modeling and fabrication of micro hole by electrochemical micromachining using retracted tip tool. *Precision Engineering*, *50*, 77–84. doi:10.1016/j.precisioneng.2017.04.015

Liu, Y., Zhu, D., Zeng, Y., & Yu, H. (2011). Development of microelectrodes for electrochemical micromachining. *International Journal of Advanced Manufacturing Technology*, *55*(1-4), 195–203. doi:10.100700170-010-3035-2

Li, Y., Yang, C., Zhao, H., Qu, S., Li, X., & Li, Y. (2014). New developments of Ti-based alloys for biomedical applications. *Materials (Basel)*, *7*(3), 1709–1800. doi:10.3390/ma7031709 PMID:28788539

Li, Z., Gu, X., Lou, S., & Zheng, Y. (2008). The development of binary Mg–Ca alloys for use as biodegradable materials within bone. *Biomaterials*, *29*(10), 1329–1344. doi:10.1016/j.biomaterials.2007.12.021 PMID:18191191

Lloyd, A. W. (2001). Interfacial bioengineering to enhance surface biocompatibility. *Medical Device Technology*, *13*(1), 18–21. PMID:11921776

Lobontiu & Garcia. (2005). Mechanics of Microelectromechanical Systems. Kluwer Academic Publishers.

Lodge, T. P., & McLeish, T. C. (2000). Self-concentrations and effective glass transition temperatures in polymer blends. *Macromolecules*, *33*(14), 5278–5284. doi:10.1021/ma9921706

Lohbauer, U., Zipperle, M., Rischka, K., Petschelt, A., & Müller, F. A. (2008). Hydroxylation of dental zirconia surfaces: Characterization and bonding potential. *Journal of Biomedical Materials Research Part B: Applied Biomaterials*, *87*(2), 461–467. PMID:18506815

Lori, A. (2003). Anatomical and biomechanical mechanisms of subacromial impingement syndrome. *Clinical Biomechanics (Bristol, Avon)*, *18*(5), 369–379. doi:10.1016/S0268-0033(03)00047-0 PMID:12763431

Lundberg, A., Goldie, I., Kalin, B., & Selvik, G. (1989). Kinematics of the Ankle/Foot Complex: Plantarflexion and Dorsiflexion. *Foot & Ankle*, *9*(4), 194–200. doi:10.1177/107110078900900409 PMID:2731829

Macke, S., Misra, R., Sharma, A., & Prahalad, C.K. (2003). *Jaipur Foot: Challenging Convention.* University of Michigan Business School Case Study Series.

Malgaigne, J. F. (1841). *The Complete Works Of Ambroise Paré: Reviews and Collations on All Previous Editions*. Paris: J. B. Baillière.

Malve, M., Pe'rez del Palomar, A., Chandra, S., Lo'pez-Villalobos, J. L., Finol A. Mena, E. A., Ginel, A., & Doblaré, M. (2011). FSI Analysis of a Healthy and a Stenotic Human Trachea Under Impedance-Based BoundaryConditions. *Journal of Biomechanical Engineering*, *133*(2), 021001–1, 12. doi:10.1115/1.4003130 PMID:21280873

Malve, M., Pe'rez del Palomar, A., Chandra, S., Lo'pez-Villalobos, J. L., & Finol, E. A. (2011). FSI Analysis of a Human Trachea Before and After Prosthesis Implantation. *Journal of Biomechanical Engineering*, *133*(7), 071003–1, 12. doi:10.1115/1.4004315 PMID:21823742

Manal, K. T., & Buchanan, T. S. (2004). *Biomechanics of Human Movement*. McGraw Hill.

Mandal, N., Doloi, B., Mondal, B., & Das, R. (2011). Optimization of flank wear using Zirconia Toughened Alumina (ZTA) cutting tool: Taguchi method and Regression analysis. *Measurement: Journal of the International Measurement Confederation*, *44*(10), 2149–2155. doi:10.1016/j.measurement.2011.07.022

Manke, A., Wang, L., & Rojanasakul, Y. (2013). Mechanisms of nanoparticle-induced oxidative stress and toxicity. *BioMed Research International*, *2013*, 15. doi:10.1155/2013/942916 PMID:24027766

Mansor, Mustafa, Hajar, Fadzullah, Omar, Salim, & Akop. (2018). *Recent advances in polyethylene-based Biocomposites*. Woodhead Publishing Series in Composites Science and Engineering.

Marks, L. J., & Michael, J. W. (2001). Artificial limbs. *BMJ (Clinical Research Ed.)*, *323*(7315), 732–735. doi:10.1136/bmj.323.7315.732 PMID:11576982

Marshall, J. (2015). *The History of Prosthetics*. Retrieved 16 April 2016 from http://unyq.com/the-history-of-prosthetics/

Martijn, D., & Horsman, K. (2007). *The Twente Lower Extremity Model, Consistent Dynamic Simulation of the Human Locomotor Apparatus* (PhD Thesis). University of Twente.

Maruo, Y., Nishigawa, G., Irie, M., Yoshihara, K., & Minagi, S. (2015). Flexural properties of polyethylene, glass and carbon fiber-reinforced resin composites for prosthetic frameworks. *Acta Odontologica Scandinavica*, *73*(8), 581–587. doi:10.3109/00016357.2014.958875 PMID:25892406

Masum, H., Bhaumik, S., & Ray, R. (2014). Conceptual Design of a Powered Ankle-Foot Prosthesis for Walking. *Procedia Technology*, *14*, 228–235. doi:10.1016/j.protcy.2014.08.030

Matthews, J. A. (2002). Electrospinning of collagen nanofibers. *Biomacromolecules*, *3*(2), 232-238.

Maurus, P. B., & Kaeding, C. C. (2004). Bioabsorbable implant material review. *Operative Techniques in Sports Medicine*, *12*(3), 158–160. doi:10.1053/j.otsm.2004.07.015

Mayer, I., Jacobsohn, O., Niazov, T., Werckmann, J., Iliescu, M., Richard-Plouet, M., ... Reinen, D. (2003). Manganese in precipitated hydroxyapatites. *European Journal of Inorganic Chemistry, 2003*(7), 1445–1451. doi:10.1002/ejic.200390188

McNally, T., Pötschke, P., Halley, P., Murphy, M., Martin, D., Bell, S. E. J., ... Quinn, J. P. (2005). Polyethylene multiwalled carbon nanotube composites. *Polymer, 46*(19), 8222–8232. doi:10.1016/j.polymer.2005.06.094

MedicalExpo. (n.d.). *K2 Prosthetic Foot* [Electronic image]. Retrieved January 2016. From http://www.medicalexpo.com/prod/college-park/product-74912-660646.html

Mekael, P., Basu, J., Syam, N., Laurencin, C., & Carter, C. B. (2010). Characterization of carbon nanotube reinforced polymer scaffold for bone tissue engineering. *Microscopy and Microanalysis, 16*(Suppl. 2), 1032–1033. doi:10.1017/S1431927610060745

Me, R. C., Ibrahim, R., & Tahir, P. M. (2012). Natural Based Biocomposite Material for Prosthetic Socket Fabrication. *ALAM CIPTA, 5*(1), 27–34.

Meredith, J., Bilson, E., & Powe, R. (2015). A performance versus cost analysis of prepeg carbon epoxy energy absorption structures. Composite Structures, 124, 206-213.

Meriç, G., Dahl, J. E., & Ruyter, I. E. (2005). Physicochemical evaluation of silica-glass fiber reinforced polymers for prosthodontic applications. *European Journal of Oral Sciences, 113*(3), 258–264. doi:10.1111/j.1600-0722.2005.00209.x PMID:15953252

Mertz, L. (2013). Dream it, design it, print it in 3-D: What can 3-D printing do for you? *IEEE Pulse, 4*(6), 15–21. doi:10.1109/MPUL.2013.2279616 PMID:24233186

Michaels, A. D., & Chatterjee, K. (2002). Angioplasty Versus Bypass Surgery for Coronary Artery Disease. *Circulation, 106*(23), e187–e190. doi:10.1161/01.CIR.0000044747.37349.64 PMID:12460885

Middleton, J. C., & Tipton, A. J. (2000). Synthetic biodegradable polymers as orthopedic devices. *Biomaterials, 21*(23), 2335–2346. doi:10.1016/S0142-9612(00)00101-0 PMID:11055281

Misagh Imani, A.M., Goudarzi, M.H., & Hojjati. (2013). Finite Element Analysis of Mechanical Behaviors of Multi-Link Stent in a Coronary Artery with Plaque. *World Applied Sciences Journal, 21*(11), 1597–1602.

Misra, S. K., & Boccaccini, A. R. (2007). Biodegradable and bioactive polymer/ceramic composite scaffolds. *Woodhead Publishing Series in Biomaterials*, 72–92.

Mohammed, M. T., Khan, Z. A., & Siddiquee, A. N. (2014a). Beta titanium alloys: the lowest elastic modulus for biomedical applications: a review. *Int. J. Chem. Mol. Nucl. Mater. Metall. Eng, 8*(8).

Mohammed, M. T., Khan, Z. A., & Siddiquee, A. N. (2014b). Surface modifications of titanium materials for developing corrosion behavior in human body environment: A review. *Procedia Materials Science, 6*, 1610-1618.

Mohan, T.P., & Kanny, K. (2012). Effect of nanoclay in HDPE_glass fiber composites on processing, structure, and properties. *Adv. Composit. Mater.*, 315-331.

Mooney, D. J., Baldwin, D. F., Suh, N. P., Vacanti, J. P., & Langer, R. (1996). Novel approach to fabricate porous sponges of poly(d,llactic- co-glycolic acid) without the use of organic solvents. *Biomaterials*, *17*(14), 1417–1422. doi:10.1016/0142-9612(96)87284-X PMID:8830969

Mountziaris, P. M., & Mikos, A. G. (2008). Modulation of the inflammatory response for enhanced bone tissue regeneration. *Tissue Engineering. Part B, Reviews*, *14*(2), 179–186. doi:10.1089/ten.teb.2008.0038 PMID:18544015

Munda, J., & Bhattacharyya, B. (2008). Investigation into electrochemical micromachining (ECMM) through response surface methodology based approach. *International Journal of Advanced Manufacturing Technology*, *35*(7-8), 821–832. doi:10.100700170-006-0759-0

Munda, J., Malapati, M., & Bhattacharyya, B. (2007). Control of micro-spark and stray-current effect during ECMM process. *Journal of Materials Processing Technology*, *194*(1-3), 151–158. doi:10.1016/j.jmatprotec.2007.04.112

Murphy, S.V., & Atala, A. (2014). 3D bioprinting of tissues and organs. *Nat. Biotechnol.*, *32*(8), 773-785.

Muschler, G. F., Nitto, H., Boehm, C. A., & Easley, K. A. (2001). Age- and gender-related changes in the cellularity of human bone marrow and the prevalence of osteoblastic progenitors. *Journal of Orthopaedic Research*, *19*(1), 117–125. doi:10.1016/S0736-0266(00)00010-3 PMID:11332607

Mwema, F. M., Oladijo, O. P., & Akinlabi, E. T. (2018). Effect of Substrate Temperature on Aluminium Thin Films Prepared byRF-Magnetron Sputtering. *Materials Today: Proceedings*, *5*(9), 20464–20473. doi:10.1016/j.matpr.2018.06.423

Mwema, F. M., Oladijo, O. P., Akinlabi, S. A., & Akinlabi, E. T. (2018). Properties of Physically Deposited Thin Aluminium Film Coatings: A Review. *Journal of Alloys and Compounds*, *747*, 306–323. doi:10.1016/j.jallcom.2018.03.006

Mwema, F. M., Oladijo, O. P., Sathiaraj, T. S., & Akinlabi, E. T. (2018). Atomic Force Microscopy Analysis of Surface Topography of Pure Thin Aluminium Films. *Material Research Express*, *5*(4), 1–15. doi:10.1088/2053-1591/aabe1b

Nagels, J., Stokdijk, M., & Rozing, P. M. (2003). Stress shielding and bone resorption in shoulder arthroplasty. *Journal of Shoulder and Elbow Surgery*, *12*(1), 35–39. doi:10.1067/mse.2003.22 PMID:12610484

Namjoshi, D. R., Good, C., Wai, H. C., Panenka, W., Richards, D., Cripton, P. A., & Wellington, C. L. (2013). Towards clinical management of traumatic brain injury: A review of models and mechanisms from a biomechanical perspective. *Disease Models & Mechanisms*, *6*(6), 1325–1338. doi:10.1242/dmm.011320 PMID:24046354

Nareliya & Kumar. (2011). Biomechanical Analysis of Human Femur Bone. *International Journal of Engineering Science and Technology*, *3*(4).

Nayak, A. A., Gangopadhyay, S., & Sahoo, D. K. (2016). Modelling, simulation and experimental investigation for generating 'I'shaped contour on Inconel 825 using electro chemical machining. *Journal of Manufacturing Processes*, *23*, 269–277. doi:10.1016/j.jmapro.2016.05.001

News Medical Life Science. (2017). *World's first split-keel fiberglass foot launched by Freedom Innovations*. Retrieved November 10, 2018, from https://www.news-medical.net/news/20170829/Worlds-first-split-keel-fiberglass-foot-launched-by-Freedom-Innovations.aspx

Nie, H., & Wang, C. H. (2007). Fabrication and characterization of PLGA/HAp composite scaffolds for delivery of BMP-2 plasmid DNA. *Journal of Controlled Release*, *120*(1-2), 111–121. doi:10.1016/j.jconrel.2007.03.018 PMID:17512077

Nigg, B., & Herzog, W. (1999). *Biomechanics of the Musculoskeletal System* (2nd ed.). John Wiley & Sons.

Nobili, M., Morbiducci, U., Ponzini, R., Del Gaudio, C., Balducci, A., Grigioni, M., ... Redaelli, A. (2008). Numerical simulation of the dynamics of a bileaflet prosthetic heartvalve using a fluid–structure interaction approach. *Journal of Biomechanics*, *41*(11), 2539–2550. doi:10.1016/j.jbiomech.2008.05.004 PMID:18579146

Norkin, C. C., & Levangie, P. K. (1992). *Joint Structure & Function: A Comprehensive Analysis* (2nd ed.). Philadelphia: F.A. Davis Co.

Norton, K. M. (2007). A Brief History of Prosthetics. *inMotion*, *17*(7), 11-13.

O'Brien, F. J., Harley, B. A., Yannas, I. V., & Gibson, L. J. (2005). The effect of pore size on cell adhesion in collagen-GAG scaffolds. *Biomaterials*, *26*(4), 433–441. doi:10.1016/j.biomaterials.2004.02.052 PMID:15275817

O'Keefe, R. J., & Mao, J. (2011). Bone tissue engineering and regeneration: From discovery to the clinicean overview. *Tissue Engineering. Part B, Reviews*, *17*(6), 389–392. doi:10.1089/ten.teb.2011.0475 PMID:21902614

Oh, S., Kleinberger, M., & McElhaney, J. H. (1994). Finite Element analysis of balloon angioplasty. *Medical & Biological Engineering & Computing*, *32*(S1), S108–S114. doi:10.1007/BF02523336 PMID:7967823

Oka, Y., Ye, M., & Zuker, C. S. (2015). Thirst driving and suppressing signals encoded by distinct neural populations in the brain. *Nature*, *520*(7547), 349–352. doi:10.1038/nature14108 PMID:25624099

Ommaya, A. K., Goldsmith, W., & Thibault, L. (2002). Biomechanics and neuropathology of adult and paediatric head injury. *British Journal of Neurosurgery*, *16*(3), 220–242. doi:10.1080/02688690220148824 PMID:12201393

OpenStax College. (n.d.). *Anatomy and Physiology*. OpenStax CNX. Retrieved from http://cnx.org/contents/14fb4ad7-39a1-4eee-ab6e-3ef2482e3e22@12.8

Orthopaedic, B. (n.d.). *Hip Abduction Brace*. Retrieved 26 July 2016 from http://www.ballert.com/pdf/HipAbductionOrthosis.pdf

Otheguy, M.E. Gibson, A.G., Robinson, M., Findon, E., Cripps, B. Ochoa, A., … Castro, A. (2001). Recycling of end-of-life thermoplastic composite boats. *Composites Structures*, 21-42.

Ozbolat, I. T., & Hospodiuk, M. (2016). Current advances and future perspectives in extrusion-based bioprinting. *Biomaterials*, *76*, 321–343. doi:10.1016/j.biomaterials.2015.10.076 PMID:26561931

Palanikumar, K. (2011). Experimental investigation and optimisation in drilling of GFRP composites. *Measurement: Journal of the International Measurement Confederation*, *44*(10), 2138–2148. doi:10.1016/j.measurement.2011.07.023

Paul E Leimkuehler Online Learning Center, American Academy of Orthotists and Prosthetists. (n.d.). Retrieved January 2016 from http://www.oandp.org/

Peterson, D. R., & Bronzino, J. D. (2008). *Biomechanics- Principles and Applications*. CRC Press.

Pezzin, A. P. T., Van Ekenstein, G. A., Zavaglia, C. A. C., Ten Brinke, G., & Duek, E. A. R. (2003). Poly (para-dioxanone) and poly (L-lactic acid) blends: Thermal, mechanical, and morphological properties. *Journal of Applied Polymer Science*, *88*(12), 2744–2755. doi:10.1002/app.11984

Phillips, S. L., & Craelius, W. (2005). Material properties of selected prosthetic laminates. *Journal of Prosthetics and Orthotics*, *17*(1), 27–34. doi:10.1097/00008526-200501000-00007

Pierce, M. C., Bertocci, G. E., Vogeley, E., & Moreland, M. S. (2004). Evaluating long bone fractures in children: A biomechanical approach with illustrative cases. *Child Abuse & Neglect*, *28*(5), 505–524. doi:10.1016/j.chiabu.2003.01.001 PMID:15206413

Pillai, H. P., Sampath, S. C., Elumalai, R., Hariharan, S., & Natarajan, Y. (2017). Influence of Process Parameters on Electrochemical Micromachining of Nimonic 75 Alloy. In *ASME 2017 International Mechanical Engineering Congress and Exposition* (pp. V002T02A007-V002T02A007). American Society of Mechanical Engineers.

Pinnoji, P. K., & Mahajan, P. (2007). Finite element modeling of helmeted head impact under frontal loading. *Sadhana*, *32*(4), 445–458. doi:10.100712046-007-0034-6

Pochrząst, M., Walke, W., & Kaczmarek, M. (2009). Biomechanical characterization of the balloon-expandable slotted tube stents. *Journal of Achievements in Materials and Manufacturing Engineering*, *3*(2), 340–347.

Polo-Corrales, L., Latorre-Esteves, M., & Ramirez-Vick, J. E. (2014). Scaffold design for bone regeneration. *Journal of Nanoscience and Nanotechnology*, *14*(1), 15–56. doi:10.1166/jnn.2014.9127 PMID:24730250

Prajer, M., & Ansell, M. P. (2014). Bio-composites for structural applications: poly-L-lactide reinforced with long sisal fiber bundles. *Journal of Applied Polymer Science*, *131*(21), 1–13. doi:10.1002/app.40999

Premraj, R., & Doble, M. (2005). Biodegradation of polymers. *Indian Journal of Biotechnology*, *4*(2), 186–193.

PrimaryL. J. (2017). *3D Printing Processes*. Retrieved from https://www.printspace3d.com/3d-printing-processes/

Prosthetics, C. (n.d.). *Multi Axis Foot* [Electronic Image]. Retrieved January 2016 from http://www.customprosthetics.com/lowerextremity.html

Prot. (2008). *Modelling and numerical analysis of the porcine and human mitral apparatus* (PhD thesis). Norwegian University of Science and Technology.

Puppi, D., Chiellini, F., Piras, A. M., & Chiellini, E. (2010). Polymeric materials for bone and cartilage repair. *Progress in Polymer Science*, *35*(4), 403–440. doi:10.1016/j.progpolymsci.2010.01.006

Pyng Medical Corp. (2011). *T-POD® Pelvic Stabilization Device Training Session*. Retrieved 25 July 2016 from www.pyng.com/wp/wp-content/uploads/2011/02/PM-088a T-POD Training PowerPoint Presentation.pdf

Qian, S., Zhu, D., Qu, N., Li, H., & Yan, D. (2010). Generating micro-dimples array on the hard chrome-coated surface by modified through mask electrochemical micromachining. *International Journal of Advanced Manufacturing Technology*, *47*(9-12), 1121–1127. doi:10.100700170-009-2246-x

Quarteroni & Formagga. (2002). Mathematical modeling and numerical simulation of the cardiovascular system. In Modeling of living systems: Handbook of numerical analysis series. Elsevier.

Raj, S. A., Muthukumaran, E. K. J., & Jayakrishna, K. (2018). A Case Study of 3D Printed PLA and Its Mechanical Properties. *Materials Today: Proceedings*, *5*(5), 11219–11226. doi:10.1016/j.matpr.2018.01.146

Ramakrishna, S., Mayer, J., Wintermantel, E., & Leong, K. W. (2001). Biomedical applications of polymer-composite materials: A review. *Composites Science and Technology*, *61*(9), 1189–1224. doi:10.1016/S0266-3538(00)00241-4

Rath, U. 2013, *Two phase flow analysis in electrochemical machining for l-shaped tool: A CFD APPROACH* (Doctoral dissertation).

Ravi Shantharaj, M. D. S., Panchali Batra, M. D. S., Pradeep Subbiah, M. D. S., & Lakshmi, B. (2014). Total Recall: An Update On Orthodontic Wires. *IJO, 25*(3).

Rebello, K. J. (2004). Applications of MEMS in Surgery. *Proceedings of the IEEE*, *92*(1), 43–55. doi:10.1109/JPROC.2003.820536

Reddy, M. M., Vivekanandhan, S., Misra, M., Bhatia, S. K., & Mohanty, A. K. (2013). Biobased plastics and bionanocomposites: Current status and future opportunities. *Progress in Polymer Science*, *38*(10-11), 1653–1689. doi:10.1016/j.progpolymsci.2013.05.006

Reilly, D. T. & Cleveland, A. H. B. (1974). The Mechanical Properties of Cortical Bone. *The Journal of Bone and Joint Surgery, 56a*(5). PMID:4603167

Robello, D. R., Eldridge, T. D., & Swanson, M. T. (1999). Degradation and stabilization of polycyanoacrylates. *Journal of Polymer Science. Part A, Polymer Chemistry, 37*(24), 4570–4581. doi:10.1002/(SICI)1099-0518(19991215)37:24<4570::AID-POLA14>3.0.CO;2-#

Robey, P. G. (2011). Cell sources for bone regeneration: The good, the bad, and the ugly (but promising). *Tissue Engineering. Part B, Reviews, 17*(6), 423–430. doi:10.1089/ten.teb.2011.0199 PMID:21797663

Rockwood, D. N., Gil, E. S., Park, S.-H., Kluge, J. A., Grayson, W., Bhumiratana, S., ... Kaplan, D. L. (2010). In growth of human mesenchymal stem cells into porous silk particle reinforced silk composite scaffolds: An in vitro study. *Acta Biomaterialia, 7*(1), 144–151. doi:10.1016/j.actbio.2010.07.020 PMID:20656075

Rosa, A. L., Beloti, M. M., & van Noort, R. (2003). Osteoblastic differentiation of cultured rat bone marrow cells on hydroxyapatite with different surface topography. *Dental Materials, 19*(8), 768–772. doi:10.1016/S0109-5641(03)00024-1 PMID:14511735

Salgado, A. J., Coutinho, O. P., & Reis, R. L. (2004). Bone tissue engineering: State of the art and future trends. *Macromolecular Bioscience, 4*(8), 743–765. doi:10.1002/mabi.200400026 PMID:15468269

Samaka & Tarlochan. (2013). Finite Element (FE) Human Head Models / Literature Review. *International Journal of Scientific & Technology Research, 2*(7).

Samanta, S., & Chakraborty, S. (2011). Parametric optimization of some non-traditional machining processes using artificial bee colony algorithm. *Engineering Applications of Artificial Intelligence, 24*(6), 946–957. doi:10.1016/j.engappai.2011.03.009

Sandino, C., & Lacroix, D. (2011). A dynamical study of the mechanical stimuli and tissue differentiation within a CaP scaffold based on micro-CT finite element models. *Biomechanics and Modeling in Mechanobiology, 10*(4), 565–576. doi:10.100710237-010-0256-0 PMID:20865437

Saunders, R. E., & Derby, B. (2014). Inkjet printing biomaterials for tissue engineering: Bioprinting. *International Materials Reviews, 59*(8), 430–448. doi:10.1179/1743280414Y.0000000040

Scattina, A., Alovisi, M., Paolino, D. S., Pasqualini, D., Scotti, N., Chiandussi, G., & Berutti, E. (2015). Prediction of Cyclic Fatigue Life of Nickel-Titanium Rotary Files by Virtual Modeling and Finite Elements Analysis. *Journal of Endodontics, 41*(11), 1867–1870. doi:10.1016/j.joen.2015.07.010 PMID:26361644

Schaffer, E., Kort, C. & Kreuter P. (2008). The Prosthetic Knee Microprocessor and Non-Microprocessor Knee Joints. *inMotion, 18*(7), 34-36.

Schantz, J. T., Chim, H., & Whiteman, M. (2007). Cell guidance in tissue engineering: SDF- 1 mediates site-directed homing of mesenchymal stem cells within threedimensional polycaprolactone scaffolds. *Tissue Engineering, 13*(11), 2615–2624. doi:10.1089/ten.2006.0438 PMID:17961003

Scheck & Siress. (n.d.). *KAFO (Knee-Ankle-Foot Orthosis)*. Retrieved 1 July 2016 from www.scheckandsiress.com

Schinhammer, M., Hänzi, A. C., Löffler, J. F., & Uggowitzer, P. J. (2010). Design strategy for biodegradable Fe-based alloys for medical applications. *Acta Biomaterialia*, *6*(5), 1705–1713. doi:10.1016/j.actbio.2009.07.039 PMID:19654056

Schmitt, O. H. (1969). Some interesting and useful biomimetic transforms. *Proc. 3rd Int. Biophysics Congress*, 297.

Scholz, M.-S., Blanchfield, J. P., Bloom, L. D., Coburn, B. H., Elkington, M., Fuller, J. D., ... Bond, I. P. (2011). The use of composite materials in modern orthopaedic medicine and prosthetic devices: A review. *Composites Science and Technology*, *71*(16), 1791–1803. doi:10.1016/j.compscitech.2011.08.017

Sen, N. (2004). Composites: Use in saucepan handles, artificial limbs and the AGNI missile. *Current Science*, *86*(3), 372–375.

Seymour, R. (2002). *Prosthetics and Orthotics: Lower Limb and Spinal*. Lippincott Williams & Wilkins.

Shackelford, J. F. (1999). Bioceramics-current status and future trends. *Materials Science Forum*, *293*, 99. doi:10.4028/www.scientific.net/MSF.293.99

Shafiee, A., & Atala, A. (2016). Printing technologies for medical applications. *Trends in Molecular Medicine*, *22*(3), 254–265. doi:10.1016/j.molmed.2016.01.003 PMID:26856235

Sheikh, Z., Najeeb, S., Khurshid, Z., Verma, V., Rashid, H., & Glogauer, M. (2015). Biodegradable materials for bone repair and tissue engineering applications. *Materials (Basel)*, *8*(9), 5744–5794. doi:10.3390/ma8095273 PMID:28793533

Shen, J., Dan, Z., Fei, H. Z., & Gan, Y. (2017). AFM Tip-Sample Convolution Effects for Cylinder Protrusions. *Applied Surface Science*, *422*, 482–491. doi:10.1016/j.apsusc.2017.06.053

Shen, J., Dan, Z., Fei, H. Z., & Gan, Y. (2018). AFM Characterization of Patterned Sapphire Substrate with Dense Cone Arrays: Image Artifacts and Tip-Cone Convolution Effect. *Applied Surface Science*, *433*, 358–366. doi:10.1016/j.apsusc.2017.10.077

Shikinami, Y., & Okuno, M. (1999). Bioresorbable devices made of forged composites of hydroxyapatite (HA) particles and poly-L-lactide (PLLA): Part I. Basic characteristics. *Biomaterials*, *20*(9), 859–877. doi:10.1016/S0142-9612(98)00241-5 PMID:10226712

Shi, S. (2009). RhBMP-2 microspheres-loaded chitosan/collagen scaffold enhanced osseointegration: An experiment in dog. *Journal of Biomaterials Applications*, *23*(4), 331–346. doi:10.1177/0885328208090013 PMID:18667455

Shi, X., Sitharaman, B., Pham, Q. P., Liang, F., Wu, K., Edward Billups, W., ... Mikos, A. G. (2007). Fabrication of porous ultra-short single-walled carbon nanotube nanocomposite scaffolds for bone tissue engineering. *Biomaterials*, *28*(28), 4078–4090. doi:10.1016/j.biomaterials.2007.05.033 PMID:17576009

Shtilman, M. I. (2015). Biodegradation of Polymers. Journal of Siberian Federal University. *Biology (Basel)*, *8*(2), 113.

Siegler, S., Chen, J., & Schnek, C. D. (1988). The Three Dimensional Kinematics and Flexibility Characteristics of the Human Ankle and Subtalar Joints-Part I: Kinematics. *Journal of Biomechanical Engineering*, *110*(4), 364–373. doi:10.1115/1.3108455 PMID:3205022

Singh, D., & Shukla, R. S. (2016). Optimization of electrochemical micromachining and electrochemical discharge machining process parameters using firefly algorithm. *International Journal of Mechatronics and Manufacturing Systems*, *9*(2), 137–159. doi:10.1504/IJMMS.2016.076169

Singh, J., Jain, V. K., & Ramkumar, J. (2016). Fabrication of complex circuit on printed circuit board (PCB) using electrochemical micro-machining. *International Journal of Advanced Manufacturing Technology*, *85*(9-12), 2073–2081. doi:10.100700170-015-7817-4

Sivanandam, S. N., & Deepa, S. N. (2008). *Introduction to genetic algorithms*. Introduction to Genetic Algorithms; doi:10.1007/978-3-540-73190-0

Slocumb, W. (2014). *Bamboo Fiber Reinforced Composites for Prosthetics and Orthotics*. Retrieved from https://www.csueastbay.edu/programs/csr/files/docs/2014%2520CSU%2520Award%2520Winner%252 0Summaries/WilliamSlocumb¬2014%2520Summary.pdf

Smith, D. G. (2005a). Higher Challenges: The Hip Disarticulation and Transpelvic Amputation Levels. *inMotion, 15*(1).

Smith, D. G. (2005b). Higher Challenges: Amputations at the Hip and Pelvis, Part 2. *inMotion, 15*(2).

Smith, S. (2006). *SCS Continuing Education, Basic Structure and Function of the Ankle and Foot*. Retrieved January 2016 From www.ceuarmy.com/BSFAFpdf.pdf

Soler-Botija, C., Bagó, J. R., Llucià-Valldeperas, A., Vallés-Lluch, A., Castells-Sala, C., Martínez-Ramos, C., ... Bayes-Genis, A. (2014). Engineered 3D bioimplants using elastomeric scaffold, self-assembling peptide hydrogel, and adipose tissue-derived progenitor cells for cardiac regeneration. *American Journal of Translational Research*, *6*(3), 291. PMID:24936221

Song, G., & Atrens, A. (2003). Understanding magnesium corrosion—a framework for improved alloy performance. *Advanced Engineering Materials*, *5*(12), 837–858. doi:10.1002/adem.200310405

SPS Co. (n.d.). *Orthotic catalogue section 7: Hip orthoses*. Retrieved from http://www.spsco.com/education/downloadable-resources/orthotic/

Stark, G. (2001). Overview of Hip Disarticulation Prostheses. *JPO*, *13*(2), 50.

Stijnen. (2004). *Interaction between the mitral and aortic heart valve- an experimental and computational study* (PhD thesis). Eindhoven University of Technology.

Stolzing, A., Jones, E., McGonagle, D., & Scutt, A. (2008). Age-related changes in human bone marrow-derived mesenchymal stem cells: Consequences for cell therapies. *Mechanisms of Ageing and Development*, *129*(3), 163–173. doi:10.1016/j.mad.2007.12.002 PMID:18241911

Sumathi, S., & Surekha, P. (2016). *Computational Intelligence Paradigms: Theory andApplications Using MATLAB*. CRC Press, Taylor & Francis Group.

Sun, C., Fang, N., Wu, D.M., & Zhang, X. (2005). Projection micro-stereolithographyusing digital micro-mirror dynamic mask. *Sensor Actuat a-Phys, 121*, 113–120.

Sun, W., Starly, B., Nam, J., & Darling, A. (2005). Bio-CAD modeling and its applications in computer-aided tissue engineering. *Comput Aided Design, 37*(11), 1097–1114.

Sung, H. J., Meredith, C., Johnson, C., & Galis, Z. S. (2004). The effect of scaffold degradation rate on three-dimensional cell growth and angiogenesis. *Biomaterials*, *25*(26), 5735–5742. doi:10.1016/j.biomaterials.2004.01.066 PMID:15147819

Sun, M., Xiao, K., Dong, C., Li, X., & Zhong, P. (2014). Effect of stress on electrochemical characteristics of pre-cracked ultrahigh strength stainless steel in acid sodium sulphate solution. *Corrosion Science*, *89*, 137–145. doi:10.1016/j.corsci.2014.08.023

Suresh, K. R., Niranjan, H. B., Martin Jebaraj, P., & Chowdiah, M. P. (2003). Tensile and wear properties of Aluminum composites. *Wear*, *255*(1-6), 638–642. doi:10.1016/S0043-1648(03)00292-8

Suthar, J., & Patel, K. M. (2018). Processing issues, machining, and applications of aluminum metal matrix composites. *Materials and Manufacturing Processes*, *33*(5), 499–527. doi:10.1080/10426914.2017.1401713

Tabassum, M., & Mathew, K. (2014). *A Genetic Algorithm Analysis towards Optimization solutions. International Journal of Digital Information and Wireless Communications*. doi:10.17781/P001091

Taïr, K., Kharoubi, O., Taïr, O. A., Hellal, N., Benyettou, I., & Aoues, A. (2016). Aluminium-induced acute neurotoxicity in rats: Treatment with aqueous extract of Arthrophytum (Hammada scoparia). *Journal of Acute Disease*, *5*(6), 470–482. doi:10.1016/j.joad.2016.08.028

Takmakov, P., Ruda, K., Phillips, K. S., Isayeva, I. S., Krauthamer, V., & Welle, C. G. (2015). Rapid evaluation of the durability of cortical neural implants using accelerated aging with reactive oxygen species. *Journal of Neural Engineering*, *12*(2), 026003. doi:10.1088/1741-2560/12/2/026003 PMID:25627426

Ţălu, Ş., Bramowicz, M., Kulesza, S., & Solaymani, S. (2018). Topographic Characterization of Thin Film Field-Effect Transistors of 2,6-Diphenyl Anthracene (DPA) by Fractal and AFM Analysis. *Materials Science in Semiconductor Processing*, *79*, 144–152. doi:10.1016/j.mssp.2018.02.008

Tambaca, Canic, Kosor, Fish, & Paniagua. (2011). Mechanical Behavior of Fully Expanded Commercially Available Endovascular Coronary Stents. Texas Heart Institute Journal, 491-501.

Tamimi, F., Le Nihouannen, D., Eimar, H., Sheikh, Z., Komarova, S., & Barralet, J. (2012). The effect of autoclaving on the physical and biological properties of dicalcium phosphate dihydrate bioceramics: Brushite vs. monetite. *Acta Biomaterialia*, *8*(8), 3161–3169. doi:10.1016/j.actbio.2012.04.025 PMID:22522010

Tang, A., Pan, F., Yang, M., & Cheng, R. (2008). Mechanical properties and microstructure of magnesium-aluminum based alloys containing strontium. *Materials Transactions*, *49*(6), 1203–1211. doi:10.2320/matertrans.MOV2007315

Tan, L., Yu, X., Wan, P., & Yang, K. (2013). Biodegradable materials for bone repairs: A review. *Journal of Materials Science and Technology*, *29*(6), 503–513. doi:10.1016/j.jmst.2013.03.002

Teramoto, H., Kawai, A., Sugihara, S., Yoshida, A., & Inoue, H. (2005). Resorption of apatite-wollastonite containing glass-ceramic and beta-tricalcium phosphate in vivo. *Acta Medica Okayama*, *59*(5), 201. PMID:16286959

Thian, E. S., Konishi, T., Kawanobe, Y., Lim, P. N., Choong, C., Ho, B., & Aizawa, M. (2013). Zinc-substituted hydroxyapatite: A biomaterial with enhanced bioactivity and antibacterial properties. *Journal of Materials Science. Materials in Medicine*, *24*(2), 437–445. doi:10.100710856-012-4817-x PMID:23160913

Ting, Z. (2017). Biomimetic design and fabrication of multilayered osteochondral scaffolds by low-temperature deposition manufacturing and thermal-induced phase-separation techniques. *Biofabrication*, *9*(2), 25–21. PMID:28462906

Torburn, L., Perry, J., & Ayyappa, E. (1990). Below-knee amputee gait with dynamic elastic response prosthetic feet: A pilot study. *Journal of Rehabilitation Research and Development*, *27*(4), 369–384. doi:10.1682/JRRD.1990.10.0369 PMID:2089148

Torii, R., Oshima, M., Kobayashi, T., Takagi, K., & Tezduyar, T. E. (2004). Computation of Cardiovascular Fluid-Structure Interactions with the DSD/SST Method. *Proceedings of the 6th World Congress on Computational Mechanics.*

Tözeren, A. (2000). *Human Body Dynamics Classical Mechanics and Human Movement.* Springer.

Tsimbouri, P. M., Childs, P. G., Pemberton, G. D., Yang, J., Jayawarna, V., Orapiriyakul, W., ... Dalby, M. J. (2017). Stimulation of 3D osteogenesis by mesenchymal stem cells using a nanovibrational bioreactor. *Nat. Biomed. Eng.*, *1*(9), 758–770. doi:10.103841551-017-0127-4

Tsuruga, E., Takita, H., Itoh, H., Wakisaka, Y., & Kuboki, Y. (1997). Pore size of porous hydroxyapatite as the cell-substratum controls BMP-induced osteogenesis. *Journal of Biochemistry*, *121*(2), 317–324. doi:10.1093/oxfordjournals.jbchem.a021589 PMID:9089406

Tyndyk, M. A., Barron, V., Mchugh, P. E., & O'mahoney, D. (2007). Generation of a finite element model of the thoracolumbar spine. *Acta of Bioengineering and Biomechanics*, *9*(1). PMID:17933103

Utzschneider, S., Harrasser, N., Schroeder, C., Mazoochian, F., & Jansson, V. (2009). Wear of contemporary total knee replacements – a knee simulator study of six current designs. *Clinical Biomechanics (Bristol, Avon)*, *24*(7), 583–588. doi:10.1016/j.clinbiomech.2009.04.007 PMID:19450910

Vaccaro, A. R. (2002). The role of the osteoconductive scaffold in synthetic bone graft. *Orthopedics*, *25*(5Suppl), 571–578. PMID:12038844

Vallittu, P. K. (2007). Effect of 10 years of in vitro aging on the flexural properties of fiber-reinforced resin composites. *The International Journal of Prosthodontics*, *20*(1), 43–45. PMID:17319361

Van De Vosse, F. N., De Hart, J., Van Oijen, C. H. G. A., Bessems, D., Gunther, T. W. M., Segal, A., ... Baaijens, F. P. T. (2003). Finite-element-based computational methods for cardiovascular fluid-structure interaction. *Journal of Engineering Mathematics*, *47*(3/4), 335–368. doi:10.1023/B:ENGI.0000007985.17625.43

van den Bogert, Samorezov, Davis, & Smith. (2012). Modeling and Optimal Control of an Energy-Storing Prosthetic Knee. *Journal of Biomechanical Engineering*, *134*. PMID:22757495

van der Waarde, T., & Michael, J. W. (2002). Hip Disarticulation and Transpelvic Amputation: Prosthetic Management. In Atlas of Limb Prosthetics: Surgical, Prosthetic, and Rehabilitation Principles. Academic Press.

van Heumen, C. C. M., Kreulen, C. M., Bronkhorst, E. M., Lesaffre, E., & Creugers, N. H. J. (2008). Fiber-reinforced dental composites in beam testing. *Dental Materials*, *24*(11), 1435–1443. doi:10.1016/j.dental.2008.06.006 PMID:18692230

van Loon, R. (2005). *A 3D method for modeling the fluid-structure interaction of heart valves* (PhD thesis). Eindhoven University of Technology.

van Loon, R., Anderson, P. D., de Hart, J., & Baaijens, F. P. T. (2004). A combined fictitious domain /adaptive meshing method for fluid–structure interaction in heart valves. *International Journal for Numerical Methods in Fluids*, *46*(5), 533–544. doi:10.1002/fld.775

van Loon, R., Anderso, P. D., & van de Vosse, F. N. (2006). A fluid–structure interaction method with solid-rigid contact for heart valve dynamics. *Journal of Computational Physics*, *217*(2), 806–823. doi:10.1016/j.jcp.2006.01.032

Vanderwerker, E. E. Jr. (1976). A Brief Review of the History of Amputations and Prostheses. *Inter-Clinic Information Bulletin*, *15*(5), 15–16.

Vanderwerker, E. E. Jr. (1976). A Brief Review of the History of Amputations and Prostheses. *Inter-Clinic Information Bulletin.*, *15*(5), 15–16.

Vena, P., Franzoso, G., Gastaldi, D., Contro, R., & Dallolio, V. (2005). A finite Element Model of the L4-L5 spinal motion segment: Biomechanical compatibility of an inter-spinous device. *Computer Methods in Biomechanics and Biomedical Engineering*, *8*(1), 7–16. doi:10.1080/10255840500062914 PMID:16154865

Ventola, C. L. (2014). Medical applications for 3D printing: Current and project uses. *Pharm. Ther., 39*(10), 704–711. PMID:25336867

Vert, M. (2009). Degradable and bioresorbable polymers in surgery and in pharmacology: Beliefs and facts. *Journal of Materials Science. Materials in Medicine, 20*(2), 437–446. doi:10.100710856-008-3581-4 PMID:18815731

Vincent, J. F. V. (2001). Stealing ideas from nature. In S. Pellegrino (Ed.), *Deployable Structures* (pp. 51–58). Vienna: Springer. doi:10.1007/978-3-7091-2584-7_3

Wahab. (2009). *Design and Implementation of MEMS Biomechanical Sensors for Real-Life Measurements of Gait Parameters* (PhD Thesis). Victoria University, Australia.

Walthers, C. M., Nazemi, A. K., Patel, S. L., Wu, B. M., & Dunn, J. C. Y. (2014). The effect of scaffold macroporosity on angiogenesis and cell survival in tissue-engineered smooth muscle. *Biomaterials, 35*(19), 5129–5137. doi:10.1016/j.biomaterials.2014.03.025 PMID:24695092

Wang, B., Li, H., Li, L., Chen, P., Wang, Z., & Gu, Q. (2013). Electrostatic adsorption method for preparing electrically conducting ultrahigh molecular weight polyethylene/graphene nanosheets composites with a segregated network. *Composites Science and Technology, 89*, 180–185. doi:10.1016/j.compscitech.2013.10.002

Wang, G., & Zreiqat, H. (2010). Functional coatings or films for hard-tissue applications. *Materials (Basel), 3*(7), 3994–4050. doi:10.3390/ma3073994 PMID:28883319

Wang, J., Tang, J., Zhang, P., Li, Y., Wang, J., Lai, Y., & Qin, L. (2012). Surface modification of magnesium alloys developed for bioabsorbable orthopedic implants: A general review. *Journal of Biomedical Materials Research. Part B, Applied Biomaterials, 100*(6), 1691–1701. doi:10.1002/jbm.b.32707 PMID:22566412

Wang, J., Zhang, J., Zong, X., Xu, C., You, Z., & Nie, K. (2015). Effects of Ca on the formation of LPSO phase and mechanical properties of Mg-Zn-Y-Mn alloy. *Materials Science and Engineering A, 648*, 37–40. doi:10.1016/j.msea.2015.09.046

Wang, S., Liu, Y., Zhang, C., Liao, Z., & Liu, W. (2014). The improvement of wettability, biotribological behavior and corrosion resistance of titanium alloy pretreated by thermal oxidation. *Tribology International, 79*, 174–182. doi:10.1016/j.triboint.2014.06.008

Wang, X. H., Ni, J. S., Cao, N. L., Yu, S., Chen, Y. G., Zhang, S. X., ... Yan, J. (2017). In vivo evaluation of Mg–6Zn and titanium alloys on collagen metabolism in the healing of intestinal anastomosis. *Scientific Reports, 7*(1), 44919. doi:10.1038rep44919 PMID:28317926

Weiler, A., Hoffmann, R. F., Stähelin, A. C., Helling, H. J., & Südkamp, N. P. (2000). Biodegradable implants in sports medicine: The biological base. *Arthroscopy, 16*(3), 305–321. doi:10.1016/S0749-8063(00)90055-0 PMID:10750011

Weiss, J. A., & Gardiner, J. C. (2001). Computational Modeling of Ligament Mechanics. *Critical Reviews in Biomedical Engineering, 29*(4), 1–70. PMID:11730098

Wernike, E. (2010). VEGF incorporated into calcium phosphate ceramics promote vascularisation and bone formation in vivo. *European Cells & Materials*, *19*, 30–40. doi:10.22203/eCM.v019a04 PMID:20178096

Whang, K., Thomas, C. H., Healy, K. E., & Nuber, G. (1995). A novel method to fabricate bioabsorbable scaffolds. *Polymer*, *36*(4), 837–842. doi:10.1016/0032-3861(95)93115-3

Williams, J. M., Adewunmi, A., Schek, R. M., Flanagan, C. L., Krebsbach, P. H., Feinberg, S. E., ... Das, S. (2005). Bone tissue engineering using polycaprolactone scaffolds fabricated via selective laser sintering. *Biomaterials*, *26*(23), 4817–4827. doi:10.1016/j.biomaterials.2004.11.057 PMID:15763261

Wintermantel, E. (2001). Composites for biomedical applications. In *Encyclopedia of materials: science and technology* (pp. 1371–1376). Oxford, UK: Elsevier. doi:10.1016/B0-08-043152-6/00255-2

Witte, F., Fischer, J., Nellesen, J., Crostack, H. A., Kaese, V., Pisch, A., ... Windhagen, H. (2006). In vitro and in vivo corrosion measurements of magnesium alloys. *Biomaterials*, *27*(7), 1013–1018. doi:10.1016/j.biomaterials.2005.07.037 PMID:16122786

Witte, F., Hort, N., Vogt, C., Cohen, S., Kainer, K. U., Willumeit, R., & Feyerabend, F. (2008). Degradable biomaterials based on magnesium corrosion. *Current Opinion in Solid State and Materials Science*, *12*(5-6), 63–72. doi:10.1016/j.cossms.2009.04.001

Wittenbrink, I., Hausmann, A., Schickle, K., Lauria, I., Davtalab, R., Foss, M., ... Fischer, H. (2015). Low-aspect ratio nanopatterns on bioinert alumina influence the response and morphology of osteoblast-like cells. *Biomaterials*, *62*, 58–65. doi:10.1016/j.biomaterials.2015.05.026 PMID:26022980

Wong, Beygi, & Zheng. (2019). Materials for Exoskeletal Orthotic and Prosthetic Systems. *Encyclopaedia of Biomedical Engineering*, 352-367.

Wood, W. (n.d.). *Pediatric SACH Foot* [Electronic image]. Retrieved January 2016 from http://www.willowwoodco.com/products-and-services/pediatric/feet/sach

Wysk, R. A., Niebel, B. W., Cohen, P. H., & Simpson, T. W. (2000). Taguchi's Robust Design Method. *Manufacturing Processes: Integrated Product and Process Design*, 1–9.

Xiaolong, F., Xianghe, Z., Pengfei, Z., Yongbin, Z., & Ningsong, Q. (2016). Improving machining accuracy in wire electrochemical micromachining using a rotary helical electrode. *International Journal of Advanced Manufacturing Technology*, *84*(5-8), 929–939.

Xia, Y. (2013). Selective laser sintering fabrication of nano-hydroxyapatite/ poly-ε-caprolactone scaffolds for bone tissue engineering applications. *International Journal of Nanomedicine*, *8*, 4197–4213. PMID:24204147

Xie, Y., Hill, C. A. S., Xiao, Z., Militz, H., & Mai, C. (2010). Silane coupling agents used for natural fiber/polymer composites: A review. *Composites. Part A, Applied Science and Manufacturing*, *41*(7), 806–819. doi:10.1016/j.compositesa.2010.03.005

Xu, Z., Smith, C., Chen, S., & Sankar, J. (2011). Development and microstructural characterizations of Mg–Zn–Ca alloys for biomedical applications. *Materials Science and Engineering B*, *176*(20), 1660–1665. doi:10.1016/j.mseb.2011.06.008

Yahyavi-Firouz-Abadi, N., Menias, C. O., Bhalla, S., Siegel, C., Gayer, G., & Katz, D. S. (2015). Imaging of cosmetic plastic procedures and implants in the body and their potential complications. *AJR. American Journal of Roentgenology*, *204*(4), 707–715. doi:10.2214/AJR.14.13516 PMID:25794060

Yakimovich, T., Lemaire, E. D., & Kofman, J. (2009). Engineering design review of stance control knee – ankle – foot orthoses. *Journal of Rehabilitation Research and Development*, *46*(2), 257–268. doi:10.1682/JRRD.2008.02.0024 PMID:19533539

Yandell, K. (2013). Organs on demand. *Science*, *27*, 38–45.

Yang, Y., Scenini, F., & Curioni, M. (2016). A study on magnesium corrosion by real-time imaging and electrochemical methods: Relationship between local processes and hydrogen evolution. *Electrochimica Acta*, *198*, 174–184. doi:10.1016/j.electacta.2016.03.043

Yap, J., Walsh, L. J., Naser-ud Din, S., Ngo, H., & Manton, D. J. (2014). Evaluation of a novel approach in the prevention of white spot lesions around orthodontic brackets. *Australian Dental Journal*, *59*(1), 70–80. doi:10.1111/adj.12142 PMID:24528001

Yeng, Y., Mahfouf, M., & Linkens, D. (2003). Parameter optimization of stress- strainconstitutive equations using genetic algorithm. *Journal of Materials Science and Technology*, *19*, 5–8.

Young, M. F. (2003). Bone matrix proteins: Their function, regulation, and relationship to osteoporosis. *Osteoporosis International*, *14*(Suppl 3), S35–S42. doi:10.100700198-002-1342-7 PMID:12730768

Yu, Y. (2016). *Three-dimensional bioprinting using self-assembling scalable scaffold-free "tissue strands" as a new bioink*. Academic Press.

Yuan, Q., Wu, D., Gotama, J., & Bateman, S. (2008). Wood fiber reinforced polyethylene and polypropylene composites with high modulus and impact strength. *J. Thermoplastic Composit. Mater.*, *21*(3), 195–208. doi:10.1177/0892705708089472

Zahedmanesh, H., & Lally, C. (2009). Determination of the influence of stent strut thickness using the finite element method: Implications for vascular injury and in-stent restenosis. *Medical & Biological Engineering & Computing*, *47*(4), 385–393. doi:10.100711517-009-0432-5 PMID:19189146

Zein, I., Hutmacher, D. W., Tan, K. C., & Teoh, S. H. (2002). Fused deposition modeling of novel scaffold architectures for tissue engineering applications. *Biomaterials*, *23*(4), 1169–1185. doi:10.1016/S0142-9612(01)00232-0 PMID:11791921

Zeltinger, J., Sherwood, J. K., Graham, D. A., Müeller, R., & Griffith, L. G. (2001). Effect of pore size and void fraction on cellular adhesion, proliferation, and matrix deposition. *Tissue Engineering*, *7*(5), 557–572. doi:10.1089/107632701753213183 PMID:11694190

Zhang, C., Hu, Y.-Y., Cui, F.-Z., Zhang, S.-M., & Ruan, D.-K. (2006). A study on a tissue-engineered bone using rhBMP-2 induced periosteal cells with a porous nano-hydroxyapatite/collagen/poly(L-lactic acid) scaffold. *Biomedical Materials (Bristol, England)*, *1*(2), 56–62. doi:10.1088/1748-6041/1/2/002 PMID:18460757

Zhang, Q., Rastogi, S., Chen, D., Lippits, D., & Lemstra, P. J. (2006). Low percolation threshold in single-walled carbon nanotube/high density polyethylene composites prepared by melt processing technique. *Carbon*, *44*(4), 778–785. doi:10.1016/j.carbon.2005.09.039

Zhang, S., Zhang, X., Zhao, C., Li, J., Song, Y., Xie, C., ... Bian, Y. (2010). Research on an Mg–Zn alloy as a degradable biomaterial. *Acta Biomaterialia*, *6*(2), 626–640. doi:10.1016/j.actbio.2009.06.028 PMID:19545650

Zhao, S., Gu, L., & Froemming, S. R. (2012). Effects of Arterial Strain and Stress in the Prediction of Restenosis Risk: Computer Modeling of Stent Trials. *Biomedical Engineering Letters*, *2*(3), 158–163. doi:10.100713534-012-0067-6

Zimmerli, W. (2014). Clinical presentation and treatment of orthopaedic implant-associated infection. *Journal of Internal Medicine*, *276*(2), 111–119. doi:10.1111/joim.12233 PMID:24605880

Zou, P., Rajora, M., Ma, M., Chen, H., Wu, W., & Liang, S. Y. (2017). January. Electrochemical Micro-Machining Process Parameter Optimization Using a Neural Network-Genetic Algorithm Based Approach. *Proceedings of the International Conference on Manufacturing Technologies*, 19-21.

About the Contributors

Kaushik Kumar, B.Tech (Mechanical Engineering, REC [Now NIT], Warangal), MBA (Marketing, IGNOU), and Ph.D (Engineering, Jadavpur University), is presently an Associate Professor in the Department of Mechanical Engineering, Birla Institute of Technology, Mesra, Ranchi, India. He has 17 years of Teaching & Research and over 11 years of industrial experience in a manufacturing unit of Global repute. His areas of teaching and research interest are Quality Management Systems, Optimization, Non-conventional machining, CAD / CAM, Rapid Prototyping and Composites. He has 9 Patents, 23 Book, 12 Edited Book, 38 Book Chapters, 131 international Journal publications, 18 International and 8 National Conference publications to his credit. He is on the editorial board and review panel of 7 International and 1 National Journals of repute. He has been felicitated with many awards and honours.

J. Paulo Davim received his Ph.D. degree in Mechanical Engineering in 1997, M.Sc. degree in Mechanical Engineering (materials and manufacturing processes) in 1991, Mechanical Engineering degree (5 years) in 1986, from the University of Porto (FEUP), the Aggregate title (Full Habilitation) from the University of Coimbra in 2005 and the D.Sc. from London Metropolitan University in 2013. He is Eur Ing by FEANI-Brussels and Senior Chartered Engineer by the Portuguese Institution of Engineers with an MBA and Specialist title in Engineering and Industrial Management. Currently, he is Professor at the Department of Mechanical Engineering of the University of Aveiro, Portugal. He has more than 30 years of teaching and research experience in Manufacturing, Materials, Mechanical and Industrial Engineering, with special emphasis in Machining & Tribology. He has also interest in Management, Engineering Education and Higher Education for Sustainability. He has guided large numbers of postdoc, Ph.D. and master's students as well as coordinated & participated in several financed research projects. He has received several scientific awards. He has worked as evaluator of projects for international research agencies as well as examiner of Ph.D. thesis for many universities. He is the Editor in Chief of several international journals, Guest Editor of journals, books Editor, book Series Editor and Scientific Advisory for many international journals and conferences. Presently, he is an Editorial Board member of 25 international journals and acts as reviewer for more than 80 prestigious Web of Science journals. In addition, he has also published as editor (and co-editor) more than 100 books and as author (and co-author) more than 10 books, 80 book chapters and 400 articles in journals and conferences (more than 200 articles in journals indexed in Web of Science core collection/h-index 45+/6000+ citations and SCOPUS/h-index 53+/8500+ citations).

* * *

Esther Titilayo Akinlabi is currently a Full Professor at the Department of Mechanical Engineering Science, University of Johannesburg, Auckland Park Kingsway Campus, Johannesburg, South Africa. She has both industrial and academic experience of about sixteen years. She completed her Doctorate degree in Mechanical Engineering in the field of Friction Stir Welding at the Nelson Mandela Metropolitan University, Port Elizabeth, South Africa; her other research areas include manufacturing processes, Laser Material Processing and materials characterization. She has more than ninety publications to her credit. She is registered with the Engineering Council of South Africa and a member of the South African Institute of Mechanical Engineers.

Dheeman Bhuyan is a graduate in Mechanical Engineering from CSVTU Bhilai and has a post graduate degree in mechanical design from Birla Institute of Technology, Mesra. He has over 4 years of experience in various fields of industry, academia and research along with multiple publications. He currently is serving as Assistant Professor in Girijananda Chowdhury Institute of Management and Technology, Guwahati.

Fredrick Mwema is a PhD student at the University of Johannesburg, Department of Mechanical Engineering Science and an assistant lecturer at Dedan Kimathi University of Technology, Kenya in the Department of Mechanical Engineering. He is a registered graduate engineer with the Engineers Board of Kenya (EBK).

Oluseyi Oladijo is a Senior Lecturer at the Department of Chemical, Material and Metallurgical Engineering, Botswana International University of Science and Technology, Palaplye, Botswana.

Nicolas Perry has a background of Manufacturing, Production and Design. He extended his research topics on the product development to focus on ecodesign of products and services since the last 10 years. This topics include the integration of environmental dimensions into product design, with a specific focus on the design for End of Life. This research addresses the evolution of the design methods of complex systems and services, with the evaluation of the value chain. He is a founding member of the French Ecodesign Sustainable Systems Network EcoSD and a member of the CIRP International Academy for Production Engineering. He also works in the field of product / material / process impacts, linking manufacturing process and parameters to material and product performance and efficiency for mechanical and composite design. Since 2001 he search in the field of ICT for enginnering, virtual engineering and Knowledge based Design methods. Ecodesign for product end of life, environmental evaluation in decision making. Since 2007 he works in the field of product / material / process impacts, linking manufacturing process and parameters to material and product performance and efficiency for mechanical and composite design. Wind turbine, high pressure hydrogen storage or tank for aerospace application are the latest domain of research activities on the carbon composite topic.

Shubhashis Sanyal is a Professor in Mechanical Engineering Department, NIT Raipur, Raipur (C.G.). Have been working as a faculty in Govt. Engg. Institutes from Nov. 1990 and has a teaching experience of more than 27 Years. Being a faculty in Design engineering, has specific interest in Structural Synthesis of Mechanism. Dr. S. Sanyal is also Life member of many Professional bodies: Life Member, Indian Society for Technical Education, Association for Machines & Mechanisms, Tribology Society of India. Fellow Member, Institution of Engineers.

Divya Zindani, (BE, Mechanical Engineering, Rajasthan Technical University, Kota), M.E. (Design of Mechanical Equipment, BIT Mesra), presently pursuing PhD (National Institute of Technology, Silchar). He has over 2 years of Industrial experience. His areas of interests are Optimization,

Product and Process Design, CAD/CAM/CAE, Rapid prototyping and Material Selection. He has 1 Patent, 4 Books, 6 Edited Books, 18 Book Chapters, 2 SCI journal, 7 Scopus Indexed international journal and 4 International Conference publications to his credit.

Index

www.ingramcontent.com/pod-product-compliance
Lightning Source LLC
LaVergne TN
LVHW081337300926
849161LV00008B/1999
* 9 7 8 1 5 2 2 5 8 2 3 5 9 *